Antibiotics: Drug Formulation, Interactions and Pharmacodynamics

Antibiotics: Drug Formulation, Interactions and Pharmacodynamics

Edited by Jack Penn

hayle
medical

New York

Hayle Medical,
750 Third Avenue, 9th Floor,
New York, NY 10017, USA

Visit us on the World Wide Web at:
www.haylemedical.com

ISBN: 978-1-63241-783-1

Cataloging-in-Publication Data

Antibiotics : drug formulation, interactions and pharmacodynamics / edited by Jack Penn.
    p. cm.
Includes bibliographical references and index.
ISBN 978-1-63241-783-1
1. Antibiotics. 2. Drug interactions. 3. Drugs--Physiological effect.
4. Pharmaceutical chemistry. I. Penn, Jack.
RM267 .A58 2019
615.792 2--dc23

Table of Contents

VI   Contents

Preface

The main aim of this book is to educate learners and enhance their research focus by presenting diverse topics covering this vast field. This is an advanced book which compiles significant studies by distinguished experts in the area of analysis. This book addresses successive solutions to the challenges arising in the area of application, along with it; the book provides scope for future developments.

The antimicrobial substances which are active in fighting against bacteria and bacterial infections are called antibiotics. They are highly effective in treating such infections, as they inhibit the growth of bacteria or kill them. Some antibiotics also possess antiprotozoal properties. Such antibiotics are useful in fighting protozoan infections. Antibiotics may also be administered as a preventive measure to at-risk individuals with a weakened immune system, cancer patients, or those undergoing surgery and taking immunosuppressive drugs. Antibiotics are usually taken orally or intravenously. They can also be taken topically in the form of ear drops for ear infections, eye drops for eye infections and in several skin infections. The interaction of alcohol with antibiotics can reduce the effectiveness of antibiotic therapy. Antibiotics are an important area of pharmaceutical science and have undergone rapid development over the past few decades. This book aims to shed light on some of the unexplored aspects of antibiotics and the recent researches in this field. The topics included in this book are of utmost significance and bound to provide incredible insights to readers.

It was a great honour to edit this book, though there were challenges, as it involved a lot of communication and networking between me and the editorial team. However, the end result was this all-inclusive book covering diverse themes in the field.

Finally, it is important to acknowledge the efforts of the contributors for their excellent chapters, through which a wide variety of issues have been addressed. I would also like to thank my colleagues for their valuable feedback during the making of this book.

Editor

Exploring Experiences of Delayed Prescribing and Symptomatic Treatment for Urinary Tract Infections among General Practitioners and Patients in Ambulatory Care

Sinead Duane [1,*], Paula Beatty [1], Andrew W. Murphy [1] and Akke Vellinga [1,2]

[1]   Discipline of General Practice, School of Medicine, National University of Ireland Galway, Galway, Ireland;
      p.beatty2@nuigalway.ie (P.B.); andrew.murphy@nuigalway.ie (A.W.M.); akke.vellinga@nuigalway.ie (A.V.)

[2]   Discipline of Bacteriology, School of Medicine, National University of Ireland Galway, Galway, Ireland

*   Correspondence: sinead.duane@nuigalway.ie

Academic Editor: Christopher Butler

Abstract: "Delayed or back up" antibiotic prescriptions and "symptomatic" treatment may help to reduce inappropriate antibiotic prescribing for Urinary Tract Infections (UTI) in the future. However, more research needs to be conducted in this area before these strategies can be readily promoted in practice. This study explores General Practitioner (GP) and patient attitudes and experiences regarding the use of delayed or back-up antibiotic and symptomatic treatment for UTI. Qualitative face to face interviews with General Practitioners (n = 7) from one urban and one rural practice and telephone interviews with UTI patients (n = 14) from a rural practice were undertaken. Interviews were analysed using framework analysis. GPs believe that antibiotics are necessary when treating UTI. There was little consensus amongst GPs regarding the role of delayed prescribing or symptomatic treatment for UTI. Delayed prescribing may be considered for patients with low grade symptoms and a negative dipstick test. Patients had limited experience of delayed prescribing for UTI. Half indicated they would be satisfied with a delayed prescription the other half would question it. A fear of missing a serious illness was a significant barrier to symptomatic treatment for both GP and patient. The findings of this research provide insight into antibiotic prescribing practices in general practice. It also highlights the need for further empirical research into the effectiveness of alternative treatment strategies such as symptomatic treatment of UTI before such strategies can be readily adopted in practice.

Keywords: Urinary tract infection; symptomatic treatment; delayed prescribing; antibiotic treatment; general practice; back-up prescribing

---

1. Introduction

With sustained spread of antibiotic resistance (ABR) and its increasing threat to public health, it is necessary to review antibiotic prescribing practices for infections. Recent NICE guidance (National Institute of Health and Care Excellence) published in the United Kingdom promote "delayed or back up" antibiotic prescriptions and "self care" with over the counter preparations when the infection is likely to be self-limiting [1]. Delayed prescribing strategies has been highlighted as an effective method of reducing ABR for acute respiratory infection [2]. In delaying a prescription the General Practitioner (GP) instructs the patient only to take the medication if there is no improvement in their condition or if their symptoms worsen [3]. While there are variations in how a delayed prescription is implemented, with the delay varying from one to seven days, it is designed to allow for the natural resolution of the illness during the specified time. Using this approach, inappropriate antibiotic consumption can potentially be greatly reduced [4,5]. The majority of evidence evaluating delayed prescribing refers to upper respiratory tract infections (URTI), otitis media and sore throats [2,4–8].

There is however an opportunity to adopt a delayed prescription strategy when treating a suspected uncomplicated urinary tract infection (UTI) in an effort to reduce inappropriate antibiotic prescriptions. For instance, though national treatment guidelines recommend empirical antibiotics, a recent study found that only 21% of patients with UTI symptoms had bacteriological confirmation of infection [9]. There is also emerging evidence that delayed prescribing in the treatment of UTI is becoming more acceptable in practice [10,11] and patients' attitudes, behaviours and expectations towards consuming antibiotics are changing. In addition to decreased antibiotic consumption, patients who received a delayed prescription for UTI were less likely to re-attend for a further consultation [12].

In addition to delayed prescribing, a number of randomised control trials (RCT) are currently evaluating symptomatic treatment of UTI (as a variation of delayed prescribing) in general practice or ambulatory care. Symptomatic treatment differs from delayed or back up treatment in that the patient is treated with pain relief only, for example ibuprofen. Studies comparing antibiotic treatment of UTI with symptomatic treatment showed better outcomes in symptom severity. Bleidorn et al. (2010) found that ibuprofen was equally as effective as ciprofloxacin in terms of the symptomatic control of UTI [13]. However, the sample size for this pilot study was small. The subsequent full trial conducted in Germany showed that two thirds of women who received symptomatic treatment recovered without any antibiotics, however, their burden of symptoms was longer. The authors of the German RCT concluded that symptomatic treatment should be used as part of a shared decision making process with a delayed prescription with women who are experiencing mild to moderate UTI symptoms [14]. To date no studies have examined the factors that influence the GP's decision to use immediate prescription, delayed prescription or symptomatic prescription for a UTI, or how a patient feels about these treatment options in ambulatory care. The aim of this feasibility study is to explore GP and patient attitudes and experiences regarding the use of delayed antibiotic and symptomatic treatment for UTI in ambulatory care. The results of this feasibility study will help identify how widespread delayed and symptomatic treatment are in practice and will inform the design of a broader RCT in the future.

2. Methods

2.1. Participant Selection and Procedure

Purposeful non-probability sampling was used to recruit participants between August and September 2014. In total, seven face to face interviews were conducted with GPs (n = 3 male and n = 4 females). All GPs from one rural practice (n = 6) were invited to participate. One declined, another GP was excluded from analysis as the dictaphone failed to record. This practice was selected as the researchers had access to it. UTI is a very common illness and all GPs should have experience treating patients with this illness. Three GPs were invited to participate from an urban practice. Both practices were selected as they had a mixture of male and female and had GPs with a range of levels of experience. Both practices welcomed private fee paying patients and public GMS (General Medical Services) patients. Within Ireland, private fee paying patients pay between €40 and €60 to consult their GP while GMS patients receive free health care with a co-payment of approximately €1.50 per prescription. Approximately 30% of the Irish population are entitled to the GMS scheme [15]. Payment of consultations and re-consultations may be one factor that influences the expected outcome of the consultation however others also exist.

Telephone interviews were conducted with female UTI patients from one rural practice. It is acknowledged that this is a limitation of the study however, the researchers had difficulty accessing patients from other practices within the time constraints of this project. Eligible patients were adult females who presented to their GP with symptoms suggestive of an UTI (dysuria, frequency, supra pubic pain, etc.) and consented to a telephone interview. Exclusion criteria included fever, known abnormality of the urinary tract, suspected pyelonephritis or insufficient comprehension of English. GPs provided the patient with an information leaflet explaining the purpose for the study and asked for consent to pass on their contact information (telephone number and name) to the researchers.

Nineteen patients were recruited to the study and a total of fourteen patient telephone interviews were completed. Five patients were excluded from the study after they consented to be contacted. One patient was difficult to comprehend due to unrelated health issues and another patient provided incorrect contact information. After several unsuccessful attempts to contact three patients they were also excluded.

Recruitment for this study continued until no new themes emerged from the interviews.

Ethical approval for the study was obtained from the Ethical committee of the Irish college of General Practitioners (1st August 2014) (ICE/2011/10).

2.2. The Interview

Semi-structured topic guides were used to achieve both flexibility of conversation and depth of content. A literature review was conducted to structure topic guides and the same researcher conducted all interviews. We employed an iterative process to ensure that any new topics emerging were fully explored.

The GP topic guide examined the factors that influence the GP's decision to use immediate prescription, delayed prescription or symptomatic treatment for a UTI. Patient interviews focused on what behaviours impacted on GP decision making and their perception of the treatment received. Table 1 outlines the key sections discussed within the interviews and a sample of the questions asked within each section.

Table 1. Sample interview questions.

GP Face to Face Interviews	UTI Patient Telephone Interviews
Section 1: Antibiotics in general	**Section 1:** Antibiotics in general
• Overall, what are your views on prescribing antibiotics? • Since you started practicing medicine have your attitudes towards prescribing antibiotics changed? Pros and cons?	• Can you describe to me what an antibiotic is? • In what sort of circumstances/situations would you expect to be prescribed an antibiotic? • Have you ever been prescribed an antibiotic in the past? For what symptoms? How did you feel about receiving the prescription?
Section 2: Delayed prescribing in general	**Section 2:** Delayed prescribing
• Have you used delayed prescribing before? • How long have you been using delayed prescribing? • What are your views on this approach? Pros and cons?	• Has your GP ever prescribed you an antibiotic, but told you only to fill the prescription if you felt no better, or felt worse after several days? • How did you feel about this approach? • Can you talk me through how the GP asked you to delay?
Section 3: Antibiotic treatment of urinary tract infections	**Section 3:** Treatment of UTI
• Can you describe a "typical" UTI patient? • Can you describe each step in your decision making process for treatment of a case like this?	• You recently attended your GP with a urinary tract infection, is this correct? • Can you describe to me the symptoms you were experiencing at the time of this consultation?
Section 4: Symptomatic Treatment	**Section 4:** Experiences of symptomatic treatment
• Have you ever used symptomatic treatment for a suspected UTI? • Can you describe the pros and cons of symptomatic treatment for a patient with a suspected UTI?	• Has your doctor ever given you an antibiotic prescription for a urinary tract infection and told you only to take it if you felt no better or felt worse after a few days? • How did you/would you feel about this? • Did you/would you follow this advice to delay?

2.3. Analysis

Framework analysis was used as a matrix to organise and analyse the themes. Framework analysis was chosen as it allowed the researchers (PB and SD) to compare the data across cases (interviewees) as well as within cases. The seven step procedure for applying Framework analysis was followed [16]. Each interview was transcribed verbatim. Three transcripts were then compared against the audio recordings and found to be accurate. All transcripts were read independently by two researchers in a process of familiarisation. The researchers recorded initial impressions of the interviews on the transcripts. The transcripts were then open coded and labelled which allowed for the identification of interesting segments related to our research objectives. Once the coding process was complete the researchers met to discuss the development of the analytical framework which emerged from the open codes and labels. A set of codes (themes) were identified and defined and these were used to undertake an in-depth analysis of the transcripts. PB applied the analytical framework within excel and SD analysed a subsample to ensure rigour within the analysis process. The GP framework contained 6 broad themes, with subthemes ranging from 2–8. The patient framework contained 4 broad themes with subthemes ranging from 2–7. Table 2 provides an example of one of the themes and sub-themes used within the analysis.

Table 2. Example of the themes and sub-themes emerging from analysis.

GP Themes and Sub-Themes	Patient Themes and Sub-Themes
Delayed prescribing for UTI	**Delayed treatment of UTI**
• Attitude to using delayed treatment in UTI	• Experience of a delayed prescription
• Influences on delaying prescription in UTI	• Attitude to delayed prescribing
• Examples of have they used delayed treatment in the past	
• Treatment given	
• Advice provided	
• Delayed prescribing UTI vs. URTI	

3. Results

3.1. GP Results

GPs Attitudes towards Delayed Prescribing in Practice

Every GP has used delayed prescribing in various circumstances. Often when the GP feels pressurized by the patient or when they feel a patient is presenting early. Most commonly, a delayed prescription was given for symptoms suggestive of upper respiratory tract infections.

> "Generally it's a parent of a child that feels that the child needs an antibiotic but the child seems reasonably well and all parameters are within normal limits. It's probably a learnt response from a previous inappropriate prescription."

> (Young Female rural GP)

The main reason a GP issues a delayed prescription is to ensure the patient will not re-consult. The GP usually has no means of knowing whether the patient consumed the antibiotic unless they ask them in a follow up consultation.

> "Delayed prescriptions are issued as a favour to the patient so they don't have to come back and pay again. It's a protective mechanism of what if."

> (GP 1, Male)

Figure 1 summarises the main motivators and influences on a GPs decision to issue a delayed prescription. Any combination could result in a delayed prescription. Children were more likely to receive a delayed prescription than elderly patients who were deemed higher risk.

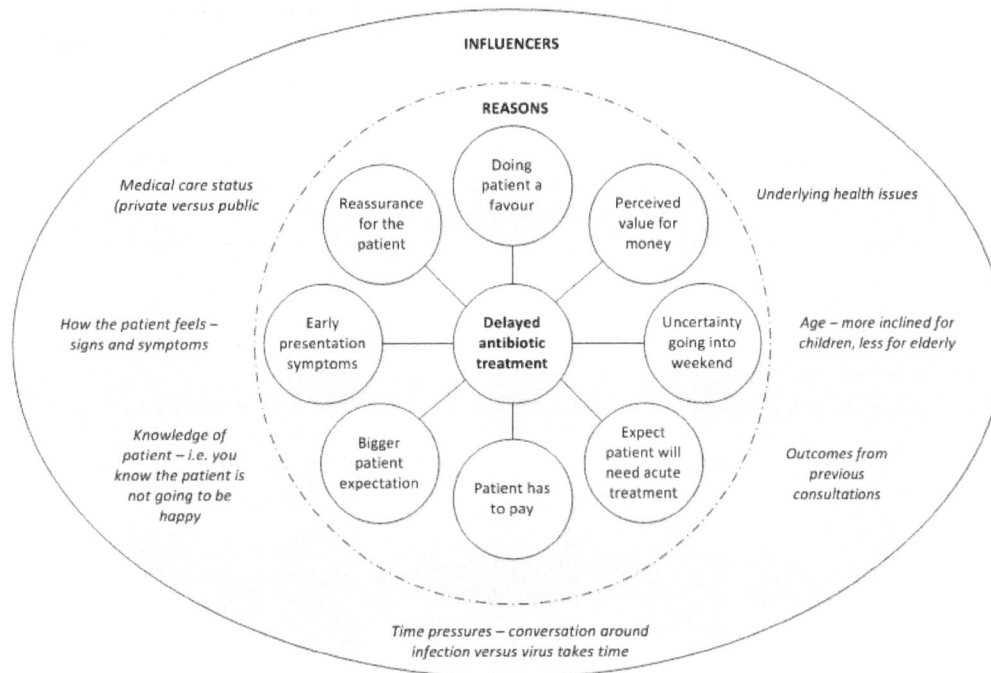

Figure 1. Motivators and Influences on GPs decision to provide a delayed antibiotic prescription.

A delayed prescription was usually verbally explained to the patient with the recommendation only to begin antibiotic treatment if symptoms worsen. Only one GP, wrote "delayed" on the prescription.

> "I have only recently started writing the delay on the prescription. I do it if I feel the patient might be more inclined to use it sooner than I would think necessary."
>
> (Female rural GP)

The majority of GPs recorded the delayed prescription in the patient notes and verbally followed up with them at their next consultation. The time suggested to delay a prescription ranged from 24 h to 72 h.

3.2. Delayed Prescribing for UTI

Most GPs believed that once they were confident the patient has a UTI, by listening to their symptoms and a positive dipstick test, the patient will 'need' antibiotic treatment.

> "I don't see the reason to wait for it to be honest. I don't see why the patient should be in pain for three days just so you can be factually correct."
>
> (Male rural GP)

> "If it's a confirmed UTI I will always treat."
>
> (Young female GP)

Two GPs also indicated that patients with past experience of a UTI will generally expect an antibiotic.

"If a patient has a past history of the infection they will expect an antibiotic. Some of them will come in and say I have cystitis and I need an antibiotic ... "

(Male urban GP)

GPs may consider delaying antibiotic treatment if the patient was symptomatic and the dipstick negative. In this scenario, the GP may be uncertain that the patient has a UTI but with a delayed antibiotic prescription, treatment is available if symptoms worsen and the patient decides the treatment is necessary.

If a patient has symptoms of a UTI, their GP may also advise to take pain relief, something GPs feel patients may not have considered.

3.3. Symptomatic Treatment for UTI

GPs said they rarely use symptomatic treatment for UTI but would consider symptomatic treatment if the patient had vague UTI symptoms. GPs agree that it is not appropriate to treat patients with antibiotics if there is a negative dipstick. Fluids and pain relief can help to manage symptoms, which patients often forget.

"I think generally people are unaware of taking pain relief for cystitis. Antibiotics don't treat pain."

(Male rural GP)

The concern with recommending symptomatic treatment only is that the symptoms become more severe and dissatisfied patients re-consult.

"The fear is always there that you miss something and you don't treat it properly and somebody gets quite sick. Then you feel a bit silly for just giving them a bit of Brufen."

(GP 1)

"For GPs the big con is that they might come back to the surgery the following day if you don't prescribe an antibiotic."

(Female rural GP)

The positive aspect of symptomatic treatment is that patients feel better and you are reducing our reliance on antibiotics.

"I think it works. You get people on board and you get less recurrent UTI. You get less people looking for antibiotic treatment. The patients are happy because they get some relief of symptoms."

(Female urban GP)

3.4. Patient Results

3.4.1. Current UTI Experience

The majority of patients attended their GP by day four of their symptoms (Table 3).

Table 3. Length of time patient waited before visiting the GP.

Days Waited	No. of Patients
First Day	4
2 days	2
3–4 days	3
5–6 days	1
One week	2
>1 week	2

Patients attended the GP because they felt their symptoms were persistent and severe.

"I was just worn out and I felt I had to put a stop to it."

(Patient 3)

All patients indicated that nothing would prevent them attending their GP with these symptoms. One patient specified that though "cost is a consideration" (Patient 6) it would not prevent her attending if she felt the symptoms were severe enough.

Some patients tried alternative self care methods to manage their symptoms before consulting their GP. These measures included drinking water or cranberry juice, taking over the counter preparations or taking pain relief. Some also reported drinking or washing with baking soda.

The majority of patients expected to be given an antibiotic prescription whilst a quarter indicated they only consulted the GP to rule out a possible infection. One patients consulted their GP to relieve their symptoms, another indicated they had no particular expectation at all on visiting her GP with symptoms of a UTI.

Ten out of the fourteen patients were prescribed an antibiotic to treat their UTI. Most were satisfied with this outcome as they felt they "needed" it at the time, they had received one before and they associated antibiotic treatment with symptom relief.

"I felt great because I didn't have pain in my lower back and it was more bearable. I found the antibiotics killed the pain in my lower back and I only needed to take one or two painkillers."

(Patient 12)

One patient however, felt she had sought antibiotic treatment too soon.

"I feel if I stayed at home a little bit more and drank more cranberry juice I might get better without antibiotics."

(Patient 13)

Two patients were prescribed an antibiotic but did not take them as their symptoms improved. Only one patient was prescribed delayed treatment with recommended pain relief, she was satisfied with this outcome.

"I was very happy with this because I'm not one for taking antibiotics if I can avoid it at all."

(Patient 6)

3.4.2. Delayed Antibiotic Prescribing for UTI

Only two of the patients interviewed had experience with delayed treatment for UTI. One eventually started treatment the other did not. Patients without experience with delayed treatment for UTI had mixed attitudes. Half of patients would follow the GPs' advice as they trusted their GP and viewed a delayed prescription as a safety net if symptoms persisted.

"I really am an anti-tablet person. I wouldn't have taken them unless I desperately needed them."

(Patient 12)

One of these patients additionally stated her acceptance would depend on how much "pain" she was in at the time.

The other half of patients felt apprehensive about delaying treatment as they perceived their symptoms to be severe enough to warrant immediate antibiotic treatment and they would not have consulted unless they needed treatment.

"I would have been a bit worried because I wouldn't have gone to the GP unless it was very severe at the time."

(Patient 5)

"I feel there wouldn't be much point in going to the doctor if you are very sick to be told to wait another few days. I wouldn't be happy about it."

(Patient 14)

3.4.3. Symptomatic Treatment for UTI

Two patients had been prescribed symptomatic treatment for UTI in the past. One patient was happy with this treatment as she trusted her GP and the GP was confident it was not a UTI. The other patient indicated she was not adverse to painkillers but she would be less satisfied if symptomatic treatment was recommended as an alternative to antibiotics.

"If it was used as an alternative to antibiotics, I don't think you would actually be treating the UTI because pain is just a symptom of it so I wouldn't be happy in that situation. It would affect my decision to return to the GP."

(Patient 10)

Overall, the patients interviewed expressed uncertainty with accepting symptomatic treatment for a UTI. They were not confident that symptomatic treatment would work as they believed an antibiotic was a necessary treatment for UTI. Some patients would trust their GPs' recommendations to treat the symptoms, others were sceptical and felt dissatisfied at the thought of treating a UTI with painkillers.

"That's fine, if they work it's good . . . It would influence my decision to return to a GP if it didn't have an effect on the symptoms."

(Patient 8)

"Sure a pain killer isn't going to cure an infection. It will only take the pain away."

(Patient 14)

4. Discussion

To our knowledge this is the first study which explored GP and patient attitudes to delayed antibiotic and symptomatic treatment for UTI. Although the generalisability of the study findings is limited by the qualitative nature of this study and the sample population, this research provides some powerful insights which need to be explored in the future if alternative treatment strategies for UTI were to be promoted. One example of an area that could be further explored is the GP and patients expectations from the consultation. GPs believed that if a patient has a positive dipstick, they need to be treated with an antibiotic and felt the patient expected one. Not all patients participating in this study sought antibiotic treatment, instead wanted relief from symptoms and/or to rule out an infection. However, the findings also revealed that from the patient perspective the appropriateness and acceptability of delayed prescribing may vary based on symptom severity and prior efforts to self-mange before consulting with a GP. It also depended on whether the GP had used a delayed prescribing strategy in the past for UTI. This research also highlighted that there was no exact exact science in the GPs decision to delay antibiotic treatment for UTI. Any combination of reasons or influencers could impact the decision ranging from the GP's past relationship with the patient (positive and negative influence), patient age or medical card status. Ultimately the GP wanted to ensure the patient did not have to re-consult whilst patients wanted to ensure that they will get back to good health.

Symptomatic treatment only was not used widely to treat UTIs by the GPs who participated in this study. However, GPs said they may recommend symptomatic treatment for patients who have a negative urinalysis and are experiencing vague symptomatic. The GPs were uncomfortable prescribing symptomatic treatment only in case a patient's symptoms become worse and they had to re-consult. Patients had little experience with symptomatic treatment for a UTI, and therefore were unsure about whether they would be comfortable accepting this treatment. Some seemed to be more willing to accept symptomatic treatment if they also had a delayed prescription.

4.1. Comparison with Existing Literature

NICE guidelines recommend "delayed or back up" antibiotic prescriptions and "self care with over the counter preparations" when the infection can be self-limiting. However this research highlights the adoption of these strategies is not as widespread in practice as other infections such as upper respiratory tract infections. GPs will consider using delayed prescribing if they feel a patient has low grade symptoms and have presented too early. Like other research studies investigating GP antibiotic prescribing behaviours [17,18], this research highlighted a multitude of motivators and influencers impacting the GPs decision to prescribe, emphasising the importance of the consultation encounter.

As observed in Leydon et al. (2009) research on UTI patient pathways to the GP [19], the majority of patients in this study had undertaken self care prior to consulting with their GP. However, this was not cited by the patients within this study as a reason not to accept a delay prescription. In another study, thirteen patients were asked to delay taking their prescription and of these thirteen, ten participants gave positive feedback. Only two patients within this study had experienced a delayed prescription, one consumed the antibiotic the other did not.

Despite its use in other areas, patients within this study had minimal experience of delayed prescribing for UTI in the past, suggesting that it is not widely in practice for UTI. However, there was a willingness to accept delayed treatment by half the patients if it had been recommended. These findings are similar to a quantitative study of 176 women, where out of 137 of those who were asked to delay antibiotic treatment, 37% reported that they were happy to accept a delayed prescription. Of those who accepted a delayed prescription, 55% reported not having used the prescription within 7 days [11]. Edwards et al. (2003) found that while two thirds of patients said they had expected an antibiotic at consultation, 92.5% of respondents said they would be happy to accept a delayed prescription in the future [20].

A recent RCT conducted by Gagyor and colleagues showed that the patients recruited to their study were biased towards women with less severe symptom scores [14]. Similarly, our study highlighted that GPs felt that antibiotic treatment was necessary for patients who present with symptoms of a UTI and who have a positive dipstick. Gagyor (2015) recommended that symptomatic treatment should be part of a shared decision making process between the GP and patient with women who are willing to avoid an antibiotic or accept a delayed prescription [14].

4.2. Strengths and Limitations

By conducting GP and patient interviews, this research adopted a holistic approach to understanding the factors affecting decisions to issue and accept delayed antibiotic prescriptions and symptomatic treatment for UTI. Qualitative research findings are limited in their generalisability, however, this research contributes to the understanding of treatment strategies and how to overcome barriers. This level of understanding cannot be achieved through quantitative research. Due to the acute nature of the UTI illness a longitudinal study of attitudes and experiences would not have been appropriate.

By interviewing female patients immediately after they consulted with a suspected UTI, patients were very aware of the type of symptoms they experienced and the impact it had on their daily lives. The group of patients were diverse in terms of their age and the length of time they waited before initially consulting the GP with their UTI. However, patient's attitudes towards delayed prescribing and symptomatic treatment may have been biased by past interactions with their GP.

5. Conclusions

This study based in ambulatory care highlights that patients presenting with a suspected UTI are more likely to be treated with an immediate antibiotic than a delay or back-up prescription. Patients are even less likely to receive symptomatic treatment only for UTI symptoms. This research provides insight into why alternative treatments have not been readily adopted into practice. At present there is insufficient evidence to change their treatment behaviours. However, there is scope for changing treatment practices with patients presenting with milder symptoms or who would like to avoid taking antibiotics unnecessarily.

Although not currently widely adopted there was support for delaying treatment for patients who are symptomatic but have a negative dipstick result. The development of guidelines could help GP become more confident in issuing delayed prescriptions for these type of patients but only if further empirical research is conducted in this area highlighting their merit. In general, patients who were given a delayed prescription were verbally advised of the delay, this recommendation could be made more powerful if it was written on prescriptions and followed up and recorded in patient notes.

Overall, GPs were reluctant to recommend symptomatic treatment only as they feared symptoms would worsen and patients would re-consult. As patients are not familiar with symptomatic treatment for UTI, patients may also need additional reassurance that by treating their symptoms with painkillers they will become more comfortable. Further research is needed to demonstrate the effectiveness of symptomatic treatment for UTI before it is adopted into practice or promoted.

Before public health messages or social marketing informed behavioural change interventions can be developed to promote the adoption of alternative treatments for UTI such as delayed and symptomatic treatment of UTI in ambulatory care, rigorous research proving the benefits of these alternative must be undertaken.

Acknowledgments: We would like to thank the GPs and patients who participated in this research and the Health Research Board in Ireland for funding it through their Summer scholarship programme 2014.

Author Contributions: Akke Vellinga and Andrew W. Murphy conceived the study and coordinated the application for funding. Paula Beatty and Sinead Duane developed the research design. Paula Beatty collected the data, Paula Beatty and Sinead Duane analysed it. Sinead Duane drafted the manuscript and Akke Vellinga, Paula Beatty and Andrew W. Murphy revised it. All authors read and approved the final version of the manuscript.

References

1. *Antimicrobial Stewardship: Systems and Processes for Effective Antimicrobial Medicine Use*; NICE: London, UK, 2015.
2. Arnold, S.R.; Straus, S.E. Interventions to improve antibiotic prescribing practices in ambulatory care. *Cochrane Database Syst. Rev.* **2005**. [CrossRef]
3. Francis, N.A.; Gillespie, D.; Nuttall, J.; Hood, K.; Little, P.; Verheij, T.; Goossens, H.; Coenen, S.; Butler, C.C. Delayed antibiotic prescribing and associated antibiotic consumption in adults with acute cough. *Br. J. Gen. Pract.* **2012**, *62*, e639–e646. [CrossRef] [PubMed]
4. Little, P. Delayed prescribing of antibiotics for upper respiratory tract infection: With clear guidance to patients and parents it seems to be safe. *BMJ* **2005**. [CrossRef] [PubMed]
5. Spurling, G.K.; Del Mar, C.B.; Dooley, L.; Foxlee, R. Delayed antibiotics for respiratory infections. *Cochrane Libr.* **2007**. [CrossRef]
6. Little, P.; Williamson, I.; Warner, G.; Gould, C.; Gantley, M.; Kinmonth, A. Open randomised trial of prescribing strategies in managing sore throat. *BMJ* **1997**. [CrossRef]
7. Dowell, J.; Pitkethly, M.; Bain, J.; Martin, S. A randomised controlled trial of delayed antibiotic prescribing as a strategy for managing uncomplicated respiratory tract infection in primary care. *Br. J. Gen. Pract.* **2001**, *51*, 200–205. [PubMed]

8. Little, P.; Gould, C.; Williamson, I.; Moore, M.; Warner, G.; Dunleavey, J. Pragmatic randomised controlled trial of two prescribing strategies for childhood acute otitis media. *BMJ* **2001**, *322*, 336–342. [CrossRef] [PubMed]

9. Vellinga, A.; Cormican, M.; Hanahoe, B.; Bennett, K.; Murphy, A.W. Antimicrobial management and appropriateness of treatment of urinary tract infection in general practice in Ireland. *BMC Fam. Pract.* **2011**. [CrossRef] [PubMed]

10. Leydon, G.; Turner, S.; Smith, H.; Little, P. Women's views about management and cause of urinary tract infection: Qualitative interview study. *BMJ* **2010**. [CrossRef] [PubMed]

11. Knottnerus, B.J.; Geerlings, S.E.; van Charante, E.P.M.; ter Riet, G. Women with symptoms of uncomplicated urinary tract infection are often willing to delay antibiotic treatment: A prospective cohort study. *BMC Fam. Pract.* **2013**. [CrossRef] [PubMed]

12. Little, P.; Moore, M.; Turner, S.; Rumsby, K.; Warner, G.; Lowes, J.; Smith, H.; Hawke, C.; Leydon, G.; Arscott, A. Effectiveness of five different approaches in management of urinary tract infection: Randomised controlled trial. *BMJ* **2010**. [CrossRef] [PubMed]

13. Bleidorn, J.; Gagyor, I.; Kochen, M.M.; Wegscheider, K.; Hummers-Pradier, E. Symptomatic treatment (ibuprofen) or antibiotics (ciprofloxacin) for uncomplicated urinary tract infection?—Results of a randomized controlled pilot trial. *BMC Med.* **2010**. [CrossRef]

14. Gágyor, I.; Bleidorn, J.; Kochen, M.M.; Schmiemann, G.; Wegscheider, K.; Hummers-Pradier, E. Ibuprofen versus fosfomycin for uncomplicated urinary tract infection in women: Randomised controlled trial. *BMJ* **2015**. [CrossRef] [PubMed]

15. McGowan, B.; Bennett, K.; Casey, M.; Doherty, J.; Silke, C.; Whelan, B. Comparison of prescribing and adherence patterns of anti-osteoporotic medications post-admission for fragility type fracture in an urban teaching hospital and a rural teaching hospital in Ireland between 2005 and 2008. *Ir. J. Med. Sci.* **2013**, *182*, 601–608. [CrossRef] [PubMed]

16. Gale, N.K.; Heath, G.; Cameron, E.; Rashid, S.; Redwood, S. Using the framework method for the analysis of qualitative data in multi-disciplinary health research. *BMC Med. Res. Methodol.* **2013**. [CrossRef] [PubMed]

17. Strandberg, E.L.; Brorsson, A.; Hagstam, C.; Troein, M.; Hedin, K. "I'm Dr Jekyll and Mr Hyde": Are GPs' antibiotic prescribing patterns contextually dependent? A qualitative focus group study. *Scand. J. Prim. Health Care* **2013**, *31*, 158–165. [CrossRef] [PubMed]

18. Duane, S.; Domegan, C.; Callan, A.; Galvin, S.; Cormican, M.; Bennett, K.; Murphy, A.W.; Vellinga, A. Using qualitative insights to change practice—Exploring the culture of antibiotic prescribing for urinary tract infections: The simple study. *BMJ Open* **2016**, *6*, e008894. [CrossRef] [PubMed]

19. Leydon, G.M.; Turner, S.; Smith, H.; Little, P. The journey from self-care to GP care: A qualitative interview study of women presenting with symptoms of urinary tract infection. *Br. J. Gen. Pract.* **2009**, *59*, e219–e225. [CrossRef] [PubMed]

20. Edwards, M.; Dennison, J.; Sedgwick, P. Patients' responses to delayed antibiotic prescription for acute upper respiratory tract infections. *Br. J. Gen. Pract.* **2003**, *53*, 845–850. [PubMed]

Antibiotic Prescribing for Oro-Facial Infections in the Paediatric Outpatient

Najla Dar-Odeh [1,2,*], Hani T. Fadel [1] ⓘ, Shaden Abu-Hammad [2], Rua'a Abdeljawad [3] and Osama A. Abu-Hammad [1,2]

[1] Dental College & Hospital, Taibah University, Al Madinah Al Munawwarah 42353, Saudi Arabia; hfadel@taibahu.edu.sa (H.T.F.); oabuhammad@taibahu.edu.sa (O.A.A.-H.)
[2] Faculty of Dentistry, University of Jordan, Amman 11942, Jordan; s.abuhammad@yahoo.com
[3] Department of Pediatrics, Ibn Alhaitham Hospital, Amman 11942, Jordan; ruaa.abdeljawad@hotmail.com
* Correspondence: ndarodeh@taibahu.edu.sa

Abstract: There are many reports on the complications associated with antibiotics abuse during the treatment of paediatric patients, particularly those related to antimicrobial resistance. The dental profession is no exception; there is growing evidence that dental practitioners are misusing antibiotics in the treatment of their paediatric patients. This review is directed to dental practitioners who provide oral healthcare to children. It is also directed to medical practitioners, particularly those working in emergency departments and encountering children with acute orofacial infections. A systematic search of literature was conducted to explore the clinical indications and recommended antibiotic regimens for orofacial infections in paediatric outpatients. The main indications included cellulitis, aggressive periodontitis, necrotizing ulcerative gingivitis, and pericoronitis. Amoxicillin was found to be the most commonly recommended antibiotic for short durations of 3–5 days, with metronidazole or azithromycin being the alternative antibiotics in penicillin-sensitive patients.

Keywords: antibiotics; prescribing; paediatric; orofacial infections; antimicrobial resistance

1. Introduction

Antibiotics continue to be the most commonly prescribed drugs in children and adults [1]. In England, for instance, it is estimated that 66.4% of dental prescriptions are antibacterial drugs [2]. Variable rates of antibiotic prescribing among European countries are attributed to cultural and social factors, in addition to variable levels of awareness about the problem of antibiotic resistance among healthcare providers [3]. Within the dental community, awareness of clinical indications of antibiotic prescriptions to the child dental patient is lacking. It was found that a substantial proportion of children who received dental treatment for pain or localized swelling under general anaesthesia had also received antibiotics, with wide variation in antibiotic regimens [4]. Further, among members of the American Academy of Pediatric Dentistry, there was a trend toward overuse of antibiotics for non-indicated clinical conditions, like pain relief, irreversible pulpitis, and localised dentoalveolar abscess [5]. Interestingly, the same study found that certain non-clinical factors initiated antibiotic prescribing for some clinicians, such as unavailability of close appointments and seeking parental satisfaction [5]. A similar trend was observed in developing countries, where a substantial proportion of dentists prescribe for non-indicated clinical conditions, such as dry socket, localised periapical infection, marginal gingivitis, periodontitis, and pulpitis [6]. This insufficient knowledge of the appropriate clinical indications is paralleled by lack of awareness of important interventions that promote the optimal use of antibiotics, such as antibiotic stewardship programs [5]. Other forms of abuse in prescribing antibiotics include prescribing broad-spectrum antibiotics for infections that can be treated by narrow-spectrum antibiotics, prescribing antibiotics for long periods, and adopting inappropriate dosing regimens.

All of the above factors might contribute to the emergence of antibiotic resistance among children. Children as young as 4 years were found to harbour multidrug resistant bacteria in their oral cavities [7,8]. Further, patients who received frequent prescriptions of amoxicillin, a common antibiotic in dental prescriptions [9], also exhibited a higher rate of amoxicillin-resistant oral streptococci [10]. In addition to the problem of antibiotic resistance, there are other complications associated with antibiotic prescribing in paediatric population. A significant proportion of practitioners prescribe mostly sugar-containing formulations at frequencies inconsistent with manufacturers' recommendations, and for prolonged periods of time, that may reach 10 days [11]. The risk of developing diabetes in children due to sugar-containing medications cannot be overlooked. Moreover, generally, there is risk of development of allergy and asthma in children treated with antibiotics [12,13]. Early-life exposure to antibiotics is also thought to change intestinal microbiota, with subsequent adverse long-term effects like obesity [13]. Other complications include superinfections with *Candida* species [14] and photosensitivity [15,16]. Children are also at risk of gastrointestinal disturbances, like diarrhoea, which is generally more frequent with three-times-daily than twice-daily regimens [17]. Furthermore, exposure to amoxicillin during early infancy may be linked to developmental enamel defects on both permanent first molars and maxillary central incisors [18].

Consequently, an urgent need arises to create more concrete and definitive guidelines for dental antibiotic prescribing in children [19], for all those involved in the management of orofacial infections in children.

This review aims at:

1. Highlighting clinical indications of therapeutic antibiotic prescribing for orofacial infections in the paediatric outpatients;
2. Presenting recommended antibiotic regimens for each clinical indication.

2. Materials and Methods

2.1. Eligibility Criteria

We used the following inclusion criteria for this review:

1. Papers published in English;
2. Papers published in the past 20 years (from January 1998 to December 2017);
3. Clinical trials;
4. Case reports and series;
5. Reviews;
6. Expert opinions;
7. Clinical guidelines;
8. Patients: paediatric outpatients having orofacial infections (odontogenic infections, periodontal infections, pericoronitis);
9. Intervention: prescribing regimen of antibiotics including: name, dose and duration.

We used the following exclusion criteria:

1. In vitro and animal studies;
2. Neonatal orofacial infections that need hospitalization;
3. Paediatric dental in-patients;
4. Prophylactic antibiotic prescribing.

2.2. Search Methodology

A literature search was conducted in MEDLINE/PubMed, Web of Science, and Google Scholar databases using the following four combinations: odontogenic OR dental AND children AND antibiotic; aggressive AND periodontitis AND antibiotics; pericoronitis AND children AND antibiotics; necrotizing AND gingivitis AND children. The search was conducted in the period up to and including December 2017. Furthermore, reference lists of included articles were searched for suitable references.

2.3. Selection Strategy

Titles and abstracts of papers were independently screened by two reviewers (Najla Dar-Odeh and Osama Abu-Hammad). If keywords and other eligibility criteria were in titles and/or abstracts, the papers were selected for full text review. Full text was critically reviewed by the same authors and papers that fulfilled all of the selection criteria were processed for data extraction. The reference lists of all selected studies were hand searched for additional relevant articles. Disagreements between the two reviewers were resolved by discussion.

2.4. Assessment of Risk of Bias

Risk of bias was assessed based on criteria for judging risk of bias according to Cochrane Handbook for systematic reviews of interventions [20].

2.5. Data Synthesis

A narrative (descriptive) synthesis of data was employed in this review, due to heterogeneity of studies. Studies were categorized according to level of evidence and the type of infection addressed in these studies. The American Academy of Pediatric Dentistry—Useful Medications for Oral Conditions [21] was further consulted for citing the antibiotic doses based on weight.

3. Results

3.1. Search and Selection

First search on facial cellulitis of odontogenic origin, identified 1124 papers. Duplicate papers and those older than 1998 were removed, producing a total of 665 papers. After initial screening of titles and abstracts, another 642 papers were excluded, as these were on:

- Prophylactic antibiotic prescribing;
- Children with chronic diseases like HIV and cardiovascular disease;
- Older guidelines when new guidelines are present;
- Non-odontogenic conditions;
- Topical use of antibiotics;
- Antimicrobials other than antibiotics;
- A recommended antibiotic regime was not mentioned.

After full text reading two references were included (Table 1).

Table 1. Recommended antibiotic regimes for indicated conditions in the paediatric dental outpatient.

Oral Infection	Author/s (Year)	Type of Study	Indicated Antibiotic Regime	Indicated Antibiotic Regime in Penicillin-Allergic Patients	Additional Measures	Comments	Quality of the Evidence
Acute odontogenic abscess associated with raised axillary temperature and diffuse swelling	Palmer (2006) [22]	Expert opinion	Amoxicillin (2–3 days, max 5 days): <12 months: 62.5 mg tds / 1–5 years: 125 mg tds / 6–12 years: 250 mg tds; Phenoxymethyl penicillin (2–3 days, max 5 days): <12 months: 62.5 mg qds / 1–5 years: 125 mg qds / 6–12 years: 250 mg qds	Metronidazole (3 days): 1–3 years: 50 mg tds / 3–7 years: 100 mg bid / 7–10 years: 100 mg tds / >10 years: 200 mg tds; Erythromycin (2–3 days, max 5 days): 1 month–2 years: 125 mg qds / 2–12 years: 250 mg qds; Azithromycin (2–3 days): 6 months–3 years: 10 mg/kg od / 3–7 years 200 mg od / 8–11 years: 300 mg od / 12–14 years: 400 mg od / >14 years: 500 mg od	Remove cause Establish drainage Review 2–3 days	Author recommends the use of these antibiotics in descending order: amoxicillin, phenoxymethyl penicillin, metronidazole and lastly erythromycin.	Low [1]
Cellulitis	SDCEP [23]	Clinical guidelines	Amoxicillin (5 days): 6 months–1 year: 62.5 mg tds / 1–5 years: 125 mg tds / 6–18 years: 250 mg tds; OR Phenoxymethyl penicillin (5 days): 6 months–1 year: 62.5 mg qds / 1–6 years: 125 mg qds / 6–12 years: 250 mg qds / 13–18 years: 500 mg qds	Metronidazole Tabs, or Oral Suspension for 5 days: 1–3 years: 50 mg tds / 4–7 years: 100 mg bid / 8–10 years: 100 mg tds / 11–18 years: 200 mg tds; OR Clarithromycin (7 days): 1–5 years: 125 g bid / 6–12 years: 187.5 mg bid / 13–18 years: 250 mg bid			Low [1]
Generalized aggressive periodontitis and localized aggressive periodontitis	Haas et al. (2008) [24]	RCT	Azithromycin 500 mg coated tablet once daily for 3 days.		Phase 1 consisted of two sessions of supragingival scaling and oral hygiene instructions. At day 15, a clinical examination was performed, and phase 2 started consisting of nonsurgical periodontal therapy with subgingival hand scaling and root planing. Phase 2 was completed within a period of 14 days. The subjects were given azithromycin the first treatment session of phase 2.	Patients were ≥13 years; One year follow up significant improvement.	Very low [2]
Localized aggressive periodontitis	Muppa et al. (2016) [25]	Case report	Amoxicillin (50 mg/kg/day) (body weight in three divided doses) AND metronidazole 30 mg/kg/day for 15 days.		Further topical application of metronidazole in chlorhexidine (Rexidin-M gel) base was advised for 2 weeks. Vitamin B complex syrup was also included.	Child was 5 years old; Regular checkups and motivation for oral hygiene were done for 1½ years.	Very low [3]

Table 1. *Cont.*

Oral Infection	Author/s (Year)	Type of Study	Indicated Antibiotic Regime	Indicated Antibiotic Regime in Penicillin-Allergic Patients	Additional Measures	Comments	Quality of the Evidence
	Beliveau et al. (2012) [26]	Retrospective analysis of clinical trial	500 mg of amoxicillin and 250 mg of metronidazole three times per day tds for 7 days.		Oral hygiene is mandatory.	Antibiotics were administered immediately after mechanical debridement.	Very low [2]
	Merchant et al. (2014) [27]	Clinical trial	Same as above			Dose modified for children less than 40 kg.	Very low [4]
Localized Aggressive periodontitis	Seremidi et al. (2012) [28]	Case report	Amoxycillin 50 mg/kg and metronidazole 30 mg/kg tds) for 2 weeks.		The oral health preventive program included oral hygiene instructions and more specifically toothbrushing twice daily with a fluoridated toothpaste, use of dental floss for interdental cleaning, and use of disclosing tablets to increase the effectiveness of plaque removal. Dietary instructions (decrease of sweets intake up to once per day) were also given. In office fluoride application was carried out every 3–4 months. Prescription of 0.2% chlorohexidine mouthrinse for 10 days.	8-year-old boy; Antibiotics were also administered at the end of the second visit of periodontal therapy which included full mouth scaling and root planing under local analgesia in two visits within a one-week interval.	Very low [3]
Ulcerative necrotizing periodontitis	SDCEP [23]	Clinical guidelines	3-day regimen Amoxicillin: 6 months–1 year: 62.5 mg tds 2–5 years: 125 mg tds 6–18 years: 250 mg tds	3-day regimen Metronidazole: 1–3 years: 50 mg tds 4–7 years: 100 mg bid 8–10 years: 100 mg tds 11–18 years: 200 mg td			Low [1]
Pericoronitis	SDCEP [23]	Clinical guidelines	3-day regimen Amoxicillin: 6 months–1 year: 62.5 mg tds 2–5 years: 125 mg tds 6–18 years: 250 mg tds	3-day regimen Metronidazole: 1–3 years: 50 mg tds 4–7 years: 100 mg bid 8–10 years: 100 mg tds 11–18 years: 200 mg td			Low [1]

RCT: randomized controlled trial; tds: three times daily; qds: four times daily; od: once daily; bid: twice daily. Quality of evidence: GRADE-Working Group [29]. [1] Expert opinion or clinical guidelines; [2] Total sample includes children and adults. Number of children was not stated; [3] Case report; [4] Small sample size (22 participants).

The second search on aggressive periodontitis in children produced a total number of 410 articles. After removal of duplicates and studies older than 1998, a total of 337 remained. After initial screening of titles and abstracts, 317 articles were excluded, leaving 20 articles based on the following exclusion criteria:

- Adult studies;
- Non-bacterial periodontal infections;
- Topical antibiotic therapy;
- Aggressive periodontitis associated with systemic diseases;
- Antimicrobials other than antibiotics.

After full text reading, 6 were included (Table 1).

The third search was on pericoronitis in children. A total of 8 studies were retrieved, 7 of them were studies for adults and children with systemic disease, and so only one study was included (Table 1).

A fourth search was on necrotizing gingivitis in children. A total of 150 studies were retrieved. After removal of studies older than 1998, 77 remained. Studies which included systemic diseases, adult patients, microbiological studies, epidemiological studies, infections of non-bacterial origin ($N = 63$) were excluded, and 14 studies remained. After full text reading, only one study was included (Table 1).

3.2. Clinical Indications and Recommendations for Paediatric Dental Antibiotic Prescribing

Children are susceptible to a number of bacterial infections in the orofacial region, and these infections are similar in most cases to adults. Figure 1 shows these orofacial bacterial infections in children with a particular focus on dental and periodontal infections.

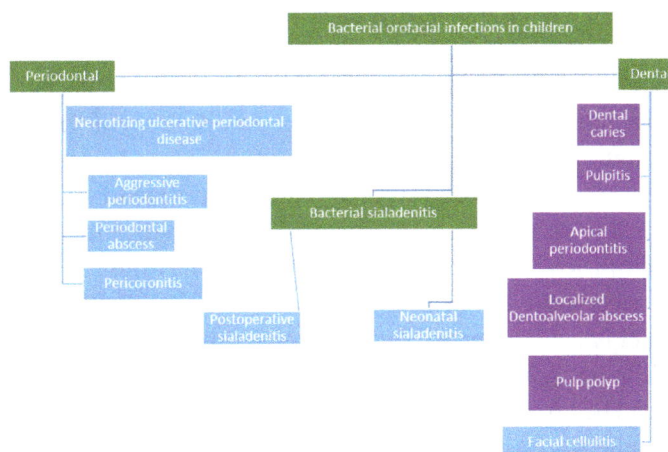

Figure 1. Orofacial infections in children. Infections quoted in blue boxes are best treated by operative intervention to remove the focus of infection in addition to adjunctive antibiotic therapy.

Although all the aforementioned infections are bacterial in origin, only a limited number require therapeutic antibiotic prescribing in paediatric dental patients, since most of these infections respond very well to operative treatment by removing the source of infection, e.g., drainage of a dentoalveolar abscess, extraction of carious tooth, or pulp therapy for teeth with necrotic pulp, pulpitis, pulp polyp, and apical periodontitis, and scaling with removal of calculus in patients with periodontitis. When antibiotics are needed, they should not be used as the only line of treatment, but rather, as an adjunct to the operative therapy [22]. These infections will be discussed below, with particular emphasis on infections that require antibiotic therapy.

3.2.1. Dentoalveolar Infections

Most orofacial infections are odontogenic in origin. The most common of these is dental caries and its complications (i.e., pulpitis, pulp necrosis, apical periodontitis, and periapical abscess). Children in many countries have high prevalence of caries, which can get to as high as 66% [30]. In his review, Finucane (2012) stresses that childhood caries (caries affecting children younger than 6 years) has to be treated, as it might be associated with pain, space loss, failure to thrive, and disruption to quality of life, among others [31]. Delay in treatment of dental decay will allow the infection to progress to cause infection of the tooth pulp (pulpitis); a bacterial infection that is associated with a more severe type of pain than dental caries. Untreated pulpitis may progress to pulpal necrosis, periapical abscess, or a dentoalveolar abscess, the latter being localised in the gingiva of the affected tooth. Chronic periapical abscess may sometimes drain in the sulcus by forming a sinus tract, and this is manifested clinically as a parulis. Another consequence of periapical infection is the formation of pulp polyp, which is a chronic hyperplastic lesion forming in the pulp chamber due to long-standing infection. Sinus tract, parulis, and pulp polyp are considered localised inflammatory lesions that are treated by operative intervention and not by antibiotic therapy. Localised infections in the form of caries, pulpitis, or periapical abscesses, are typically treated by operative intervention, either by pulp therapy, abscess drainage, or extraction, depending on the restorability of the tooth and the stage of development of the successor permanent tooth.

Sepsis is a serious complication of carious primary teeth, and this can progress to cellulitis. A substantial proportion of facial cellulites can be attributed to odontogenic infections [32]. If not properly treated, cellulitis can spread to the floor of mouth, leading to Ludwig's angina, compromising the airway [32], or it can lead to blindness and involvement of mediastinum and spinal column [33–35]. Early treatment of odontogenic infections can prevent these morbidities. When infection becomes severe, the need for antibiotic administration may arise. Therefore, it is important to treat carious lesions in primary dentition, even if they become temporarily asymptomatic after pulpal necrosis. Dental anxiety—or fear from dental chair—in children has a prevalence that can get to as high as 39% [36], and is an important factor contributing to delayed treatment of localized odontogenic infections. Delayed treatment may also be related to parents' dental fear [37], which may further complicate the problem.

When antibiotics are indicated for the treatment of an odontogenic infection, empiric therapy with a broad-spectrum antibiotic is recommended. For abscesses larger than 5 cm, cellulitis or conditions with mixed abscess-cellulitis, drainage and administration of antibiotics are indicated [38]. Some studies have recommended the use of amoxicillin and metronidazole, or amoxicillin with clavulanic acid, as an empiric treatment for odontogenic infections. However, a recent report showed a reduction in susceptibility of oral streptococci to amoxicillin [39]. Holmes and Pelleschia (2016) recommend amoxicillin, clindamycin, and azithromycin as empiric antibiotics for odontogenic infections [40]. Amoxicillin has good characteristics to be the drug of choice for orofacial infections; it is readily absorbed, it can be taken with food, and it is capable of resisting damage caused by gastric acidity [41]. In patients allergic to penicillin, researchers recommend clindamycin, azithromycin, metronidazole and moxifloxacin [40]. The latter has been found to be effective in severe odontogenic infections [42]. As for the duration of therapy, it is recommended to use short courses, particularly in children, to overcome the problem of compliance. In adults, the antibiotic regime of 1 g amoxicillin for 3 days was reported to be as clinically effective as long courses extending up to 7 days [39]. In children, the use of 2–3 day courses is recommended. This is supported by the findings that low daily dose or long duration of treatment with an oral beta-lactam (more than 5 days) can contribute to the appearance of penicillin-resistant pneumococci [43]. Recommended antibiotic regimens for odontogenic infections in children are explained in Table 1.

3.2.2. Periodontal Diseases

There is growing evidence on the link of periodontitis and important systemic diseases, like cardiovascular disease and diabetes [44,45]. The problem is complicated by the high prevalence of periodontitis in the community with noticeable predilection to adult populations; as it is estimated to affect 85% of those older than 65 years of age [46]. The paediatric population are also susceptible to periodontal diseases, and these can be classified into [47]:

1. Plaque-induced periodontal diseases;
2. Aggressive periodontal disease;
3. Periodontal disease as a manifestation of systemic diseases;
4. Necrotizing periodontal diseases;
5. Abscesses of the periodontium;
6. Periodontal disease associated with endodontic lesions;
7. Developmental or acquired periodontal deformities and conditions.

The most common of the abovementioned conditions are related to bacterial plaque and poor oral hygiene, hence, the appropriate treatment is the operative intervention by scaling and oral hygiene measures to achieve mechanical removal of plaque and calculus. Plaque-induced gingivitis, i.e., reversible bleeding from the gingiva with no loss of periodontal attachment, demonstrated a prevalence among children and adolescents between 36% and 97% [48]. Periodontitis, which involves irreversible loss of attachment of mild, moderate, or severe intensities, can generally present in children in the following main forms [47]:

1. Chronic periodontitis;
2. Aggressive periodontitis;
3. Necrotizing ulcerative periodontitis;
4. Periodontitis associated with systemic diseases

Chronic periodontitis is closely associated with bacterial plaque, and occurs almost exclusively in adults [49]. It may also be observed in childhood or adolescence [49], although severe attachment loss in such a young age suggests a more aggressive form of periodontal disease [50]. Chronic periodontitis can be treated successfully via mechanical means, deeming the routine use of antimicrobials and antibiotics during treatment of questionable benefit, as opposed to the undeniable risks [51]. Aggressive periodontitis and necrotizing ulcerative periodontitis, on the other hand, are more characteristic entities that significantly benefit from adjunctive antibiotic therapy, in addition to operative intervention [52]. Management of periodontitis associated with systemic diseases broadly involves cause-related periodontal therapy through effective plaque removal and the control of the underlying systemic condition [52]. Whether this includes the adjunctive use of systemic antibiotics is dependent on a number of factors related to the specific condition, the host defences, and the physician's opinion [52]. In this review, two types of periodontal diseases affecting children were considered: aggressive periodontitis and necrotizing ulcerative periodontal disease. These diseases may be encountered in the paediatric outpatient community as localised entities that require antibiotic therapy

Aggressive Periodontitis

Aggressive periodontitis, previously known as juvenile periodontitis, develops relatively early in life, and is characterised by rapid periodontal destruction [53]. Other possible features include possible familial aggregation, inconsistent low visible plaque deposits with advanced periodontal destruction, and elevated levels of certain specific microbial species [54]. When compared to other forms of periodontal diseases, aggressive periodontitis has a relatively low prevalence in populations. A recent study found that the prevalence among school children aged 13–19 is estimated to be 3.4% [55]. However, the importance of these diseases stems from their significant impact on patients' quality of life, as they are characterised by a relatively rapid course of tissue destruction, with which timely intervention is crucial [53].

Aggressive periodontitis is best described as being multifactorial in nature, where genetic, microbiologic, immunologic, and environmental factors contribute to the initiation and progression of the disease [56]. The ideal treatment plan for managing aggressive periodontitis constitutes early diagnosis, mechanical, and chemical periodontal treatment, coupled with adjunctive antibiotic therapy, and long-term follow-up [25]. Mechanical treatment may involve nonsurgical as well as surgical procedures. Adjunctive use of systemic antibiotics in the treatment of aggressive periodontitis has yielded significant benefits [57]. The rational for using antibiotics in this context originates from the fact that aggressive forms of periodontitis represent a notable threat to oral and systemic health, making the prudent use of effective antibiotics ethically permissible in appropriately selected cases [58].

The most commonly used antibiotics for aggressive periodontitis include tetracyclines, amoxicillin, metronidazole, macrolides (spiramycin, erythromycin, and azithromycin), clindamycin, and ciprofloxacin, with the most common antibiotic combination regimen being metronidazole and amoxicillin [59]. Azithromycin (500 mg once daily for 3 days) has also been recommended [24]. Recommended antibiotic regimens are explained in Table 1.

While there is no consensus on the ideal regimen, it is important to prescribe an antibiotic in sufficient dose for adequate duration [59]. Another important clinical question is when it is best to start administering antibiotics in relation to the mechanical phase of treatment. Indirect evidence suggests that antibiotic intake should start on the day debridement is completed, and debridement should be completed within a short period of time, of less than one week [60].

Necrotizing Periodontal Lesions

Necrotizing periodontal diseases are a group of infectious diseases that include necrotizing ulcerative gingivitis, necrotizing ulcerative periodontitis, and necrotizing stomatitis. These diseases share common clinical features consisting of an acute inflammatory process and the presence of periodontal destruction [61]. In developing countries, the reported prevalence of necrotizing periodontal diseases is higher than that of developed countries, especially in children [62]. In South Africa, 73% of patients with necrotizing gingivitis were 5–12 years of age [63]. It affects predominantly young children in undeveloped countries, particularly in sub-Saharan Africa, and is caused by a mixed anaerobic bacterial infection in subjects with pre-existing debilitating conditions, mainly malnutrition, and less frequently, malaria, measles, and/or AIDS [64].

Clinically, necrotizing ulcerative gingivitis is characterized by the appearance of necrotic ulcers of the interdental papillae, associated with pain and halitosis. Necrotizing periodontal diseases can progress rapidly, causing severe tissue destruction. Accordingly, necrotizing gingivitis which is confined to the gingiva, can progress to necrotizing periodontitis to involve the alveolar bone. It is therefore important for these conditions to be managed promptly. Treatment includes gentle removal of hard and soft deposits, and the use of antiseptic mouth washes and oxygen–releasing agents [61]. In cases that show unsatisfactory response to debridement or if systemic signs and symptoms (fever and/or malaise) appear, the use of systemic antimicrobials may be considered [61]. Metronidazole is the first drug of choice, because of its activity against strict anaerobes. However, for aggressive oral infections, metronidazole may be used in combination with amoxicillin (metronidazole 250 mg 3 times/day with amoxicillin 250–375 mg 3 times/day for 7–10 days) as shown in Table 1. Other systemic drugs have also been proposed with acceptable results, including penicillin, tetracyclines, clindamycin, or amoxicillin plus clavulanate [61].

3.3. Recommended Antibiotic Regimens

Recommended antibiotic regimens are presented in Table 2, according to the references cited in Table 1. Duration of antibiotic therapy varied between studies addressing aggressive periodontitis. The case reports [25,28] recommended a 15-day duration, whilst the clinical trials [26,27] recommended a 7-day duration.

Table 2. Recommended antibiotic regimens for orofacial infections in children.

Infection	Recommended Antibiotic Regimen	Recommended Antibiotic Regimen for Penicillin-Allergic Patient
Cellulitis	Amoxicillin (2–3 days, max 5 days): Children >3 months and <40 kg: 20–40 mg/kg/day in divided doses 8 hourly OR 25–45 mg/kg/day in divided doses 12 hourly Children >40 kg: 250–500 mg 8 hourly OR 500–875 mg 12 hourly OR Phenoxymethyl penicillin: (2–3 days, max 5 days) Children <12 years: 25–50 mg/kg/day in divided doses 6 hourly (max 3 g/day) Children ≥12 years: 250–500 mg 6 hourly	Metronidazole (3 days): Children: 30 mg/kg/day in divided doses 6 hourly (max 4 g/24 h) Adolescents and adults: 7.5 mg/kg 6 hourly (max 4 g/24 h) OR Azithromycin: Children >6 months up to 16 years: 5–12 mg/kg daily for 3 days (max 500 mg/day) OR 30 mg/kg as a single dose (max 1500 mg) OR Clarithromycin (7 days): 7.5 mg/kg 12 hourly 13–18 years: 250 mg 12 hourly
Aggressive periodontitis	Amoxicillin (50 mg/kg/day) AND Metronidazole 30 mg/kg/day 8 hourly for 7 days	Azithromycin (3 days): 10 mg/kg daily OR Metronidazole: 30 mg/kg/day 8 hourly for 7 days
Necrotizing ulcerative gingivitis	Amoxicillin (3 days): Children >3 months and <40 kg: 20–40 mg/kg/day in divided doses 8 hourly OR 25–45 mg/kg/day in divided doses 12 hourly Children >40 kg: 250–500 mg 8 hourly OR 500–875 mg 12 hourly	Metronidazole (3 days): Children: 30 mg/kg/day in divided doses 6 hourly (max 4 g/24 h) Adolescents: 250 mg 6 hourly OR 500 mg 8 hourly
Pericoronitis	Amoxicillin (3 days): Children >3 months and <40 kg: 20–40 mg/kg/day in divided doses 8 hourly OR 25–45 mg/kg/day in divided doses 12 hourly Children >40 kg: 250–500 mg 8 hourly OR 500–875 mg 12 hourly	Metronidazole (3 days): Children: 30 mg/kg/day in divided doses 6 hourly (max 4 g/24 h) Adolescents: 250 mg 6 hourly OR 500 mg 8 hourly

3.4. Assessment of Risk of Bias

Only one randomised controlled trial was included in this review [24]. Risk of bias for this study was judged to be low. More details are presented in Table 3.

Table 3. Assessment of risk of bias for Haas et al. (2008) [24].

Domain	Support for Judgment	Authors' Judgment
Selection bias		
Random sequence generation	Participants were randomly assigned by means of a draw	Low risk of bias
Allocation concealment	Medications were stored in opaque-coloured bottles identified only by the respective code of each participant	Low risk of bias
Performance bias		
Blinding of participants	Participants were masked from medications types	Low risk of bias
Blinding of personnel	Both periodontists involved in the treatment and clinical examination were masked from the identity of participants	Low risk of bias
Detection bias		
Blinding of outcome assessor	Blinding was ensured	Low risk of bias
Attrition bias		
Incomplete outcome data	There was no drop out of participants	Low risk of bias
Reporting bias		
Selective reporting	The article includes all expected outcomes, including those that were pre-specified	Low risk of bias

4. Discussion

In the pre-antibiotic era, odontogenic infections were challenging to the oral surgeon, who had to deal with the frequently associated septic complications and fatal consequences [65]. Historically, the introduction of antibiotics in dental practice had a strong impact on the successful outcome of some critical dental treatments. From the year 1940 onwards, antibiotics have allowed for performing more apicectomies [66], and during World War II, penicillin and other antibiotics were introduced into surgeries, making maxillofacial surgeries much safer [67]. Those (and other) achievements should not be overturned because of malpractice in antibiotic prescribing. Whilst it is important to understand factors influencing the practitioners' attitudes towards antibiotic prescribing, it is also necessary to provide clear guidelines based on sound clinical knowledge. Unfortunately, there is scarcity of resources on dental antibiotic prescribing for children. As can be noticed by this review, there are no clinical trials on antibiotic prescribing for facial cellulitis and pericoronitis in children, in contrast to other infections that received better attention, like otitis media and pharyngitis [17]. Further, studies that addressed aggressive periodontitis have pooled children and adults in the same patient group, and recruited a small sample size, which provides a very low level of evidence. Another important aspect is improving access to guidelines, and making these guidelines available to improve practitioners' knowledge and practices. The planning and preparation of these guidelines should take into consideration that antibiotic prescribing for children is different to adults in a number of aspects. Medication intake in children remains a challenge. However, no matter how effective medication regimens are, treatment outcomes would be compromised if children and parents do not follow instructions adequately. Children's behaviour may be characterised by lack of adherence to the prescription itself, so it is important that adherence and parents' cooperation is guaranteed, for successful treatment. Prescribing medications that can be given once or twice daily, will improve patient's compliance to the treatment [68]. Sugar-containing medications are expected to increase the patients' adherence. However, sugar increases susceptibility to dental decay, tooth erosion, and associated complications, such as pulpitis and dentoalveolar abscess, emphasizing the importance of performing optimum oral hygiene activities during antibiotic therapy and beyond. Children may also show lack of cooperation when receiving dental treatment. Operative interventions should remain the first line of treatment for management of dental/periodontal infections in children. However, these interventions are highly resisted by children especially when treatment entails performing local anaesthetic injections, extractions, and preparing cavities or root canals for fillings. The situation may get complicated when parents' faulty beliefs and perceptions encourage children's dental phobic attitudes. All the aforementioned factors may help initiate antibiotic prescriptions by dentists, particularly those who lack patience and training in dealing with difficult children. Other inappropriate clinical practices that must be avoided are antibiotic prescribing for viral infections. Although many childhood diseases, like primary herpetic gingivostomatitis and infectious mononucleosis, may present with oral and systemic manifestations, they are still viral infections that should be treated by palliative treatment, rather than antibiotics. Worried parents may sometimes complicate the problem by expecting antibiotics and putting pressure on dentists to meet their expectations. In addition, parents' lack of understanding of the diagnosis might hinder children's intake of medications [68].

For children with little compliance, antibiotics with a long half-life like azithromycin become useful, as they only need to be taken once daily for three days and are well tolerated in children. On the other hand, azithromycin is more expensive than amoxicillin and clindamycin [40]. Furthermore, care should be taken when prescribing azithromycin, as it may lead to growth of azithromycin-resistant bacteria [69], and it may be associated with pro-arrhythmic effects [70]. Amoxicillin, on the other hand, is considered safer, especially when less frequent doses are used. A recent study found that using once or twice daily doses of amoxicillin, with or without clavulanate, were comparable with three doses for the treatment of acute otitis media in children [71]. The applicability of this finding in the treatment of dental infections needs to be further explored.

It was reported that physicians are more likely than dentists to prescribe antibiotics for dental problems [72]. Indeed, orofacial infections in children may be considered a common domain between dentistry, otolaryngology, and paediatrics, among others. This fact should encourage practitioners of different specialties to embrace the concept of interprofessional education and practice, so that medical and dental practitioners gain more knowledge about the correct clinical indications for antibiotic prescriptions.

Choice of the antibiotic and the appropriate dosing regimen may be challenging to the dentist. Certain antibiotics should be avoided in children, like fluoroquinolones, which can lead to chondrotoxicity in growing cartilage [40], and tetracycline, which can cause discoloration of permanent teeth. Further, choosing amoxicillin-clavulanic acid should cover a broader spectrum than amoxicillin. However, the use of clavulanic acid in the paediatric population has been associated with gastrointestinal disturbances (diarrhoea), but these can be reduced by using the two-daily rather than the three-daily regimen [73].

This review focused on the paediatric dental outpatient, so infections that require hospitalization for the treatment, like suppurative sialadenitis, were excluded. However, practitioners should be aware of the clinical presentation of sialadenitis since it may mimic other orofacial infections. Viral sialadenitis and juvenile recurrent parotitis represent the most common salivary gland diseases in children and adolescents [74]. The literature revealed a few types that can be described as suppurative sialadenitis. This bacterial infection may be attributed to sialolithiasis, a rare disease in children [75]. Acute postoperative sialadentitis has been described as a rare entity occurring after general anaesthesia in children, or following prolonged neurosurgical procedures with extreme positioning of the head and neck [76]. Due to the severity of infection and high possibility of compromising the airway, these children are usually hospitalised, and usually, clindamycin is prescribed [76]. Others prefer ampicillin with a beta lactamase inhibitor, third generation cephalosporins, vancomycin, and fluoroquinolones [77].

Recommendations

When prescribing to children, it is important to follow certain measures to improve treatment outcomes. It will be beneficial to educate caregivers on the uses and potential side effects of antibiotics if the correct dosing regimen and treatment duration were not followed. This will help guarantee adherence by both caregivers and children. Health care professionals prescribing to children whether they are dentists or physicians are advised to consider the following when prescribing:

- Proper diagnosis is mandatory to design an appropriate treatment plan. To achieve the accurate diagnosis, history collection and clinical examination should be appropriately performed. Adjunctive diagnostic tools, like radiographs, can be of benefit, and should be used when indicated;
- It may seem more suitable to prescribe analgesics to supplement operative treatment for patients in pain;
- In case antibiotics were prescribed, children should be followed up for a few days to evaluate response to treatment, and the development of unwanted side effects;
- Dosing regimens for children can generally be estimated from their weight in kilograms, or from age, using the formula $((age + 4) \times 2)$ if the child's weight is unknown. In any case, the dose should not exceed the maximum adult dose;
- Treatment of orofacial infections entails collaborative efforts from all practitioners involved in the child's healthcare.

Author Contributions: N.D.-O. and O.A.A.-H. screened the list of titles and abstracts resulting from the search, created an overview of the papers selected for full text reading, performed the full text reading, made a selection of the papers that fulfilled the eligibility criteria, collected the data, worked on the interpretation of the data, assisted in the analysis of the data, drafted and designed the manuscript. S.A.-H and R.A. participated in the design, and helped in the drafting of the manuscript. H.T.F. revised the manuscript critically for important intellectual content, and helped by the interpretation of the data, participated in the design and the drafting of the manuscript. All authors read and approved the final manuscript.

Funding: This research received no external funding.

Acknowledgments: We acknowledge the library department of Taibah University, Al Madinah Al Munawwarah, Saudi Arabia for providing full text articles during the literature review.

References

1. Esposito, S.; Castellazzi, L.; Tagliabue, C.; Principi, N. Allergy to antibiotics in children: An overestimated problem. *Int. J. Antimicrob. Agents* **2016**, *48*, 361–366. [CrossRef] [PubMed]
2. Hurley, S.; Westgarth, D. When David met Sara Part 2. *Br. Dent. J.* **2015**, *219*, 477–478. [PubMed]
3. Cars, O.; Molstad, S.; Melander, A. Variation in antibiotic use in the European Union. *Lancet* **2001**, *357*, 1851–1853. [CrossRef]
4. Harte, H.; Palmer, N.O.; Martin, M.V. An investigation of therapeutic antibiotic prescribing for children referred for dental general anaesthesia in three community national health service trusts. *Br. Dent. J.* **2005**, *198*, 227–231. [CrossRef] [PubMed]
5. Sivaraman, S.S.; Hassan, M.; Pearson, J.M. A national survey of pediatric dentists on antibiotic use in children. *Pediatr. Dent.* **2013**, *35*, 546–549. [PubMed]
6. Kouidhi, B.; Zmantar, T.; Hentati, H.; Najjari, F.; Mahdouni, K.; Bakhrouf, A. Molecular investigation of macrolide and Tetracycline resistances in oral bacteria isolated from Tunisian children. *Arch. Oral Boil.* **2011**, *56*, 127–135. [CrossRef] [PubMed]
7. Ready, D.; Bedi, R.; Spratt, D.A.; Mullany, P.; Wilson, M. Prevalence, proportions, and identities of antibiotic-resistant bacteria in the oral microflora of healthy children. *Microb. Drug Resist.* **2003**, *9*, 367–372. [CrossRef] [PubMed]
8. Abu-zineh, R.; Dar-Odeh, N.; Shehabi, A. Macrolide Resistance Genes and Virulence Factors of Common Viridans Streptococci Species Colonizing Oral Cavities of Patients in Jordan. *Oral Health Dent. Manag.* **2015**, *14*, 337–341.
9. Dar-Odeh, N.S.; Al-Abdalla, M.; Al-Shayyab, M.H.; Obeidat, H.; Obeidat, L.; Abu Kar, M.; Abu-Hammad, O.A. Prescribing Antibiotics for pediatric dental patients in Jordan; knowledge and attitudes of dentists. *Int. Arab. J. Antimicrob. Agents* **2013**, *3*, 1–6.

10. Nemoto, H.; Nomura, R.; Ooshima, T.; Nakano, K. Distribution of amoxicillin-resistant oral streptococci in dental plaque specimens obtained from Japanese children and adolescents at risk for infective endocarditis. *J. Cardiol.* **2013**, *62*, 296–300. [CrossRef] [PubMed]

11. Palmer, N.O.; Martin, M.V.; Pealing, R.; Ireland, R.S. Paediatric antibiotic prescribing by general dental practitioners in England. *Int. J. Paediatr. Dent.* **2001**, *11*, 242–248. [CrossRef] [PubMed]

12. Droste, J.H.; Wieringa, M.H.; Weyler, J.J.; Nelen, V.J.; Vermeire, P.A.; Van Bever, H.P. Does the use of antibiotics in early childhood increase the risk of asthma and allergic disease? *Clin. Exp. Allergy* **2000**, *30*, 1547–1553. [CrossRef] [PubMed]

13. Yallapragada, S.G.; Nash, C.B.; Robinson, D.T. Early-Life Exposure to Antibiotics, Alterations in the Intestinal Microbiome, and Risk of Metabolic Disease in Children and Adults. *Pediatr. Ann.* **2015**, *44*, e265–e269. [CrossRef] [PubMed]

14. Al-Shayyab, M.H.; Abu-Hammad, O.A.; Al-Omiri, M.K.; Dar-Odeh, N.S. Antifungal prescribing pattern and attitude towards the treatment of oral candidiasis among dentists in Jordan. *Int. Dent. J.* **2015**, *65*, 216–226. [CrossRef] [PubMed]

15. Ferguson, J.; McEwen, J.; Al-Ajmi, H.; Purkins, L.; Colman, P.J.; Willavize, S.A. A comparison of the photosensitizing potential of trovafloxacin with that of other quinolones in healthy subjects. *J. Antimicrob. Chemother.* **2000**, *45*, 503–509. [CrossRef] [PubMed]

16. Verdugo, F.; Laksmana, T.; Uribarri, A. Systemic antibiotics and the risk of superinfection in peri-implantitis. *Arch. Oral Boil.* **2016**, *64*, 39–50. [CrossRef] [PubMed]

17. Easton, J.; Noble, S.; Perry, C.M. Amoxicillin/clavulanic acid: A review of its use in the management of paediatric patients with acute otitis media. *Drugs* **2003**, *63*, 311–340. [CrossRef] [PubMed]

18. Hong, L.; Levy, S.M.; Warren, J.J.; Dawson, D.V.; Bergus, G.R.; Wefel, J.S. Association of amoxicillin use during early childhood with developmental tooth enamel defects. *Arch. Pediatr. Adolesc. Med.* **2005**, *159*, 943–948. [CrossRef] [PubMed]

19. Cherry, W.R.; Lee, J.Y.; Shugars, D.A.; White, R.P., Jr.; Vann, W.F., Jr. Antibiotic use for treating dental infections in children: A survey of dentists' prescribing practices. *J. Am. Dent. Assoc.* **2012**, *143*, 31–38. [CrossRef] [PubMed]

20. Higgins, J.P.T.; Altman, D.G.; Sterne, J.A.C. Chapter 8: Assessing risk of bias in included studies. In *Cochrane Handbook for Systematic Reviews of Interventions*; Version 5.1.0; Higgins, J.P.T., Green, S., Eds.; The Cochrane Collaboration: London, UK, 2011.

21. The American Academy of Pediatric Dentistry-Useful Medications for Oral Conditions. Available online: http://www.aapd.org/media/policies_guidelines/rs_commonmeds.pdf (accessed on 9 March 2018).

22. Palmer, N.O. Pharmaceutical prescribing for children. Part 3. Antibiotic prescribing for children with odontogenic infections. *Prim. Dent. Care* **2006**, *13*, 31–35. [CrossRef] [PubMed]

23. Scottish Dental Clinical Effectiveness Programme DPFD, Dental Clinical Guidance, Third Edition. Available online: http://www.sdcep.org.uk/wp-content/uploads/2016/03/SDCEP-Drug-Prescribing-for-Dentistry-3rd-edition.pdf (accessed on 25 December 2016).

24. Haas, A.N.; de Castro, G.D.; Moreno, T.; Susin, C.; Albandar, J.M.; Oppermann, R.V.; Rosing, C.K. Azithromycin as an adjunctive treatment of aggressive periodontitis: 12-months randomized clinical trial. *J. Clin. Periodontol.* **2008**, *35*, 696–704. [CrossRef] [PubMed]

25. Muppa, R.; Nallanchakrava, S.; Chinta, M.; Manthena, R.T. Nonsyndromic localized aggressive periodontitis of primary dentition: A rare case report. *Contemp. Clin. Dent.* **2016**, *7*, 262–264. [CrossRef] [PubMed]

26. Beliveau, D.; Magnusson, I.; Bidwell, J.A.; Zapert, E.F.; Aukhil, I.; Wallet, S.M.; Shaddox, L.M. Benefits of early systemic antibiotics in localized aggressive periodontitis: A retrospective study. *J. Clin. Periodontol.* **2012**, *39*, 1075–1081. [CrossRef] [PubMed]

27. Merchant, S.N.; Vovk, A.; Kalash, D.; Hovencamp, N.; Aukhil, I.; Harrison, P.; Zapert, E.; Bidwell, J.; Varnado, P.; Shaddox, L.M. Localized aggressive periodontitis treatment response in primary and permanent dentitions. *J. Periodontol.* **2014**, *85*, 1722–1729. [CrossRef] [PubMed]

28. Seremidi, K.; Gizani, S.; Madianos, P. Therapeutic management of a case of generalised aggressive periodontitis in an 8-year old child: 18-month results. *Eur. Arch. Paediatr. Dent.* **2012**, *13*, 266–271. [CrossRef] [PubMed]

29. GRADE-Working Group. Available online: http://training.cochrane.org/path/grade-approach-evaluating-quality-evidence-pathway (accessed on 9 March 2018).

30. Sayegh, A.; Dini, E.L.; Holt, R.D.; Bedi, R. Oral cleanliness, gingivitis, dental caries and oral health behaviours in Jordanian children. *J. Int. Acad. Periodontol.* **2002**, *4*, 12–18. [PubMed]

31. Finucane, D. Rationale for restoration of carious primary teeth: A review. *Eur. Arch. Paediatr. Dent.* **2012**, *13*, 281–292. [CrossRef] [PubMed]

32. Olsen, I.; van Winkelhoff, A.J. Acute focal infections of dental origin. *Periodontology 2000* **2014**, *65*, 178–189. [CrossRef] [PubMed]

33. Lewandowski, B.; Pakla, P.; Wolek, W.; Jednakiewicz, M.; Nicpon, J. A fatal case of descending necrotizing mediastinitis as a complication of odontogenic infection. A case report. *Kardiochirurgia i Torakochirurgia Polska = Pol. J. Cardio-Thorac. Surg.* **2014**, *11*, 324–328. [CrossRef] [PubMed]

34. Dhariwal, D.K.; Patton, D.W.; Gregory, M.C. Epidural spinal abscess following dental extraction—A rare and potentially fatal complication. *Br. J. Oral Maxillofac. Surg.* **2003**, *41*, 56–58. [CrossRef]

35. Zachariades, N.; Vairaktaris, E.; Mezitis, M.; Rallis, G.; Kokkinis, C.; Moschos, M. Orbital abscess: Visual loss following extraction of a tooth—Case report. *Oral Surg. Oral Med. Oral Pathol. Oral Radiol. Endod.* **2005**, *100*, e70–e73. [CrossRef] [PubMed]

36. Colares, V.; Franca, C.; Ferreira, A.; Amorim Filho, H.A.; Oliveira, M.C. Dental anxiety and dental pain in 5- to 12-year-old children in Recife, Brazil. *Eur. Arch. Paediatr. Dent.* **2013**, *14*, 15–19. [CrossRef] [PubMed]

37. Coric, A.; Banozic, A.; Klaric, M.; Vukojevic, K.; Puljak, L. Dental fear and anxiety in older children: An association with parental dental anxiety and effective pain coping strategies. *J. Pain Res.* **2014**, *7*, 515–521. [PubMed]

38. Long, S.S. Optimizing antimicrobial therapy in children. *J. Infect.* **2016**, *72*, S91–S97. [CrossRef] [PubMed]

39. Chardin, H.; Yasukawa, K.; Nouacer, N.; Plainvert, C.; Aucouturier, P.; Ergani, A.; Descroix, V.; Toledo-Arenas, R.; Azerad, J.; Bouvet, A. Reduced susceptibility to amoxicillin of oral streptococci following amoxicillin exposure. *J. Med. Microbiol.* **2009**, *58 Pt 8*, 1092–1097. [CrossRef] [PubMed]

40. Holmes, C.J.; Pellecchia, R. Antimicrobial Therapy in Management of Odontogenic Infections in General Dentistry. *Dent. Clin. N. Am.* **2016**, *60*, 497–507. [CrossRef] [PubMed]

41. Segura-Egea, J.J.; Gould, K.; Sen, B.H.; Jonasson, P.; Cotti, E.; Mazzoni, A.; Sunay, H.; Tjaderhane, L.; Dummer, P.M. Antibiotics in Endodontics: A review. *Int. Endod. J.* **2016**, *50*, 1169–1184. [CrossRef] [PubMed]

42. Gomez-Arambula, H.; Hidalgo-Hurtado, A.; Rodriguez-Flores, R.; Gonzalez-Amaro, A.M.; Garrocho-Rangel, A.; Pozos-Guillen, A. Moxifloxacin versus Clindamycin/Ceftriaxone in the management of odontogenic maxillofacial infectious processes: A preliminary, intrahospital, controlled clinical trial. *J. Clin. Exp. Dent.* **2015**, *7*, e634–e639. [CrossRef] [PubMed]

43. Guillemot, D.; Carbon, C.; Balkau, B.; Geslin, P.; Lecoeur, H.; Vauzelle-Kervroedan, F.; Bouvenot, G.; Eschwege, E. Low dosage and long treatment duration of beta-lactam: Risk factors for carriage of penicillin-resistant Streptococcus pneumoniae. *JAMA* **1998**, *279*, 365–370. [CrossRef] [PubMed]

44. Widen, C.; Holmer, H.; Coleman, M.; Tudor, M.; Ohlsson, O.; Sattlin, S.; Renvert, S.; Persson, G.R. Systemic inflammatory impact of periodontitis on acute coronary syndrome. *J. Clin. Periodontol.* **2016**, *43*, 713–719. [CrossRef] [PubMed]

45. Mesia, R.; Gholami, F.; Huang, H.; Clare-Salzler, M.; Aukhil, I.; Wallet, S.M.; Shaddox, L.M. Systemic inflammatory responses in patients with type 2 diabetes with chronic periodontitis. *BMJ Open Diabetes Res. Care* **2016**, *4*, e000260. [CrossRef] [PubMed]

46. White, D.A.; Tsakos, G.; Pitts, N.B.; Fuller, E.; Douglas, G.V.; Murray, J.J.; Steele, J.G. Adult Dental Health Survey 2009: Common oral health conditions and their impact on the population. *Br. Dent. J.* **2012**, *213*, 567–572. [CrossRef] [PubMed]

47. Clerehugh, V.; Kindelan, S. Guidelines for periodontal screening and management of children and adolescents under 18 years of age. British Society of Periodontology and The British Society of Paediatric Dentistry. Available online: https://www.bsperio.org.uk/publications/downloads/53_085556_executive-summary-bsp_bspd-perio-guidelines-for-the-under-18s.pdf (accessed on 9 February 2018).

48. Jenkins, W.M.; Papapanou, P.N. Epidemiology of periodontal disease in children and adolescents. *Periodontology 2000* **2001**, *26*, 16–32. [CrossRef] [PubMed]

49. Califano, J.V. Position paper: Periodontal diseases of children and adolescents. *J. Periodontol.* **2003**, *74*, 1696–1704. [PubMed]

50. Demmer, R.T.; Papapanou, P.N.; Jacobs, D.R., Jr.; Desvarieux, M. Evaluating clinical periodontal measures as surrogates for bacterial exposure: The Oral Infections and Vascular Disease Epidemiology Study (INVEST). *BMC Med. Res. Methodol.* **2010**, *10*, 2. [CrossRef] [PubMed]

51. Jepsen, K.; Jepsen, S. Antibiotics/antimicrobials: Systemic and local administration in the therapy of mild to moderately advanced periodontitis. *Periodontology 2000* **2016**, *71*, 82–112. [CrossRef] [PubMed]

52. Clerehugh, V.; Tugnait, A. Periodontal diseases in children and adolescents: 2. Management. *Dent. Update* **2001**, *28*, 274–281. [CrossRef] [PubMed]

53. Albandar, J.M. Aggressive periodontitis: Case definition and diagnostic criteria. *Periodontology 2000* **2014**, *65*, 13–26. [CrossRef] [PubMed]

54. Armitage, G.C. Development of a classification system for periodontal diseases and conditions. *Ann. Periodontal.* **1999**, *4*, 1–6. [CrossRef] [PubMed]

55. Elamin, A.M.; Skaug, N.; Ali, R.W.; Bakken, V.; Albandar, J.M. Ethnic disparities in the prevalence of periodontitis among high school students in Sudan. *J. Periodontol.* **2010**, *81*, 891–896. [CrossRef] [PubMed]

56. Roshna, T.; Nandakumar, K. Generalized aggressive periodontitis and its treatment options: Case reports and review of the literature. *Case Rep. Med.* **2012**, *2012*, 535321. [CrossRef] [PubMed]

57. Rabelo, C.C.; Feres, M.; Goncalves, C.; Figueiredo, L.C.; Faveri, M.; Tu, Y.K.; Chambrone, L. Systemic antibiotics in the treatment of aggressive periodontitis. A systematic review and a Bayesian Network meta-analysis. *J. Clin. Periodontol.* **2015**, *42*, 647–657. [CrossRef] [PubMed]

58. Slots, J.; Ting, M. Systemic antibiotics in the treatment of periodontal disease. *Periodontology 2000* **2002**, *28*, 106–176. [CrossRef] [PubMed]

59. Heitz-Mayfield, L.J. Systemic antibiotics in periodontal therapy. *Aust. Dent. J.* **2009**, *54* (Suppl. 1), S96–S101. [CrossRef] [PubMed]

60. Herrera, D.; Alonso, B.; Leon, R.; Roldan, S.; Sanz, M. Antimicrobial therapy in periodontitis: The use of systemic antimicrobials against the subgingival biofilm. *J. Clin. Periodontol.* **2008**, *35* (Suppl. 8), 45–66. [CrossRef] [PubMed]

61. Herrera, D.; Alonso, B.; de Arriba, L.; Santa Cruz, I.; Serrano, C.; Sanz, M. Acute periodontal lesions. *Periodontology 2000* **2014**, *65*, 149–177. [CrossRef] [PubMed]

62. Albandar, J.M.; Tinoco, E.M. Global epidemiology of periodontal diseases in children and young persons. *Periodontology 2000* **2002**, *29*, 153–176. [CrossRef] [PubMed]

63. Arendorf, T.M.; Bredekamp, B.; Cloete, C.A.; Joshipura, K. Seasonal variation of acute necrotising ulcerative gingivitis in South Africans. *Oral Diseases* **2001**, *7*, 150–154. [CrossRef] [PubMed]

64. Feller, L.; Altini, M.; Chandran, R.; Khammissa, R.A.; Masipa, J.N.; Mohamed, A.; Lemmer, J. Noma (cancrum oris) in the South African context. *J. Oral Pathol. Med.* **2014**, *43*, 1–6. [CrossRef] [PubMed]

65. Dalla Torre, D.; Brunold, S.; Kisielewsky, I.; Kloss, F.R.; Burtscher, D. Life-threatening complications of deep neck space infections. *Wiener Klinische Wochenschrift* **2013**, *125*, 680–686. [CrossRef] [PubMed]

66. Gelbier, S. 125 years of developments in dentistry, 1880–2005. Part 4: Clinical dentistry. *Br. Dent. J.* **2005**, *199*, 615–619. [CrossRef] [PubMed]

67. Gelbier, S. 125 years of developments in dentistry, 1880–2005. Part 7: War and the dental profession. *Br. Dent. J.* **2005**, *199*, 794–798. [CrossRef] [PubMed]

68. Gardiner, P.; Dvorkin, L. Promoting medication adherence in children. *Am. Fam. Phys.* **2006**, *74*, 793–798.

69. Serisier, D.J. Risks of population antimicrobial resistance associated with chronic macrolide use for inflammatory airway diseases. *Lancet Respir. Med.* **2013**, *1*, 262–274. [CrossRef]

70. Zhang, M.; Xie, M.; Li, S.; Gao, Y.; Xue, S.; Huang, H.; Chen, K.; Liu, F.; Chen, L. Electrophysiologic Studies on the Risks and Potential Mechanism Underlying the Proarrhythmic Nature of Azithromycin. *Cardiovasc. Toxicol.* **2017**, *17*, 434–440. [CrossRef] [PubMed]

71. Thanaviratananich, S.; Laopaiboon, M.; Vatanasapt, P. Once or twice daily versus three times daily amoxicillin with or without clavulanate for the treatment of acute otitis media. *Cochrane Database Syst. Rev.* **2013**, CD004975. [CrossRef] [PubMed]

72. Anderson, R.; Calder, L.; Thomas, D.W. Antibiotic prescribing for dental conditions: General medical practitioners and dentists compared. *Br. Dent. J.* **2000**, *188*, 398–400. [PubMed]

73. Bax, R. Development of a twice daily dosing regimen of amoxicillin/clavulanate. *Int. J. Antimicrob. Agents* **2007**, *30* (Suppl. 2), S118–S121. [CrossRef] [PubMed]

74. Francis, C.L.; Larsen, C.G. Pediatric sialadenitis. *Otolaryngol. Clin. N. Am.* **2014**, *47*, 763–778. [CrossRef] [PubMed]

75. Chung, M.K.; Jeong, H.S.; Ko, M.H.; Cho, H.J.; Ryu, N.G.; Cho, D.Y.; Son, Y.I.; Baek, C.H. Pediatric sialolithiasis: What is different from adult sialolithiasis? *Int. J. Pediatr. Otorhinolaryngol.* **2007**, *71*, 787–791. [CrossRef] [PubMed]

76. Yim, M.T.; Liu, Y.C.; Ongkasuwan, J. A review of acute postoperative sialadenitis in children. *Int. J. Pediatr. Otorhinolaryngol.* **2017**, *92*, 50–55. [CrossRef] [PubMed]

77. Stong, B.C.; Sipp, J.A.; Sobol, S.E. Pediatric parotitis: A 5-year review at a tertiary care pediatric institution. *Int. J. Pediatr. Otorhinolaryngol.* **2006**, *70*, 541–544. [CrossRef] [PubMed]

3

Fosfomycin: Pharmacological, Clinical and Future Perspectives

Anneke Corinne Dijkmans [1,2], Natalia Veneranda Ortiz Zacarías [1], Jacobus Burggraaf [1],
Johan Willem Mouton [3,4], Erik Bert Wilms [5], Cees van Nieuwkoop [6] (iD),
Daniel Johannes Touw [7] (iD), Jasper Stevens [1] and Ingrid Maria Catharina Kamerling [1,*]

[1]   Centre for Human Drug Research, Leiden, 2333 CL, The Netherlands;
      annekedijkmans@hotmail.com (A.C.D.); n.v.ortiz.zacarias@lacdr.leidenuniv.nl (N.V.O.Z.); kb@chdr.nl (J.B.);
      j.stevens@umcg.nl (J.S.)
[2]   Department of Medical Microbiology, Albert Schweitzer Hospital, Dordrecht, 3318 AT, The Netherlands
[3]   Department of Medical Microbiology, Radboud University Medical Center,
      Nijmegen, 6500 HB, The Netherlands; jwmouton@gmail.com
[4]   Department of Medical Microbiology and Infectious Diseases, Erasmus Medical Center,
      Rotterdam, 3015 CN, The Netherlands
[5]   Hospital Pharmacy, The Hague Hospitals, The Hague, 2545 AB, The Netherlands; e.wilms@ahz.nl
[6]   Department of Internal Medicine, Haga Teaching Hospital, The Hague, 2566 MJ, The Netherlands;
      c.vannieuwkoop@hagaziekenhuis.nl
[7]   Groningen Research Institute for Asthma and COPD, Department of Clinical Pharmacy and Pharmacology,
      University Medical Center Groningen, University of Groningen, Groningen, 9713 GZ, The Netherlands;
      d.j.touw@umcg.nl
*   Correspondence: annekedijkmans@hotmail.com

Academic Editor: Christopher C. Butler

Abstract: Fosfomycin is a bactericidal, low-molecular weight, broad-spectrum antibiotic, with putative activity against several bacteria, including multidrug-resistant Gram-negative bacteria, by irreversibly inhibiting an early stage in cell wall synthesis. Evidence suggests that fosfomycin has a synergistic effect when used in combination with other antimicrobial agents that act via a different mechanism of action, thereby allowing for reduced dosages and lower toxicity. Fosfomycin does not bind to plasma proteins and is cleared via the kidneys. Due to its extensive tissue penetration, fosfomycin may be indicated for infections of the CNS, soft tissues, bone, lungs, and abscesses. The oral bioavailability of fosfomycin tromethamine is <50%; therefore, oral administration of fosfomycin tromethamine is approved only as a 3-gram one-time dose for treating urinary tract infections. However, based on published PK parameters, PK/PD simulations have been performed for several multiple-dose regimens, which might lead to the future use of fosfomycin for treating complicated infections with multidrug-resistant bacteria. Because essential pharmacological information and knowledge regarding mechanisms of resistance are currently limited and/or controversial, further studies are urgently needed, and fosfomycin monotherapy should be avoided.

Keywords: fosfomycin; pharmacokinetics; multidrug resistance; antimicrobial activity

1. Introduction

The discovery of antibiotics in the 1920s was one of the greatest breakthroughs in the history of healthcare, leading to a marked decrease in both morbidity and mortality associated with bacterial infections [1]. However, the intensive and extensive use and misuse of antibiotics over the past 50 years has contributed to the emergence and spread of antibiotic-resistant bacterial strains [2–4]. This increase and global spread of multidrug-resistant (MDR) bacteria is particularly alarming [3,5], and the World Health Organization has identified antibacterial drug resistance as a major threat to global public health.

The decrease in the number of effective antibiotics—together with a relative paucity of new antimicrobial drugs—is particularly relevant for treating infections with Gram-negative MDR bacteria [6–8]. To overcome this problem, the reassessment and reintroduction of "old" antibiotics has emerged as a viable strategy [9,10]. However, these antibiotics were never subjected to the rigorous drug development program that is currently mandatory for receiving marketing authorization. Thus, the pharmacological information needed in order to develop optimal dosing regimens with maximal activity and minimal toxicity is limited [9,11]. One such "old" antibiotic is fosfomycin, a broad-spectrum antibiotic that was originally developed more than 45 years ago. Because it has both in vitro and in vivo activity against a wide range of MDR bacteria, as well as XDR (extensively drug-resistant) and PDR (pan-drug-resistant) bacteria, fosfomycin is potentially a good candidate for treating infections with these bacteria [12–18].

In this review, we discuss the potential for using fosfomycin to treat MDR bacterial infections. Specifically, we review the currently available pharmacological data, with a focus on the chemistry, pharmacokinetics, pharmacodynamics, and clinical use of fosfomycin.

2. Methods

2.1. Systematic Search Strategy

The PUBMED/MEDLINE and OVID/EMBASE databases were searched systematically in February 2016 to identify all published relevant articles regarding fosfomycin. To be as comprehensive as possible, the search terms included synonyms of fosfomycin in the article titles.

The search strategies were designed and performed by a specialist librarian and were restricted to journals published in English or Dutch. No other publication or date restrictions were applied. A comprehensive database of the retrieved articles was created, and duplicate publications were removed. The abstract of each identified publication was then independently reviewed by the first author (A.C. Dijkmans) and last author (I.M.C. Kamerling). We then obtained and reviewed the full-text version of all articles that focused on multidrug-resistant Gram-negative bacteria (e.g., Enterobacteriaceae, *A. baumannii*, and *P. aeruginosa*), pharmacokinetics, pharmacodynamics, critically ill patients, treatment outcome, and/or mode of action. To search for any additional relevant articles, we screened the reference lists of the full-text articles, as well as relevant guidelines and references from the cited product information.

A final check was performed prior to submission of the manuscript in order to update the systematic search and include any new publications.

2.2. PUBMED/MEDLINE

PUBMED/MEDLINE was searched using the following terms: ("Fosfomycin"[Majr] OR phosphomycin[ti] OR fosfomycin[ti] OR phosphonomycin[ti] OR fosfonomycin[ti] OR monuril[ti] OR tromethamine[ti] OR trometamine[ti] OR trometamol[ti] OR tromethamol[ti]) AND (eng[la] OR dut[la]).

2.3. OVID/EMBASE

OVID/EMBASE was searched using the following terms: (exp *fosfomycin/ OR phosphomycin.ti. OR fosfomycin.ti. OR phosphonomycin.ti. OR fosfonomycin.ti. OR monuril.ti. OR tromethamine.ti. OR trometamine.ti. OR trometamol.ti. OR tromethamol.ti.) AND (english.lg. OR dutch.lg.).

3. Results

In total, our combined search of the databases PUBMED/MEDLINE and OVID/EMBASE retrieved 3422 records; after 2135 duplicates were removed, 1287 unique publications were screened

(Figure 1). Of the remaining 1287 records that were screened by title and abstract, 975 were excluded as they were judged not relevant to the topic. The remaining 312 records were examined as full-text articles, and an additional 251 were excluded, leaving 61 articles. An additional 31 articles were identified by manually checking the included publications and product information. Thus, a total of 92 articles were included in our analysis.

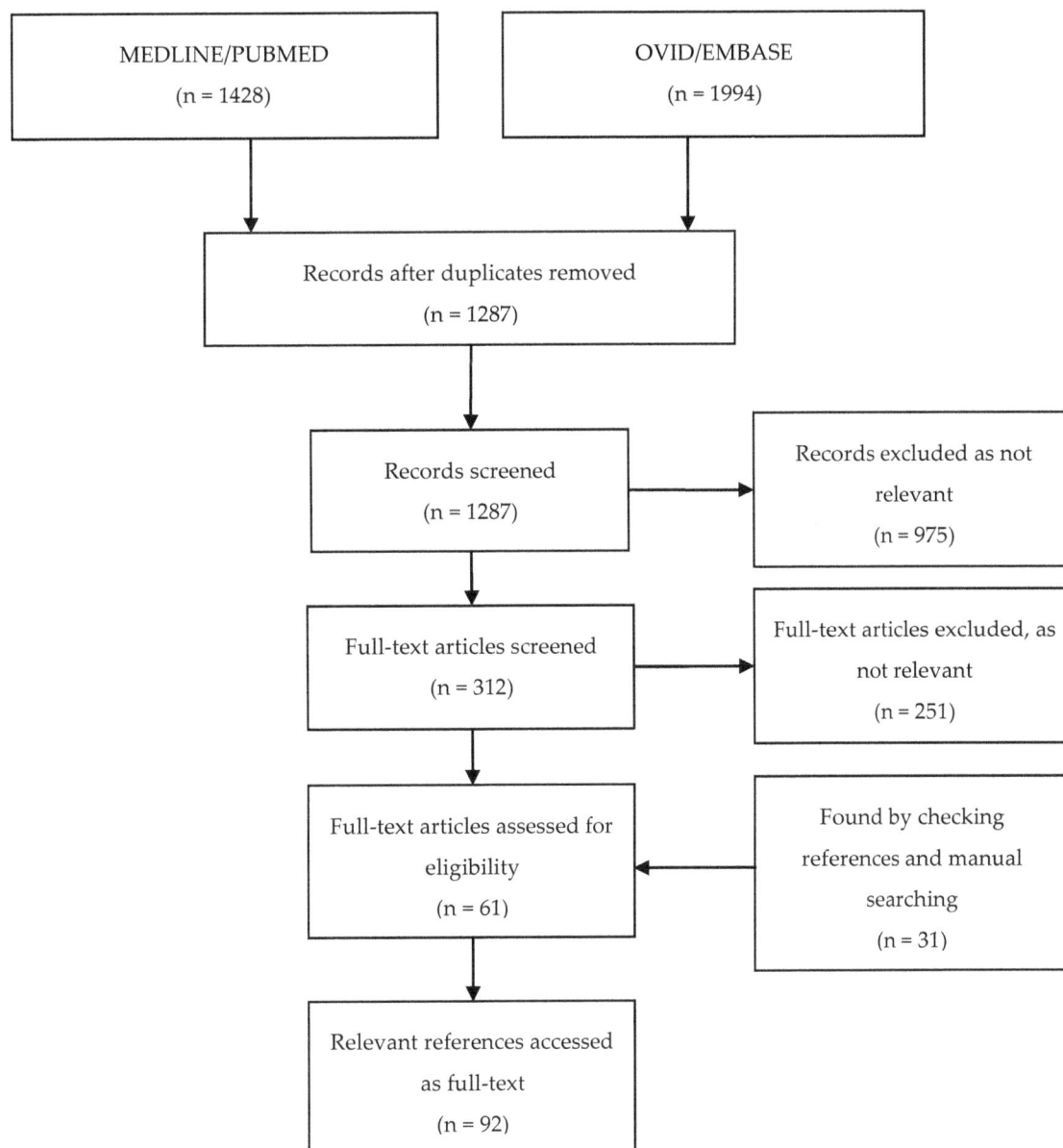

Figure 1. Flow-chart depicting the systematic search process and articles included.

4. Pharmacology of Fosfomycin for Treating MDR Bacteria

4.1. Chemistry

Fosfomycin is a bactericidal broad-spectrum antibiotic first isolated in 1969 from cultures of *Streptomyces* spp. [19]. Fosfomycin, which is currently produced using a synthetic process, is a low-molecular weight (138 g/mol), highly polar phosphonic acid derivative (cis–1,2-epoxypropyl phosphonic acid) that represents its own class of antibiotics [20]. Fosfomycin was initially marketed as both a calcium salt formulation (fosfomycin calcium) for oral administration and a more hydrophilic disodium salt (fosfomycin disodium) for parenteral administration. Later, because of its improved bioavailability, fosfomycin tromethamine became the standard formulation for oral administration [20,21]. The chemical structures of the various formulations of fosfomycin are shown in Figure 2.

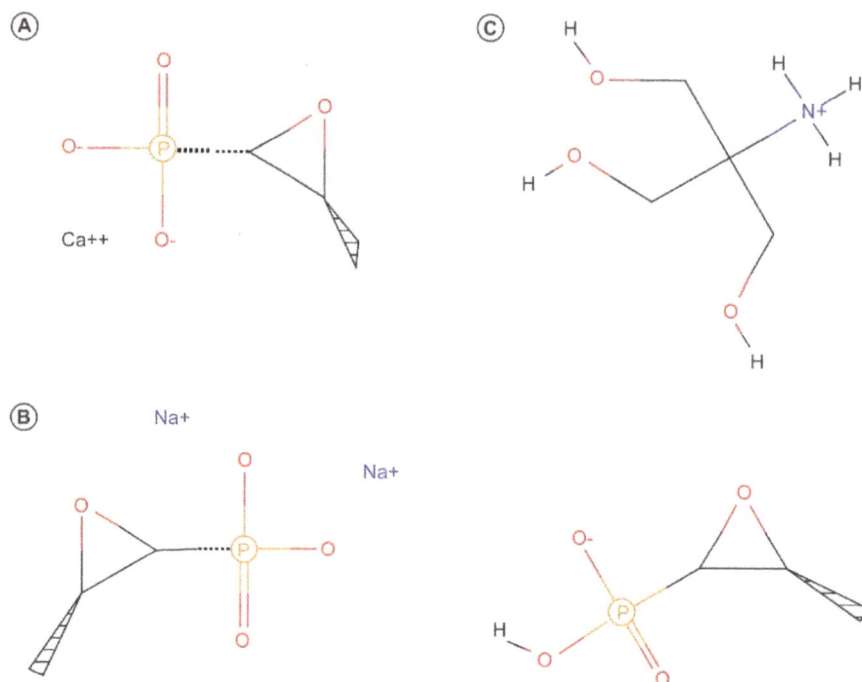

Figure 2. Chemical structures of fosfomycin calcium (**A**), fosfomycin disodium (**B**) and fosfomycin tromethamine (**C**).

4.2. Pharmacokinetics of Fosfomycin

4.2.1. Absorption

Orally administered fosfomycin is absorbed partially in the small intestine via two proposed mechanisms: (*i*) a saturable carrier-mediated system associated with a phosphate transport system, and (*ii*) a non-saturable process with first-order kinetics [22]. Studies with fosfomycin calcium have shown that before reaching the small intestine, fosfomycin undergoes acid-catalyzed hydrolysis in the stomach, where intragastric acidity and gastric emptying rate can affect the extent of fosfomycin's hydrolytic degradation and—consequently—its bioavailability [23]. Variations between individuals with respect to intragastric acidity and gastric emptying rate may also explain the high variability in serum levels achieved after oral administration of fosfomycin [23,24].

Tromethamine is a pH-elevating (i.e., alkaline) organic compound believed to slow acid-catalyzed hydrolysis. As mentioned above, fosfomycin tromethamine is now the preferred oral formulation due to its improved properties compared to fosfomycin calcium, including higher bioavailability (F) which ranges from 33% to 44% [21,25,26] (compared to 12–37% for the calcium salt [21,27,28]). When bioavailability was calculated from urinary excretion data following oral and IV administration of fosfomycin tromethamine, values as high as 58% have been calculated [25]. Although the bioavailability of both salts is reduced when taken orally following food [24,29], when taken under fasting conditions, serum concentrations of the tromethamine salt are approximately 2–4-fold higher than the calcium formulation [21,30]. However, because no cross-over study has been performed, a systematic study of bioavailability is recommended.

Despite the improved bioavailability achieved with orally administered fosfomycin tromethamine, maximum concentrations (C_{max}) of fosfomycin are still well below the C_{max} values achieved following

IV administration [21,31]. For example, 2–2.5 h after a single fasting oral dose of fosfomycin tromethamine at 3 g (approximately 50 mg/kg body weight), C_{max} is 21.8–32.1 mg/L, with a total area under the serum concentration-time curve (AUC) of 145–193 mg·h/L [21,25,26]. In contrast, after IV administration of the same dose of fosfomycin disodium, C_{max} was 276–370 mg/L, with an AUC of 405–448 mg·h/L [21,25,26].

4.2.2. Distribution and Tissue Penetration

Fosfomycin binds to plasma proteins at only negligible levels [31] and is distributed widely into a variety of tissues; in addition to serum, biologically relevant concentrations of fosfomycin have been measured in the kidneys, bladder, prostate, lungs, bone, and cerebrospinal fluid, as well as in inflamed tissues and abscess fluid [32–40].

The apparent volume of distribution (V_d/F) following oral administration of fosfomycin tromethamine is approximately 100–170 L for a 70-kg individual [29,30]. In contrast, because of its higher bioavailability, IV-administered fosfomycin disodium has a reported V_d of 9–30 L at steady state, and values of 3–12 L have been reported for both the central (Vc) and peripheral (Vp) compartments [25,27,28,32,36,41,42].

4.2.3. Metabolism and Excretion

Approximately 90% of an IV dose of 3 g fosfomycin disodium is recovered unchanged in the urine 36–48 h after dosing [21,25,26]. In contrast, only 40–50% of a 3 g oral dose of fosfomycin disodium is recovered; this difference compared to an IV dose is due primarily to incomplete absorption of oral fosfomycin disodium [21,25,26,29]. Following an oral dose of fosfomycin tromethamine, approximately 10% of the original dose is recovered unchanged in the feces [29].

Segre et al. reported that the fraction of the original dose excreted in the urine decreases as the oral dose increases [25], suggesting decreased absorption at higher doses. However, their study used a relatively limited range of doses (2, 3, and 4 g) in a small number of individuals ($n = 12$). On the other hand, urinary concentrations >128 mg/L are maintained 24–48 h after an oral dose of 2, 3, or 4 g and 12–24 h after an IV dose of 3 g [26].

In general, the total clearance rate ranges from 5 to 10 L/h, whereas renal clearance ranges from 6 to 8 L/h [25,27,31,32,35,36,41,43]. Fosfomycin has also been detected in the bile, with biliary concentrations of approximately 20% of the serum concentration [31,44,45]. Given this finding, Segre et al. suggested that fosfomycin undergoes biliary recirculation, based on the presence of secondary peaks in serum drug concentration following oral administration and based on the concentrations of fosfomycin measured in the bile [25,31,38,44,45].

In healthy individuals, IV fosfomycin is distributed in and eliminated from the serum in a bi-exponential manner; the serum disposition half-life ($t_{1/2\alpha}$) of fosfomycin is 0.18–0.38 h [28,43], and the terminal (or elimination) half-life ($t_{1/2\beta}$) of fosfomycin is 1.9–3.9 h [21,25–28,32,35,36,43]. In contrast, the $t_{1/2\beta}$ is longer following an oral dose of fosfomycin tromethamine (3.6–8.28 h [21,26,30]), which can be explained by a longer absorption phase. In patients who have renal failure and/or are receiving hemodialysis, the $t_{1/2\beta}$ of fosfomycin can be as long as 50 h, depending on the level of renal function; therefore, the dosing schedule should be adjusted accordingly, particularly if creatinine clearance (CL_{CR}) drops below 40 mL/min [43,44,46].

An overview of the farmacokinetics is given in Table 1.

Table 1. Overview of the reported pharmacokinetic properties of fosfomycin calcium, fosfomycin tromethamine, and fosfomycin disodium.

Ref	Dose	Study Group (N)	T_{max} (h)	$t_{1/2\beta}$ (h)	V_d (L)	CL (L/h)	CL_R	F (%)	k_a	k_{el}	Q
				Fosfomycin calcium							
Cadorniga et al., 1977 [28]	500 mg	HV (6)	2–2.5	2.04	20.7	ND	ND	37	ND	0.12	NA
Goto et al., 1981 [27]	20 mg/kg	HV (7)	2.3 (0.3)	3.01 (0.67)[g]	30.1 (4.6)	7.1 (1.5)	ND	28 (7.0)	1.03 (0.38)	0.24 (0.05)	NA
	40 mg/kg	HV (7)	2.7 (0.2)	5.05 (0.81)[g]	60.2 (17.4)	9.0 (1.7)	ND	28 (8.0)	0.92 (0.40)	0.14 (0.02)	NA
Borsa et al., 1988 [30]	40 mg/kg SD	Young HV (5)	1.41 (0.67)	4.81 (1.90)[g]	435.0 (144.0)	59.3 (23.3)[a]	5.0 (1.1)[a]	ND	ND	0.170 (0.084)	NA
		Elderly HV (8)	2.58 (0.54)	11.80 (6.86)[g]	409.4 (100.4)	33.4 (23.1)[a]	3.3 (1.1)[a]	ND	ND	0.082 (0.047)	NA
Bergan et al., 1990 [21]	50 mg/kg	HV (8)	2.9 (0.6)	5.6 (1.8)[g]	ND	ND	ND	12.0 (7.5)	ND	0.135 (0.053)	NA
				Fosfomycin tromethamine							
Segre et al., 1987 [25]	50 mg/kg	HV (5)	2.2 (0.44)	2.43 (0.31)	10.4 (1.5)	8.3 (1.6)	7.0 (0.9)	0.44 (0.09) 0.58 (0.04)[e]	Transit model k_{10}: 1.24 (0.55) k_{12}: 1.69 (0.62) k_{23}: 0.34 (0.10)	k_{35}: 0.69 (0.07)[f]	NA
Borsa et al., 1988 [30]	25 mg/kg SD	Young HV (5)	1.61 (0.23)	5.37 (2.56)[g]	186.3 (129.4)	19.4 (8.4)[a]	10.8 (1.5)[a]	ND	ND	0.156 (0.073)	NA
		Elderly HV (8)	2.16 (0.72)	8.28 (5.51)[g]	101.1 (61.2)	9.7 (4.2)[a]	2.9 (1.0)[a]	ND	ND	0.124 (0.078)	NA
Bergan et al., 1990 [21]	25 mg/kg	HV (8)	2.6 (0.5)	3.9 (0.65)[g]	ND	ND	ND	ND	ND	0.183 (0.031)	NA
	50 mg/kg	HV (8)	2.5 (0.8)	3.6 (0.44)[g]	ND	ND	ND	40.6 (17.9)	ND	0.197 (0.024)	NA
Bergan et al., 1993 [26]	2 g	HV (12)	2.2 (0.9)	4.1 (0.8)[g]	ND	ND	ND	ND	ND	0.17b	NA
	3 g	HV (12)	2.0 (0.6)	4.5 (2.1)[g]	ND	ND	ND	32.9 (7.9)	ND	0.15b	NA
	4 g	HV (12)	2.0 (0.0)	3.9 (0.7)[g]	ND	ND	ND	ND	ND	0.18b	NA
				Fosfomycin disodium							
Kwan et al., 1971 [42]	250 or 500 mg, 10-min infusion, Single dose 500 mg every 6 h, 8 times.	HV (17)	NA	1.1[c]	V_c: 12.9	7.5	7.1	NA	NA	K13: 0.62	12.4[b] k_{12}: 0.96 k_{21}: 1.19
Cadorniga et al., 1977 [28]	500 mg, 5-min infusion	HV (6)	NA	$t_{1/2\alpha}$: 0.38 $t_{1/2\beta}$: 2.04	V_c: 12.9 V_p: 7.8 V_{dss}: 20.7	ND	ND	NA	NA	K13: 0.67	6.9[b] k_{12}: 0.54 k_{21}: 0.88

Table 1. *Cont.*

Ref	Dose	Study Group (N)	T_{max} (h)	$t_{1/2\beta}$ (h)	V_d (L)	CL (L/h)	CL_R	F (%)	k_a	k_{el}	Q
Goto et al., 1981 [27]	20 mg/kg, 5-min infusion	HV (7)	NA	2.25 (0.74)	V_c: 8.7 (2.9) V_p: 9.8 (1.7) V_{dss}: 18.5 (4.6)	7.2 (1.6)	6.0 (2.2)	NA	NA	β: 0.34 (0.12) k_{10}: 0.92 (0.31)	14.2 [b] k_{12}: 1.62 (0.76) k_{21}: 1.45 (0.75)
	40 mg/kg, 5-min infusion	HV (7)	NA	2.22 (0.46)	V_c: 8.7 (2.9) V_p: 12.7 (2.9) V_{dss}: 20.8 (3.5)	8.0 (0.8)	6.6 (0.9)	NA	NA	β: 0.32 (0.06) k_{10}: 0.99 (0.22)	16.2 [b] k_{12}: 1.84 (0.85) k_{21}: 1.30 (0.49)
Lastra et al., 1983 [43]	30 mg/kg	Patients with normal renal function (9)	NA	$t_{1/2\alpha}$: 0.18 (0.09) $t_{1/2\beta}$: 1.91 (0.50)	21.2 (10.4)	7.9 (3.2)	ND	NA	NA	k_{13}: 1.91 (1.29)	k_{12}: 2.22 (1.49) k_{21}: 1.18 (0.68)
		Patients with impaired renal function (8)	NA	$t_{1/2\alpha}$: 0.61 (0.18) $t_{1/2\beta}$: 16.3 (11.9)	17.8 (6.8)	1.1 (0.8)	ND	NA	NA	k_{13}: 0.21 (0.17)	k_{12}: 0.66 (0.38) k_{21}: 0.43 (0.13)
Segre et al., 1987 [25]	50 mg/kg, Single injection	HV (5)	NA	2.43 (0.31)	10.4 (1.5)	8.3 (1.6)	7.0 (0.9)	NA	NA	k_{35}: 0.69 (0.07) [f]	10.6 [b] k_{34}: 1.00 (0.92) k_{43}: 1.40 (0.91)
Bergan et al., 1990 [21]	50 mg/kg, 5-min infusion	HV (8)	NA	3.4 (1.1)	ND	ND	ND	NA	NA	0.206 (0.048)	ND
Bergan et al., 1993 [26]	3 g	HV (12)	0.02 (0.0)	2.1 (0.1)	ND	ND	ND	NA	NA	0.33 [b]	ND
Joukhadar et al., 2003 [35]	8 g, 20-min infusion	Critically ill patients (9)	0.4 (0.1)	3.9 (0.9)	31.5 (4.5)	7.2 (1.3)	ND	NA	NA	0.18 [b]	ND
Pfausler et al., 2004 [32]	8 g, 30-min infusion, Single dose	Patients requiring extraventricular drainage (6)	1.2 (0.4)	3.0 (1.0)	30.8 (10.2)	7.4 (2.3)	ND	NA	NA	ND	ND
	8 g, 30-min infusion, every 8 h for 5 days	Patients requiring EVD	1.5 (1.2)	4.0 (0.5)	26.3 (9.7)	5.0 (2.0)	ND	NA	NA	ND	ND
Sauermann et al., 2005 [36]	8 g, 30-min infusion, Single dose	Patients (12)	0.47 (0.12)	3.7 (2.2)	V_c: 15.5 (4.5) V_{dss}: 28.6 (9.9)	7.6 (4.1)	ND	NA	NA	0.19 [b]	ND
Kjellsson et al., 2009 [41]	8 g, 30-min infusion, Single dose	Patients (12)	NA	1.2 [c]	V_c: 10.1 (5.4–14.8) V_p: 9.80 (5.7–13.9)	5.8 (3.8–7.8)	ND	NA	NA	0.58 [d]	15.4 (9.1–21.6)

HV, healthy volunteers; N, number of subjects; V_d, apparent volume of distribution (unless specified as another reported volume); CL_R, renal clearance; F, bioavailability; k_a, apparent first-order absorption rate constant; k_{el}, apparent first-order elimination rate constant; Q, intercompartmental clearance. [a] Calculated in L/h per 1.73 m^2. [b] Calculated from kel and k_{12}. k_{21}. Q = k_{12}*V1 and Q = k_{21}*V2. [c] Calculated using the equation $t_{1/2}$ = 0.693/kel. [d] Calculated from CL and central V_d the equations Kel = CL/Vc and Kel = 0.693/$t_{1/2}$. [e] Bioavailability calculated using the PK model (F = k_{12}/(k_{12}+k10)) and the ratio of the amount excreted in the urine after oral and IV administration, [f] Rate of elimination in the urine, [g] Apparent terminal half-life.

4.3. Pharmacodynamics of Fosfomycin

4.3.1. Mechanism of Action

In general, antibiotics exert their bactericidal or bacteriostatic activity by targeting the microorganism's essential physiological and/or metabolic functions, including protein, DNA, RNA, or cell wall synthesis and cell membrane organization. Fosfomycin has a unique mechanism of action in which it irreversibly inhibits an early stage of bacterial cell wall biosynthesis.

In order to exert its bactericidal activity, fosfomycin must reach the bacterial cytoplasm. To enter the cell, fosfomycin uses the active transport proteins GlpT and UhpT by mimicking both glucose-6-P (G6P) and glycerol-3-P (G3P). Thus, fosfomycin can be imported into the bacterial cell via the hexose monophosphate transport system (which is induced by G6P) and via the L-a-glycerophosphate transport system (which is induced by G3P) [20,47]. Once in the cytoplasm, fosfomycin acts as an analog of phosphoenolpyruvate (PEP) and binds MurA (UDP-GlcNAc enopyruvyl transferase), thereby inactivating the enzyme enolpyruvyl transferase, an essential enzyme in peptidoglycan biosynthesis [48]. Thus, fosfomycin prevents the formation of UDP-GlcNac-3-O-enolpyruvate from UDP-GlcNAc and PEP during the first step in peptidoglycan biosynthesis, thereby leading to bacterial cell lysis and death (Figure 3) [47]. In addition, fosfomycin also decreases penicillin-binding proteins [49].

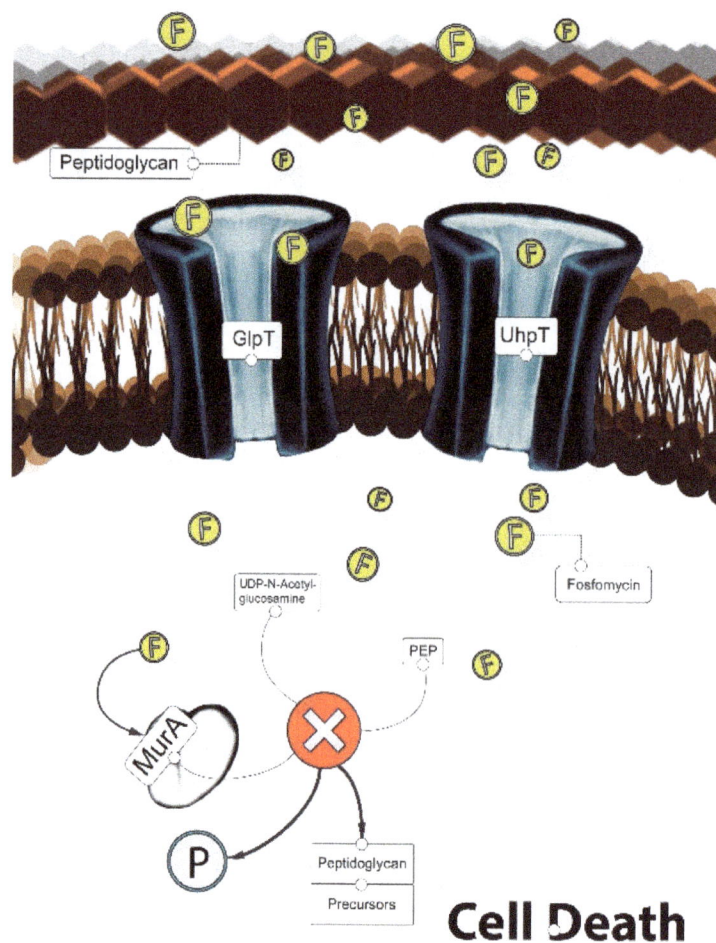

Figure 3. Mechanism of action of fosfomycin ("F").

4.3.2. Antibacterial Activity

Because both Gram-negative and Gram-positive bacteria require N-acetylmuramic acid for cell wall synthesis, fosfomycin is as a broad-spectrum antibiotic with activity against a wide range of bacteria, including *Escherichia coli*, *Proteus mirabilis*, *Klebsiella pneumoniae*, *Enterobacter* spp., *Citrobacter* spp., and *Salmonella typhi* [12,20,50–52]. However, due to a paucity of preclinical and clinical data, no universally accepted minimum inhibitory concentration (MIC) values have been defined for the susceptibility and resistance to fosfomycin; overall, the MIC for susceptibility ranges from ≤ 32 to ≤ 64 mg/L, and the MIC for resistance ranges from >32 to >256 mg/L, according to the Clinical and Laboratory Standards Institute (CLSI) and the European Committee on Antimicrobial Susceptibility Testing (EUCAST) [14,53].

Several studies have investigated the microbiological activity and efficacy of fosfomycin against several MDR, XDR, and PDR strains of Gram-negative bacteria. In this respect, fosfomycin has been reported to have both in vitro and in vivo activity against several MDR and XDR species of Enterobacteriaceae, including species that express extended-spectrum β-lactamases (ESBL) and metallo-β-lactamases (MBL) [14–18]. Due to the broad range of MIC values and differences in methods used to test susceptibility (e.g., agar dilution, microdilution, E-test), it is difficult to compare the results of different studies. However, given that some studies found that more than 90% of MDR and XDR isolates are susceptible to fosfomycin, fosfomycin is a promising candidate for treating infections with these pathogens [15,16], provided that in vivo results support the in vitro data.

MDR *P. aeruginosa* and *A. baumannii* are Gram-negative pathogens primarily responsible for nosocomial (i.e., hospital-acquired) infections, particularly in intensive care units [54]. A systematic review of microbiological, animal, and clinical studies using non-fermenting Gram-negative bacilli concluded that using fosfomycin in combined therapy may provide a safe and effective therapeutic option for treating infections due to MDR *P. aeruginosa* [13]. The clinical efficacy of fosfomycin against MDR-bacteria, including *P. aeruginosa*, has been suggested in patients with severe infections and critical conditions [18], and in cystic fibrosis patients with infective pulmonary exacerbations [55,56]. However, when used as monotherapy, *P. aeruginosa* should generally be regarded resistant to fosfomycin [57] and its use in *P. aeruginosa* infections should ideally be reversed for additional evaluation in clinical studies because the increased bacterial killing of combination therapy does not prevent the emergence of fosfomycin resistance [58]. In contrast, nearly all isolates of *A. baumannii* are resistant to fosfomycin, with a MIC_{90} value higher than 512 mg/L and there are no data on its use in combination therapy [14].

5. Fosfomycin Resistance

Three separate mechanisms of fosfomycin resistance have been reported [59]. The first mechanism is based on decreased uptake by the bacterium due to mutations in the genes that encode the glycerol-3-phosphate transporter or the glucose-6-phosphate transporter [47,60,61]. The second mechanism is based on point mutations in the binding site of the targeted enzyme (MurA) [62], and several isolates of *E. coli* have clinical resistance levels (32 mg/L) due to increased expression of the *murA* gene [63].The third mechanism of resistance is based on the inactivation of fosfomycin either by enzymatic cleavage of the epoxide ring or by phosphorylation of the phosphonate group. In the presence of the metalloenzymes FosA, FosB, and FosX, the epoxide structure is cleaved, with glutathione (FosA), bacillithiol and other thiols (FosB), or water (FosX) serving as the nucleophile [64]. With respect to the phosphorylation of the phosphonate group, FomA and FomB are kinases that catalyze the phosphorylation of fosfomycin to the diphosphate and triphosphate states, respectively [65,66]. Fosfomycin dosing regimens that include a total daily dose of up to 24 g per day resulted in the emergence of a resistant subpopulation within 30–40 h of drug exposure, suggesting that resistance can occur rapidly.

5.1. In Vitro Synergy between Fosfomycin and Other Antibiotics

The use of combined antimicrobial therapy is recommended in specific patient populations and indications, including critically ill patients who are at high risk for developing an MDR bacterial infection and patients with a *P. aeruginosa* infection [11,67,68]. In this regard, fosfomycin has an in vitro synergistic effect of up to 100% when combined with other antimicrobial agents [69].

The synergistic effect between fosfomycin and β-lactam antibiotics is proposed to arise from the inhibition of cell wall synthesis at separate steps; fosfomycin inhibits the first enzymatic step, whereas β-lactam antibiotics inhibit the final stage in the cell wall synthesis process [70]. In addition, fosfomycin may modify the activity of penicillin-binding proteins, which may account for the synergistic effect between fosfomycin and β-lactam antibiotics [49,71,72]. Another study found that the synergistic effect between fosfomycin and ciprofloxacin is due to ciprofloxacin-mediated damage to the outer membrane, which increases the penetration and activity of fosfomycin [73]. With respect to *P. aeruginosa*, several in vitro studies found synergy between fosfomycin and a variety of other antibiotics, including aztreonam, cefepime, meropenem, imipenem, ceftazidime, gentamycin, amikacin, ciprofloxacin, and others [70,74,75]. In addition, a few studies measured the synergistic effect of combining fosfomycin with amikacin or sulbactam against *A. baumannii* strains, providing evidence that these drugs might provide an effective combination therapy for infections with this pathogen [76,77]. Fosfomycin also has synergistic effects when combined with other antibiotics for treating methicillin-resistant *S. aureus*, *Streptococcus*, *Enterococcus*, and Enterobacteriaceae species [69,70]. In addition to increasing antibacterial efficacy, fosfomycin can also reduce toxicity associated with other antibiotics such as aminoglycosides, glycopeptides, and polymyxin B, as lower doses of these drugs can be prescribed [78–80].

5.2. Properties of Fosfomycin

The reintroduction of "old" antimicrobial agents to treat MDR bacteria requires optimization of the dosing regimen. This optimization includes obtaining a thorough understanding of the drug's pharmacokinetic (PK) and pharmacodynamic (PD) properties, thereby providing maximal antibacterial activity while minimizing toxicity and the development of resistance [11]. However, some "old" antibiotics, including fosfomycin, are currently used clinically despite uncertainty regarding the required and/or optimal exposure [11]. Therefore, it is essential to determine a rational dosing regimen based on the drug's PK/PD properties when introduced as a therapy against MDR bacteria.

5.3. PK/PD Properties

Because the exposure-response relationship can differ between antibiotics, it is important to define the correct PK/PD index for each antibiotic in order to establish the PK/PD target value that will maximize clinical efficacy [11,81,82]. With respect to antimicrobials, three PK/PD indices are commonly used: $T_{>MIC}$, which is the duration of time in which the drug concentration remains above the MIC during a dose interval; C_{max}/MIC, which is the drug's C_{max} divided by the MIC; and AUC/MIC, which is the AUC measured over a 24-h period divided by the MIC.

Relatively few in vitro studies have been performed to characterize fosfomycin's PK/PD properties. Some such studies suggest that fosfomycin has a time-dependent bactericidal activity, specifically against the Gram-positive *S. aureus* and *S. pyogenes* strains [32,35]; therefore, based on these results $T_{>MIC}$ should be optimized. However, in vitro studies by Mazzei et al. [83] and VanScoy et al. [84] suggest that fosfomycin shows a tendency towards a concentration-dependent bactericidal activity against *E.coli* and *P. mirabilis* strain, achieving complete sterilization at concentrations ≥4X MIC and ≥8X MIC, respectively. Moreover, an in vitro concentration-dependent post-antibiotic effect (PAE) was observed for both *E.coli* and *P. mirabilis* 3.2–3.4 h at 0.25X MIC and 3.5–4.7 h at 8X MIC [83]. However, with respect to these studies, it is not clear whether the bactericidal activity is concentration-dependent and/or time-dependent [85]. These studies however, do not provide conclusive data on the concentration- or time depending nature of bactericidal activity.

Therefore, the target PK/PD to achieve during therapy remains unknown, which is a major hurdle that must be overcome in order to optimize therapy.

5.4. Current Clinical Indications for Fosfomycin and Potential Future Applications

5.4.1. Intravenous Administration

Fosfomycin disodium is currently available in only a few European countries—namely, Spain, France, Germany, the United Kingdom, the Netherlands, Austria, and Greece—where it is approved for the treatment of soft-tissue infection and sepsis. A Fosfomycin disodium adult dose of 12–24 g daily is commonly administered in 2–4 separate infusions [51].

Due to is extensive tissue penetration, fosfomycin has emerged as a potential therapy for treating infections in the central nervous system (CNS) [32], soft tissues [33,39,40], bone [39], lungs [34], and abscesses [36]. Fosfomycin has high penetration into the interstitial fluid of soft tissues [40], reaching 50–70% of the levels measured in plasma, reaching sufficiently high levels to eliminate relevant pathogens [33,40]. Moreover, Schintler et al. reported that fosfomycin might also be effective in treating "deep" infections involving the osseous matrix [39].

With respect to CNS infections, Pfausler et al. reported that three daily IV doses of 8 g provided a steady-state concentration of 16 mg/L in the cerebrospinal fluid (CSF) for more than 90% of the interval between doses [32]. Moreover, the concentration of fosfomycin in the CSF can increase by nearly threefold with meningeal inflammation [86]. With respect to suppurative lesions, Sauermann et al. reported that repeated doses of IV fosfomycin can yield a concentration of 32 mg/L fosfomycin in the abscess, albeit with high inter-individual variability in the PK of fosfomycin in the abscess fluid [36,41].

MDR bacteria such as ESBL-producing bacteria and carbapenem-resistant bacteria are still susceptible to fosfomycin [17,18], and fosfomycin is used in combination therapy for treating these infections.

The repurposing of fosfomycin based on its activity against MDR Enterobacteriaceae is an important strategy for addressing the ever-present threat of antimicrobial resistance. The AUC/MIC seems to be the dynamically linked index for determining resistance suppression. In this respect, it is essential to develop optimal dosing strategies for each MDR Enterobacteriaceae species based on PK/PD data; moreover, additional dosing regimens may need to be developed for targeting different tissue sites of infection in order to prevent the development of resistance. Another promising approach is the use of combination therapy; for example, combining fosfomycin and meropenem yielded a significant synergistic effect, but also yielded a significantly additive effect in the fosfomycin-resistant subpopulation [87].

Currently, the FOREST study group is comparing the efficacy of combining fosfomycin with meropenem in treating urinary tract infections (UTIs) with ESBL-producing *E. coli* [88].

5.4.2. Oral Administration

Fosfomycin tromethamine is currently approved for use in several European countries and is only approved as a single 3-g dose for treating uncomplicated UTIs in women, specifically UTIs due to *E. coli* infection [29]. Fosfomycin tromethamine has also been investigated as a potential therapy for surgical prophylaxis in order to prevent prostate infection and even as a treatment for prostatitis due to MDR Gram-negative bacteria [37]. The use of a multiple-dose regimen with fosfomycin tromethamine has emerged as a potential strategy for treating of complicated and/or recurrent UTI, as well as infections due to MDR bacteria [89–91]. In this respect, simulations of the urinary concentrations of fosfomycin have been developed in order to determine the optimum dosing regimen that can provide a urinary concentration above the MIC (i.e., >16 mg/L) for seven days [89]; these simulations suggest that a single dose of 3 g administered every 72 h is sufficient to achieve the appropriate concentration. In addition, an uncontrolled, open-label, multicenter study conducted in China found that a regimen of single 3-g doses of fosfomycin tromethamine administered at two-day intervals might provide a safe, effective, and well-tolerated option for treating recurrent and/or complicated lower UTIs [90]. Thus, although the currently approved 3-g single dose of fosfomycin tromethamine is sufficient to reach efficacious concentrations in the urine, it might not be sufficient to achieve serum and/or tissue concentrations that are relevant for a clinical cure. A multiple-dose regimen of fosfomycin tromethamine might therefore be warranted for the oral treatment of more severe infections.

Ortiz et al. conducted simulations of several multiple-dose regimens using a wide range of daily doses of fosfomycin tromethamine and fosfomycin disodium [92]. The authors calculated PK/PD indices, including C_{max}/MIC, AUC/MIC, and %$T_{>MIC}$, for each dosing regimen using a MIC of 8 mg/L. They concluded that a total daily dose of 6–12 g for microorganisms with a MIC of 8 mg/L well exceeds the currently approved single dose of 3 g. However, the safety and tolerability of fosfomycin tromethamine at such high doses has not been investigated. Nevertheless, further studies are urgently needed in order to assess the PK, safety, tolerability, and efficacy of fosfomycin in both multiple-dose regimens and synergistic combinations.

6. Conclusions

The World Health Organization currently recognizes that antibacterial drug resistance is one of the major threats facing global public health, particularly given the reduction in the number of effective antibiotics. In this respect, reassessing and reevaluating "old" antibiotics such as fosfomycin has been proposed as a possible strategy in treating drug-resistant bacterial infections. Fosfomycin is a broad-spectrum antibiotic with both in vivo and in vitro activity against a wide range of bacteria, including MDR, XDR, and PDR bacteria. Thanks to its high tissue penetration, fosfomycin may be used in a broad range of tissues and targets, including the CNS, soft tissue, bone, lungs, and abscess fluid. Oral fosfomycin in a multiple-dose regimen has emerged as a potential strategy for treating complicated UTIs and prostatitis; however, given the relative lack of essential information regarding the pharmacological properties and mechanisms of resistance, additional studies are urgently needed. In the meantime, using fosfomycin as a monotherapy should be avoided due to the rapid development of resistance in vitro.

Acknowledgments: We acknowledge Thomas Vissers and Annemarie van der Velden, Librarians at Medical Center Haaglanden and Bronovo-Nebo (The Hague, the Netherlands) for helping with the literature search. We are also grateful to Folkert van Meurs at the Centre for Human Drug Research (Leiden, the Netherlands) for help preparing the figures in this review.

Author Contributions: Data collection: Anneke Corinne Dijkmans and Ingrid Maria Catharina Kamerling; manuscript preparation: Anneke Corinne Dijkmans; contributions to manuscript: Anneke Corinne Dijkmans, Natalia Veneranda Ortiz Zacarías, Jacobus Burggraaf, Johan Willem Mouton, Erik Bert Wilms, Cees van Nieuwkoop, Daniel Johannes Touw, Jasper Stevens and Ingrid Maria Catharina Kamerling; review of the manuscript: Anneke Corinne Dijkmans, Natalia Veneranda Ortiz Zacarías, Jacobus Burggraaf, Johan Willem Mouton, Erik Bert Wilms, Cees van Nieuwkoop, Daniel Johannes Touw, Jasper Stevens and Ingrid Maria Catharina Kamerling. All authors read and approved the final manuscript.

References

1.   Rice, L.B. Federal funding for the study of antimicrobial resistance in nosocomial pathogens: No ESKAPE. *J. Infect. Dis.* **2008**, *197*, 1079–1081. [CrossRef] [PubMed]
2.   Spellberg, B.; Guidos, R.; Gilbert, D.; Bradley, J.; Boucher, H.W.; Scheld, W.M.; Bartlett, J.G.; Edwards, J., Jr.; The Infectious Diseases Society of America. The epidemic of antibiotic-resistant infections: A call to action for the medical community from the Infectious Diseases Society of America. *Clin. Infect. Dis.* **2008**, *46*, 155–164. [CrossRef] [PubMed]
3.   Alanis, A.J. Resistance to Antibiotics: Are We in the Post-Antibiotic Era? *Arch. Med. Res.* **2005**, *36*, 697–705. [CrossRef] [PubMed]

4. Laxminarayan, R.; Duse, A.; Wattal, C.; Zaidi, A.K.M.; Wertheim, H.F.L.; Sumpradit, N.; Vlieghe, E.; Hara, G.L.; Gould, I.M.; Goossens, H.; et al. Antibiotic resistance—The need for global solutions. *Lancet Infect. Dis.* **2013**, *13*, 1057–1098. [CrossRef]

5. World Health Organization. *Antimicrobial Resistance: Global Report on Surveillance 2014*; World Health Organization: Geneva, Switzerland, 2014.

6. Boucher, H.W.; Talbot, G.H.; Bradley, J.S.; Edwards, J.E.; Gilbert, D.; Rice, L.B.; Scheld, M.; Spellberg, B.; Bartlett, J. Bad bugs, no drugs: No ESKAPE! An update from the Infectious Diseases Society of America. *Clin. Infect. Dis.* **2009**, *48*, 1–12. [CrossRef] [PubMed]

7. ECDC; EMEA. *The Bacterial Challenge: Time to React. Joint Technical Report*; European Centre for Disease Prevention and Control: Stockholm, Sweden; European Medicines Agency: London, UK, 2009.

8. Freire-Moran, L.; Aronsson, B.; Manz, C.; Gyssens, I.C.; So, A.D.; Monnet, D.L.; Cars, O.; the ECDC-EMA Working Group. Critical shortage of new antibiotics in development against multidrug-resistant bacteria—Time to react is now. *Drug Resist. Updates* **2011**, *14*, 118–124. [CrossRef] [PubMed]

9. Bergen, P.J.; Landersdorfer, C.B.; Lee, H.J.; Li, J.; Nation, R.L. "Old" antibiotics for emerging multidrug-resistant bacteria. *Curr. Opin. Infect. Dis.* **2012**, *25*, 626–633. [CrossRef] [PubMed]

10. Bush, K.; Courvalin, P.; Dantas, G.; Davies, J.; Eisenstein, B.; Huovinen, P.; Jacoby, G.A.; Kishony, R.; Kreiswirth, B.N.; Kutter, E.; et al. Tackling antibiotic resistance. *Nat. Rev. Microbiol.* **2011**, *9*, 894–896. [CrossRef] [PubMed]

11. Mouton, J.W.; Ambrose, P.G.; Canton, R.; Drusano, G.L.; Harbarth, S.; MacGowan, A.; Theuretzbacher, U.; Turnidge, J. Conserving antibiotics for the future: New ways to use old and new drugs from a pharmacokinetic and pharmacodynamic perspective. *Drug Resist. Updates* **2011**, *14*, 107–117. [CrossRef] [PubMed]

12. Falagas, M.E.; Giannopoulou, K.P.; Kokolakis, G.N.; Rafailidis, P.I. Fosfomycin: Use beyond urinary tract and gastrointestinal infections. *Clin. Infect. Dis.* **2008**, *46*, 1069–1077. [CrossRef] [PubMed]

13. Falagas, M.E.; Kastoris, A.C.; Karageorgopoulos, D.E.; Rafailidis, P.I. Fosfomycin for the treatment of infections caused by multidrug-resistant non-fermenting Gram-negative bacilli: A systematic review of microbiological, animal and clinical studies. *Int. J. Antimicrob. Agents* **2009**, *34*, 111–120. [CrossRef] [PubMed]

14. Falagas, M.E.; Kanellopoulou, M.D.; Karageorgopoulos, D.E.; Dimopoulos, G.; Rafailidis, P.I.; Skarmoutsou, N.D.; Papafrangas, E.A. Antimicrobial susceptibility of multidrug-resistant Gram negative bacteria to fosfomycin. *Eur. J. Clin. Microbiol. Infect. Dis.* **2008**, *27*, 439–443. [CrossRef] [PubMed]

15. Falagas, M.E.; Maraki, S.; Karageorgopoulos, D.E.; Kastoris, A.C.; Mavromanolakis, E.; Samonis, G. Antimicrobial susceptibility of multidrug-resistant (MDR) and extensively drug-resistant (XDR) Enterobacteriaceae isolates to fosfomycin. *Int. J. Antimicrob. Agents* **2010**, *35*, 240–243. [CrossRef] [PubMed]

16. Falagas, M.E.; Kastoris, A.C.; Kapaskelis, A.M.; Karageorgopoulos, D.E. Fosfomycin for the treatment of multidrug-resistant, including extended-spectrum b-lactamase producing, Enterobacteriaceae infections: A systematic review. *Lancet Infect. Dis.* **2010**, *10*, 43–50. [CrossRef]

17. Michalopoulos, A.; Virtzili, S.; Rafailidis, P.; Halevelakis, G.H.; Damala, M.; Falagas, M. Intravenous fosfomycin for the treatment of nosocomial infections caused by carbapenem-resistant Klebsiella pneumoniae in critically ill patients: A prospective evaluation. *Clin. Microbiol. Infect.* **2010**, *16*, 184–186. [CrossRef] [PubMed]

18. Dinh, A.; Salomon, J.; Bru, J.P.; Bernard, L. Fosfomycin: Efficacy against infections caused by multidrug-resistant bacteria. *Scand. J. Infect. Dis.* **2012**, *44*, 182–189. [CrossRef] [PubMed]

19. Hendlin, D.; Stapley, E.O.; Jackson, M.; Wallick, H.; Miller, A.K.; Wolf, F.J.; Miller, T.W.; Chaiet, L.; Kahan, F.M.; Foltz, E.L.; et al. Phosphonomycin, a new antibiotic produced by strains of Streptomyces. *Science* **1969**, *166*, 122–123. [CrossRef] [PubMed]

20. Popovic, M.; Steinort, D.; Pillai, S.; Joukhadar, C. Fosfomycin: An old, new friend? *Eur. J. Clin. Microbiol. Infect. Dis.* **2010**, *29*, 127–142. [CrossRef] [PubMed]

21. Bergan, T. Degree of absorption, pharmacokinetics of fosfomycin trometamol and duration of urinary antibacterial activity. *Infection* **1990**, *18*, S65–S69. [CrossRef] [PubMed]

22. Ishizawa, T.; Sadahiro, S.; Hosoi, K.; Tamai, I.; Terasaki, T.; Tsuji, A. Mechanisms of intestinal absorption of the antibiotic, fosfomycin, in brush-border membrane vesicles in rabbits and humans. *J. Pharm. Dyn.* **1992**, *15*, 481–489. [CrossRef]

23. Bundgaard, H. Acid-catalyzed hydrolysis of fosfomycin and its implication in oral absorption of the drug. *Int. J. Pharm.* **1980**, *6*, 1–9. [CrossRef]

24. Shimizu, K. Fosfomycin: Absorption and excretion. *Chemotherapy* **1977**, *23*, 153–158. [CrossRef] [PubMed]

25. Segre, G.; Bianchi, E.; Cataldi, A.; Zannini, G. Pharmacokinetic profile of fosfomycin trometamol (Monuril). *Eur. Urol.* **1986**, *13*, 56–63. [CrossRef]

26. Bergan, T.; Thorsteinsson, S.B.; Albini, E. Pharmacokinetic profile of fosfomycin trometamol. *Chemotherapy* **1993**, *39*, 297–301. [CrossRef] [PubMed]

27. Goto, M.I.T.S.; Sugiyama, M.A.S.A.; Nakajima, S.H.I.N.; Yamashina, H. Fosfomycin kinetics after intravenous and oral administration to human volunteers. *Antimicrob. Agents Chemother.* **1981**, *20*, 393–397. [CrossRef] [PubMed]

28. Cadorniga, R.; Diaz Fierros, M.; Olay, T. Pharmacokinetic study of fosfomycin and its bioavailability. *Chemotherapy* **1977**, *23*, 159–174. [CrossRef] [PubMed]

29. Zambon Switzerland Ltd. *Monurol® (Fosfomycin Tromethamine): US Prescribing Information*; Zambon Switzerland Ltd.: Cadempino, Switzerland, 2011.

30. Borsa, F.; Leroy, A.; Fillastre, J.P.; Godin, M.; Moulin, B. Comparative pharmacokinetics of tromethamine fosfomycin and calcium fosfomycin in young and elderly adults. *Antimicrob. Agents Chemother.* **1988**, *32*, 938–941. [CrossRef] [PubMed]

31. Kirby, W.M.M. Pharmacokinetics of fosfomycin. *Chemotherapy* **1977**, *23*, 141–151. [CrossRef] [PubMed]

32. Pfausler, B.; Spiss, H.; Dittrich, P.; Zeitlinger, M.; Schmutzhard, E.; Joukhadar, C. Concentrations of fosfomycin in the cerebrospinal fluid of neurointensive care patients with ventriculostomy-associated ventriculitis. *J. Antimicrob. Chemother.* **2004**, *53*, 848–852. [CrossRef] [PubMed]

33. Frossard, M.; Joukhadar, C.; Erovic, B.M.; Dittrich, P.; Mrass, P.E.; van Houte, M.; Burgmann, H.; Georgopoulos, A.; Müller, M. Distribution and antimicrobial activity of fosfomycin in the interstitial fluid of human soft tissues. *Antimicrob. Agents Chemother.* **2000**, *44*, 2728–2732. [CrossRef] [PubMed]

34. Matzi, V.; Lindenmann, J.; Porubsky, C.; Kugler, S.A.; Maier, A.; Dittrich, P.; Smolle-Jüttner, F.M.; Joukhadar, C. Extracellular concentrations of fosfomycin in lung tissue of septic patients. *J. Antimicrob. Chemother.* **2010**, *65*, 995–998. [CrossRef] [PubMed]

35. Joukhadar, C.; Klein, N.; Dittrich, P.; Zeitlinger, M.; Geppert, A.; Skhirtladze, K.; Frossard, M.; Heinz, G.; Müller, M. Target site penetration of fosfomycin in critically ill patients. *J. Antimicrob. Chemother.* **2003**, *51*, 1247–1252. [CrossRef] [PubMed]

36. Sauermann, R.; Karch, R.; Langenberger, H.; Kettenbach, J.; Mayer-Helm, B.; Petsch, M.; Wagner, C.; Sautner, T.; Gattringer, R.; Karanikas, G.; et al. Antibiotic abscess penetration: Fosfomycin levels measured in pus and simulated concentration-time profiles. *Antimicrob. Agents Chemother.* **2005**, *49*, 4448–4454. [CrossRef] [PubMed]

37. Gardiner, B.J.; Mahony, A.A.; Ellis, A.G.; Lawrentschuk, N.; Bolton, D.M.; Zeglinski, P.T.; Frauman, A.G.; Grayson, M.L. Is fosfomycin a potential treatment alternative for multidrug-resistant gram-negative prostatitis? *Clin. Infect. Dis.* **2014**, *58*, e101–e105. [CrossRef] [PubMed]

38. Müller, O.; Rückert, P.D.D.; Walter, W.; Haag, R.; Sauer, W. Fosfomycin-Konzentrationen im Serum und in der Galle. *Infection* **1982**, *10*, 18–20. [CrossRef] [PubMed]

39. Schintler, M.V.; Traunmller, F.; Metzler, J.; Kreuzwirt, G.; Spendel, S.; Mauric, O.; Popovic, M.; Scharnagl, E.; Joukhadar, C. High fosfomycin concentrations in bone and peripheral soft tissue in diabetic patients presenting with bacterial foot infection. *J. Antimicrob. Chemother.* **2009**, *64*, 574–578. [CrossRef] [PubMed]

40. Legat, F.J.; Maier, A.; Dittrich, P.; Zenahlik, P.; Kern, T.; Nuhsbaumer, S.; Frossard, M.; Salmhofer, W.; Kerl, H.; Müller, M. Penetration of fosfomycin into inflammatory lesions in patients with cellulitis or diabetic foot syndrome. *Antimicrob. Agents Chemother.* **2003**, *47*, 371–374. [CrossRef] [PubMed]

41. Kjellsson, M.C.; Kern, S.; Sauermann, R.; Dartois, V.; Pillai, G. Modeling the permeability of fosfomycin into abscess fluid. In Proceedings of the 18th Meeting of the Population Approach Group in Europe PAGE, St. Petersburg, Russia, 23–26 June 2009.

42. Kwan, K.C.; Wadke, D.A.; Foltz, E.L. Pharmacokinetics of phosphonomycin in man I: Intravenous administration. *J. Pharm. Sci.* **1971**, *60*, 678–685. [CrossRef] [PubMed]

43. Lastra, C.F.; Marino, E.L.; Dominguez-Gil, A.; Tabernero, J.M.; Lope, A.G.; Chaves, M.Y. The influence of uremia on the accessibility of phosphomycin into interstitial tissue fluid. *Eur. J. Clin. Pharmacol.* **1983**, *25*, 333–338. [CrossRef]

44. Bergan, T. Pharmacokinetic comparison between fosfomycin and other phosphonic acid derivatives. *Chemotherapy* **1990**, *36*, 10–18. [CrossRef] [PubMed]

45. Woodruff, H.B.; Mata, J.M.; Agravendez, S.; Mochales, S.; Rodríguez, A.; Stapley, E.O.; Wallick, H.; Miller, A.K.; Hendlin, D. Fosfomycin: Laboratory studies. *Chemotherapy* **1977**, *23*, 1–22. [CrossRef] [PubMed]

46. Neuman, M.; Fluteau, G. Blood and urinary concentrations of fosfomycin as a function of the renal function value. *Chemotherapy* **1977**, *23*, 196–199. [CrossRef] [PubMed]

47. Kahan, F.M.; Kahan, J.S.; Cassidy, P.J.; Kropp, H. The Mechanism of Action of Fosfomycin (Phosphonomycin). *Ann. N. Y. Acad. Sci.* **1974**, *235*, 364–386. [CrossRef] [PubMed]

48. Brown, E.D.; Vivas, E.I.; Walsh, C.T.; Kolter, R. MurA (MurZ), the enzyme that catalyzes the first committed step in peptidoglycan biosynthesis, is essential in Escherichia coli. *J. Bacteriol.* **1995**, *177*, 4194–4197. [CrossRef] [PubMed]

49. Utsui, Y.; Ohya, S.; Magaribuchi, T.; Tajima, M.; Yokota, T. Antibacterial activity of cefmetazole alone and in combination with fosfomycin against methicillin- and cephem-resistant *Staphylococcus aureus*. *Antimicrob. Agents Chemother.* **1986**, *30*, 917–922. [CrossRef] [PubMed]

50. Frimodt-Moller, N. Fosfomycin. In *Kucers' the Use of Antibiotics*; Grayson, M.L., Crowe, S.M., McCarthy, J.S., Mills, J., Mouton, J.M., Norrby, S.R., Paterson, D.L., Pfaller, M.A., Eds.; Hodder Arnold/ASM Press: London, UK, 2010; pp. 935–944.

51. Michalopoulos, A.S.; Livaditis, I.G.; Gougoutas, V. The revival of fosfomycin. *Int. J. Infect. Dis.* **2011**, *15*, e732–e739. [CrossRef] [PubMed]

52. Barry, A.L.; Brown, S.D. Antibacterial spectrum of fosfomycin trometamol. *J. Antimicrob. Chemother.* **1995**, *35*, 228–230. [CrossRef] [PubMed]

53. European Committee on Antimicrobial Susceptibility Testing. *Fosfomycin: Rationale for the Clinical Breakpoints, Version 1.0*; European Committee on Antimicrobial Susceptibility Testing: Växjö, Sweden, 2013.

54. Paterson, D.L. Serious infections in the intensive care unit: Pseudomonas aeruginosa and Acinetobacter baumannii. *Clin. Infect. Dis.* **2006**, *43*, S41–S42. [CrossRef]

55. Faruqi, S.; McCreanor, J.; Moon, T.; Meigh, R.; Morice, A.H. Fosfomycin for Pseudomonas-related exacerbations of cystic fibrosis. *Int. J. Antimicrob. Agents* **2008**, *32*, 461–463. [CrossRef] [PubMed]

56. Mirakhur, A.; Gallagher, M.J.; Ledson, M.J.; Harta, C.A.; Walshawa, M.J. Fosfomycin therapy for multiresistant Pseudomonas aeruginosa in cystic fibrosis. *J. Cyst. Fibros.* **2003**, *2*, 19–24. [CrossRef]

57. Lu, C.L.; Liu, C.Y.; Huang, Y.T.; Liao, C.H.; Teng, L.J.; Turnidge, J.D.; Liao, C.H.; Teng, L.J.; Turnidge, J.D.; Hsueh, P.R. Antimicrobial Susceptibilities of commonly encountered bacterial isolates to fosfomycin determined by agar dilution and disk diffusion methods. *Antimicrob. Agents Chemother.* **2011**, *55*, 4295–4301. [CrossRef] [PubMed]

58. Walsh, C.C.; Landersdorfer, C.B.; McIntosh, M.P.; Peleg, A.Y.; Hirsch, E.B.; Kirkpatrick, C.M.; Bergen, P.J. Clinically relevant concentrations of fosfomycin combined with polymyxin B, tobramycin or ciprofloxacin enhance bacterial killing of Pseudomonas aeruginosa, but do not suppress the emergence of fosfomycin resistance. *J. Antimicrob. Chemother.* **2016**, *71*, 2218–2229. [CrossRef] [PubMed]

59. Castaneda-Garcia, A.; Blazquez, J.; Rodriguez-Rojas, A. Molecular Mechanisms and Clinical Impact of Acquired and Intrinsic Fosfomycin Resistance. *Antibiotics* **2013**, *2*, 217–236. [CrossRef] [PubMed]

60. Tsuruoka, T.; Yamada, Y. Charactertization of spontaneous fosfomycin (phosphonomycin)-resistant cells of Escherichia coli B in vitro. *J. Antibiot.* **1975**, *28*, 906–911. [CrossRef] [PubMed]

61. Kadner, R.J.; Winkler, H.H. Isolation and characterization of mutations affecting the transport of hexose phosphates in Escherichia coli. *J. Bacteriol.* **1973**, *113*, 895–900. [PubMed]

62. Kim, D.H.; Lees, W.J.; Kempsell, K.E.; Lane, W.S.; Duncan, K.; Walsh, C.T. Characterization of a Cys115 to Asp substitution in the Escherichia coli cell wall biosynthetic enzyme UDP-GlcNAc enolpyruvyl transferase (MurA) that confers resistance to inactivation by the antibiotic fosfomycin. *Biochemistry* **1996**, *35*, 4923–4928. [CrossRef] [PubMed]

63. Horii, T.; Kimura, T.; Sato, K.; Shibayama, K.; Ohta, M. Emergence of fosfomycin-resistant isolates of Shiga-like toxin-producing Escherichia coli O26. *Antimicrob. Agents Chemother.* **1999**, *43*, 789–793. [PubMed]

64. Rigsby, R.E.; Fillgrove, K.L.; Beihoffer, L.A.; Armstrong, R.N. Fosfomycin resistance proteins: A nexus of glutathione transferases and epoxide hydrolases in a metalloenzyme superfamily. *Methods Enzymol.* **2005**, *401*, 367–379. [PubMed]

65. Kobayashi, S.; Kuzuyama, T.; Seto, H. Characterization of the fomA and fomB gene products from Streptomyces wedmorensis, which confer fosfomycin resistance on Escherichia coli. *Antimicrob. Agents Chemother.* **2000**, *44*, 647–650. [CrossRef] [PubMed]

66. Kuzuyama, T.; Kobayashi, S.; O'Hara, K.; Hidaka, T.; Seto, H. Fosfomycin monophosphate and fosfomycin diphosphate, two inactivated fosfomycin derivatives formed by gene products of fomA and fomB from a fosfomycin producing organism Streptomyces wedmorensis. *J. Antibiot.* **1996**, *49*, 502–504. [CrossRef] [PubMed]

67. Dellit, T.H.; Owens, R.C.; McGowan, J.E.; Gerding, D.N.; Weinstein, R.A.; Burke, J.P.; Huskins, W.C.; Paterson, D.L.; Fishman, N.O.; Brennan, C.F.C.P.J. Infectious Diseases Society of America and the Society for Healthcare Epidemiology of America guidelines for developing an institutional program to enhance antimicrobial stewardship. *Clin. Infect. Dis.* **2007**, *44*, 159–177. [CrossRef] [PubMed]

68. Safdar, N.; Handelsman, J.; Maki, D.G. Does combination antimicrobial therapy reduce mortality in Gram-negative bacteraemia? A meta-analysis. *Lancet Infect. Dis.* **2004**, *4*, 519–527. [CrossRef]

69. Kastoris, A.C.; Rafailidis, P.I.; Vouloumanou, E.K.; GkegkesMatthew, I.D.; Falagas, E. Synergy of fosfomycin with other antibiotics for Gram-positive and Gram-negative bacteria. *Eur. J. Clin. Pharmacol.* **2010**, *66*, 359–368. [CrossRef] [PubMed]

70. Samonis, G.; Maraki, S.; Karageorgopoulos, D.E.; Vouloumanou, E.K.; Falagas, M.E. Synergy of fosfomycin with carbapenems, colistin, netilmicin, and tigecycline against multidrug-resistant Klebsiella pneumoniae, Escherichia coli, and Pseudomonas aeruginosa clinical isolates. *Eur. J. Clin. Microbiol. Infect. Dis.* **2012**, *31*, 695–701. [CrossRef] [PubMed]

71. Grossato, A.; Sartori, R.; Fontana, R. Effect of non-b-lactam antibiotics on penicillin-binding protein synthesis of Enterococcus hirae ATCC 9790. *J. Antimicrob. Chemother.* **1991**, *27*, 263–271. [CrossRef] [PubMed]

72. Totsuka, K.; Uchiyama, T.; Shimizu, K.; Kanno, Y.; Takata, T.; Yoshida, T. In vitro combined effects of fosfomycin and b-lactam antibiotics against penicillin-resistant *Streptococcus pneumoniae. J. Infect. Chemother.* **1997**, *3*, 49–54. [CrossRef]

73. Yamada, S.; Hyo, Y.; Ohmori, S.; Ohuchi, M. Role of ciprofloxacin in its synergistic effect with fosfomycin on drug-resistant strains of *Pseudomonas aeruginosa. Chemotherapy* **2007**, *53*, 202–209. [CrossRef] [PubMed]

74. Okazaki, M.; Suzuki, K.; Asano, N.; Araki, K.; Shukuya, N.; Egami, T.; Higurashi, Y.; Morita, K.; Uchimura, H.; Watanabe, T. Effectiveness of fosfomycin combined with other antimicrobial agents against multidrug-resistant *Pseudomonas aeruginosa* isolates using the efficacy time index assay. *J. Infect. Chemother.* **2002**, *8*, 37–42. [CrossRef] [PubMed]

75. Tessier, F.; Quentin, C. In vitro activity of fosfomycin combined with ceftazidime, imipenem, amikacin, and ciprofloxacin against Pseudomonas aeruginosa. *Eur. J. Clin. Microbiol. Infect. Dis.* **1997**, *16*, 159–162. [CrossRef] [PubMed]

76. Martinez-Martinez, L.; Rodriguez, G.; Pascual, A.; Suárez, A.I.; Perea, E.J. In Vitro activity of antimicrobial agent combinations against multiresistant *Acinetobacter baumannii. J. Antimicrob. Chemother.* **1996**, *38*, 1107–1108. [CrossRef] [PubMed]

77. Santimaleeworagun, W.; Wongpoowarak, P.; Chayakul, P.; Pattharachayakul, S.; Tansakul, P.; Garey, K.W. In vitro activity of colistin or sulbactam in combination with fosfomycin or imipenem against clinical isolates of carbapenem-resistant Acinetobacter baumannii producing OXA-23 carbapenemases. *Southeast Asian J. Trop. Med. Public Health* **2011**, *42*, 890–900. [PubMed]

78. Inouye, S.; Watanabe, T.; Tsuruoka, T.; Kitasato, I. An increase in the antimicrobial activity in vitro of fosfomycin under anaerobic conditions. *J. Antimicrob. Chemother.* **1989**, *24*, 657–666. [CrossRef] [PubMed]

79. Yanagida, C.; Ito, K.; Komiya, I.; Horie, T. Protective effect of fosfomycin on gentamicin-induced lipid peroxidation of rat renal tissue. *Chem. Biol. Interact.* **2004**, *148*, 139–147. [CrossRef] [PubMed]

80. Nakamura, T.; Kokuryo, T.; Hashimoto, Y.; Inui, K.I. Effects of fosfomycin and imipenem-cilastatin on the nephrotoxicity of vancomycin and cisplatin in rats. *J. Pharm. Pharmacol.* **1999**, *51*, 227–232. [CrossRef] [PubMed]

81. Craig, W.A. Pharmacokinetic/pharmacodynamic parameters: Rationale for antibacterial dosing of mice and men. *Clin. Infect. Dis.* **1998**, *26*, 1–10. [CrossRef] [PubMed]

82. Mouton, J.W.; Brown, D.F.J.; Apfalter, P.; Cantón, R.; Giske, C.G.; Ivanova, M.; MacGowan, A.P.; Rodloff, A.; Soussy, C.J.; Steinbakk, M.; et al. The role of pharmacokinetics/pharmacodynamics in setting clinical MIC breakpoints: The EUCAST approach. *Clin. Microbiol. Infect.* **2012**, *18*, E37–E45. [CrossRef] [PubMed]

83. Mazzei, T.; Cassetta, M.I.; Fallani, S.; Arrigucci, S.; Novelli, A. Pharmacokinetic and pharmacodynamic aspects of antimicrobial agents for the treatment of uncomplicated urinary tract infections. *Int. J. Antimicrob. Agents* **2006**, *28*, 35–41. [CrossRef] [PubMed]

84. VanScoy, B.; McCauley, J.; Bhavnani, S.M.; Ellis-Grosseb, E.J.; Ambrosea, P.G. Relationship between Fosfomycin Exposure and Amplification of Escherichia coli Subpopulations with Reduced Susceptibility in a Hollow-Fiber Infection Model. *Antimicrob. Agents Chemother.* **2016**, *60*, 5141–5145. [CrossRef] [PubMed]

85. Roussos, N.; Karageorgopoulos, D.E.; Samonis, G.; Falagas, M.E. Clinical significance of the pharmacokinetic and pharmacodynamic characteristics of fosfomycin for the treatment of patients with systemic infections. *Int. J. Antimicrob. Agents* **2009**, *34*, 506–515. [CrossRef] [PubMed]

86. Kühnen, E.; Pfeifer, G.; Frenkel, C. Penetration of fosfomycin into cerebrospinal fluid across non-inflamed and inflamed meninges. *Infection* **1987**, *15*, 422–424. [CrossRef] [PubMed]

87. Docobo-Perez, F.; Drusano, G.L.; Johnson, A.; Goodwin, J.; Whalley, S.; Ramos-Martín, V.; Ballestero-Tellez, M.; Rodriguez-Martinez, J.M.; Conejo, M.C.; van Guilder, M.; et al. Pharmacodynamics of fosfomycin: Insights into clinical use for antimicrobial resistance. *Antimicrob. Agents Chemother.* **2015**, *59*, 5602–5610. [CrossRef] [PubMed]

88. Rosso-Fernandez, C.; Sojo-Dorado, J.; Barriga, A.; Lavín-Alconero, L.; Palacios, Z.; López-Hernández, I.; Merino, V.; Camean, M.; Pascual, A.; Rodríguez-Baño, J. Fosfomycin versus meropenem in bacteraemic urinary tract infections caused by extended-spectrum beta-lactamase-producing *Escherichia coli* (FOREST): Study protocol for an investigator-driven randomised controlled trial. *BMJ Open* **2015**, *5*, e007363. [CrossRef] [PubMed]

89. Sádaba-Díaz De Rada, B.; Azanza-Perea, J.R.; García-Quetglas, E.; Honorato-Pérez, J. Fosfomicina trometamol. Dosis múltiples como pauta larga en el tratamiento de las infecciones urinarias bajas. *Enferm. Infect. Microbiol. Clin.* **2006**, *24*, 546–550. [CrossRef]

90. Qiao, L.D.; Zheng, B.; Chen, S.; Yang, Y.; Zhang, K.; Guo, H.F.; Yang, B.; Niu, Y.J.; Wang, Y.; Shi, B.K.; et al. Evaluation of three-dose fosfomycin tromethamine in the treatment of patients with urinary tract infections: An uncontrolled, open-label, multicentre study. *BMJ Open* **2013**, *3*, e004157. [CrossRef] [PubMed]

91. Shrestha, N.K.; Amuh, D.; Goldman, M.P.; Riebel, W.J.; Tomford, W.J. Treatment of a complicated vancomycin-resistant enterococcal urinary tract infection with fosfomycin. *Infect. Dis. Clin. Pract.* **2000**, *9*, 368–371. [CrossRef]

92. Multiple-Dose Regimen Of Intravenous and Oral Fosfomycin Tromethamine as a Potential Therapy for the Treatment of Systemic Infections Due to Multidrug-Resistantbacteria. Available online: https://www.escmid.org/research_projects/escmid_conferences/past_escmid_conferences/reviving_old_antibiotics/poster_presentations/ (accessed on 17 October 2017).

4

Dual Regulation of the Small RNA MicC and the Quiescent Porin OmpN in Response to Antibiotic Stress in *Escherichia coli*

Sushovan Dam, Jean-Marie Pagès and Muriel Masi * (iD)

UMR_MD1, Aix-Marseille Univ & Institut de Recherche Biomédicale des Armées, 27 Boulevard Jean Moulin, 13005 Marseille, France; sushovan.dam@etu.univ-amu.fr (S.D.); jean-marie.pages@univ-amu.fr (J.-M.P.)
* Correspondence: muriel.masi@univ-amu.fr

Academic Editor: Leonard Amaral

Abstract: Antibiotic resistant Gram-negative bacteria are a serious threat for public health. The permeation of antibiotics through their outer membrane is largely dependent on porin, changes in which cause reduced drug uptake and efficacy. *Escherichia coli* produces two major porins, OmpF and OmpC. MicF and MicC are small non-coding RNAs (sRNAs) that modulate the expression of OmpF and OmpC, respectively. In this work, we investigated factors that lead to increased production of MicC. *micC* promoter region was fused to *lacZ*, and the reporter plasmid was transformed into *E. coli* MC4100 and derivative mutants. The response of *micC–lacZ* to antimicrobials was measured during growth over a 6 h time period. The data showed that the expression of *micC* was increased in the presence of β-lactam antibiotics and in an *rpoE* depleted mutant. Interestingly, the same conditions enhanced the activity of an *ompN–lacZ* fusion, suggesting a dual transcriptional regulation of *micC* and the quiescent adjacent *ompN*. Increased levels of OmpN in the presence of sub-inhibitory concentrations of chemicals could not be confirmed by Western blot analysis, except when analyzed in the absence of the sigma factor σ^E. We suggest that the MicC sRNA acts together with the σ^E envelope stress response pathway to control the OmpC/N levels in response to β-lactam antibiotics.

Keywords: *Escherichia coli*; outer membrane porins; regulatory small RNAs; membrane transport; antibiotic susceptibility

1. Introduction

Antibacterial resistance is broadly recognized as a growing threat for human health [1–3]. As such, increasing antibiotic treatment failures due to multidrug resistant (MDR) bacteria have stirred the urgent need to better understand the underlying molecular mechanisms and promote innovation, with the development of new antibiotics and alternative therapies [4,5]. The efficacy of antibacterial compounds depends on their capacity to reach inhibitory concentrations at the vicinity of their target. This is particularly challenging for drugs directed against Gram-negative bacteria, which exhibit a complex envelope comprising two membranes and transmembrane efflux pumps [6]. The Gram-negative envelope comprises an inner membrane (IM), which is a symmetric phospholipid bilayer; a thin peptidoglycan (PG) layer ensuring the cell shape; and an outer membrane (OM) that is an asymmetric bilayer, composed of an inner phospholipid leaflet and an outer leaflet of lipopolysaccharide (LPS) [7]. First, the OM is a barrier to both hydrophobic and hydrophilic compounds, including necessary nutrients, metabolic substrates and antibiotics, but access is provided by the water filled β-barrel channels called porins [8,9]. In *Escherichia coli*, the channels of the general porins OmpF and OmpC, are size restricted, and show a preference for passage of hydrophilic charged compounds, including antibiotics such as β-lactams and fluoroquinolones. Second, constitutive tripartite RND (resistance–nodulation–cell division) efflux pumps, such as the AcrAB–TolC pump of *E. coli*, play a major role in removing antibiotics from the periplasm [10]. Importantly, it has been noted that the efflux pumps are synergized by the OM, since, once ejected into the extracellular space, compounds must re-traverse the restricted-permeability OM barrier [10]. Not surprisingly, MDR clinical isolates of *Enterobacteriaceae* generally exhibit porin loss and/or increased efflux, which both contribute to reduce the intracellular accumulation of antibiotics below the threshold that would be efficient for activity [9–11].

Given the importance of the OM in controlling the uptake of beneficial as well as toxic compounds, one can expect that the expression of porins depends on environmental factors, and is well-coordinated at the transcriptional and post-transcriptional levels. Best studied transcriptional regulators are the IM sensor kinase EnvZ and its cognate response regulator OmpR [12]. EnvZ autophosphorylates in response to a specific envelope stress, such as high osmolarity, then transfers its phosphate group to OmpR. OmpR and OmpR-P have different binding affinities to the porin promoters. At low osmolarity, OmpR activates *ompF* transcription, whereas at high osmolarity, OmpR-P represses *ompF* transcription and activates *ompC* transcription. This differential regulation of OmpF and OmpC is consistent with that in high osmolarity environments, such as in a host where nutrients are abundant, the small pore porin OmpC is predominant, thus limiting the uptake of toxic bile salts; whereas in low osmolarity environments where nutrients are scarce, the large pore porin OmpF is expressed [8]. EnvZ–OmpR [12] and CpxA–CpxR [13] are the main two-component systems involved in the transcriptional control of OmpF and OmpC. Interestingly, the two systems are interconnected [14], and mutations have been found in response to antibiotic stresses [15] (Masi M, Pagès J.-M and Kohler T, personal observations).

The post-transcriptional repression of OmpF by the small regulatory RNA (sRNA) MicF has been discovered in 1984 [16–18]. This 93 nucleotide (nt) RNA is divergent to the *ompC* gene, and acts by direct base-pairing to a region that encompasses the ribosome binding site (RBS) and the start codon of the *ompF* mRNA, thus preventing translation initiation [19]. The expression of the MicF sRNA is subjected to multiple signals and regulatory pathways [20]. Positive regulation includes EnvZ–OmpR in high osmolarity conditions [21], SoxS in response to oxidative stress [22], and MarA in response to antibiotic stress [23]. The 109 nt MicC sRNA has been discovered more recently, and shown to repress OmpC by direct base-pairing to a 5′ untranslated region of the *ompC* mRNA [24]. Interestingly, MicC is transcribed clockwise, and is opposite to the adjacent *ompN* gene that encodes a quiescent porin homologous to OmpF and OmpC [25]. Due to the similar genetic organization of *ompN–micC* and *ompC–micF*, and the co-induction of *ompC* and *micF* under specific conditions (i.e., high osmolarity via EnvZ–OmpR), it has been suggested that *ompN* and *micC* could also be subjected to dual regulation [24]. With the recent interest in post-transcriptional regulators, additional sRNAs that modulate expression of abundant OM proteins have been found. As yet, the *ompC* mRNA is targeted by multiple sRNAs MicC [24], RybB [26], RseX [27], and IpeX [28–30]. To date, external growth conditions and regulatory factors that control the expression of MicC and/or OmpN remain largely unknown.

In this work, we first examined the transcription of *micC* and *ompN* in *E. coli* MC4100 cells grown under a series of external conditions by using *lacZ* transcriptional fusions and β-galactosidase assays. We optimized the assay by using 96-well microtiter plates, and screened the entire collection of compounds provided by the Biolog Phenotype MicroArrays™ for bacterial chemical susceptibility, in order to extend the range of putative inducing cues. Results showed that high concentrations of carbapenems and cephalosporins, two clinically relevant classes of β-lactams, induce both *micC* and *ompN*. Then, the impact of carefully chosen inducing conditions on the expression levels of OmpC and OmpN was tested by Western blotting with appropriate antisera. Because the OmpN protein was undetectable in the presence of mild antibiotic stress conditions, we reasoned to investigate the transcription of *micC* and *ompN* in a series of MC4100 derivatives carrying null mutations or multicopy plasmids in order to identify putative transcriptional regulators. Interestingly, we found that OmpN was specifically expressed when the envelope stress sigma factor σ^E was depleted by the overexpression of the anti-sigma RseA, or when the *hns* gene encoding the histone nucleoid structuring protein, H-NS, was inactivated. Finally, we examined the functional relevance of OmpN as compared to OmpC and OmpF, with respect to drug translocation.

All these data are discussed considering the current knowledge on the Gram-negative envelope stress response pathways.

2. Results

2.1. Screening of MicC and OmpN Inducing Conditions Using LacZ Transcriptional Fusions and Biolog^TM Plates

Changes in porin expression play a major role in the development of antibacterial resistance. Because increased levels of MicC are associated with a decreased expression of OmpC, we aimed to examine the expression profile of the MicC sRNA by using a *micC–lacZ* transcriptional fusion in MC4100 cells grown under a series of growth conditions and β-galactosidase assays. First, we selected a number of representative growth conditions, some of which are sensed by known regulatory factors: growth phase (stationary phase accumulates RpoS), exposure to heat shock, high osmolarity (activates EnvZ–OmpR), iron or nitrogen starvation, or exposure to chemicals, such as salicylate (activates MarA), paraquat (activates SoxR/S), or different classes of antibiotics (β-lactams and fluoroquinolones). To determine whether MicC and OmpN are co-regulated, the β-galactosidase activity of an *ompN–lacZ* transcriptional fusion was also tested in MC4100 grown under the same conditions. These preliminary assays showed that growth conditions that are known to induce specific regulatory factors, such as RpoS, EnvZ–OmpR, MarA and SoxR/S, do not significantly affect the activity of the *micC–* and *ompN–lacZ* fusions, suggesting that the expression of MicC and OmpN is not controlled by these regulators. Instead, these assays allowed the identification of β-lactams potent inducers of both the *micC–* and *ompN–lacZ* fusions. As an example, Figure 1a shows that increasing concentrations of the carbapenem biapenem were accompanied with increased β-galactosidase activities. In order to extend the range of putative inducing compounds, we optimized the β-galactosidase assay using preloaded 96-well microtiter plates, and then screened Phenotype MicroArrays^TM plates (Biolog PM11 to PM19) for bacterial chemical susceptibility (Supplementary Data 1). A total of 18 compounds were found to increase the activity of the *micC–* and *ompN–lacZ* fusions more than 10 times, and 6 of them were selected for further investigations. Concentrations of compounds for β-galactosidase assays adapted to microtiter plates were determined with respect to their MICs (Supplementary Data 2). The data showed that the activity of the *micC–* and *ompN–lacZ* fusions were strongly increased when cells were exposed to carbapenems (i.e., biapenem and ertapenem) or cephalosporins (i.e., ceftazidime and cefepime) (Figure 1b). Interestingly, these compounds belong to the most potent subclasses of clinically used β-lactams used for treating Gram-negative infections. Other strong inducers include antiseptics (e.g., benzalkonium chloride and benzethonium chloride) and anesthetics (e.g., chlorpromazine HCl), which are also used in the clinics (Figure 1b).

2.2. Effects of MicC and OmpN Inducing Conditions on the Expression Levels of OmpC and OmpN

The effect of MicC overexpression on *ompC* expression was first examined by monitoring OmpC protein levels directly. MC4100 was transformed with the MicC overexpression plasmid (pSD01) and the corresponding empty vector (pDrive). Cultures were induced with IPTG to allow MicC expression, OM extracts were prepared, and levels of OmpC were analyzed by Western blot (WB) with specific anti-peptide antibodies. As shown in Figure 2a, the overexpression of MicC clearly resulted in reduced OmpC levels, confirming that the MicC sRNA represses *ompC* expression. As noted in the section above, high *micC–lacZ* activities were obtained in the presence of high concentrations of compounds, which were detrimental for the cell growth. Therefore, MC4100 was cultured in the presence of sub-inhibitory concentrations of inducing compounds—namely biapenem, imipenem, ertapenem, ceftazidime, cefepime, and chlorpromazine HCl—in order to obtain exponentially grown cells and examine their effect on OmpC protein levels. As shown in Figure 2a, these conditions only weakly altered OmpC levels.

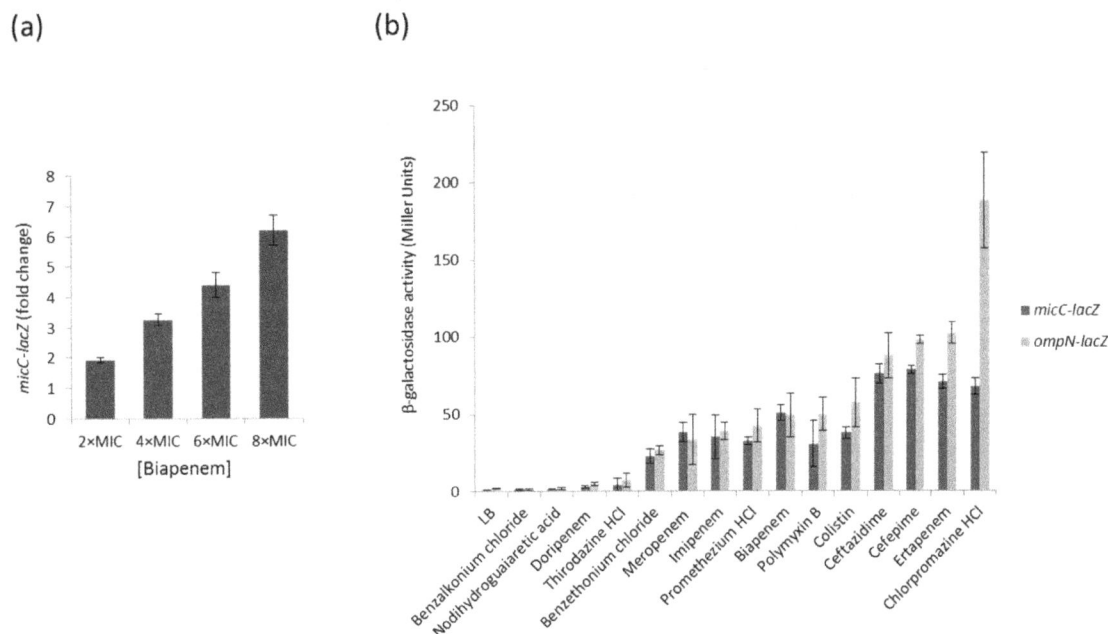

Figure 1. (a) Dose dependent *micC–lacZ* activity in presence of increasing concentrations of biapenem (MIC of 0.32 μg/mL); (b) β-galactosidase activity of the *micC*- and *ompN-lacZ* fusions in the presence of selected compounds. Values are means from three independent determinations, and standard deviation is represented.

Given the co-induction of *micC* and *ompN*, we also tested whether OmpN expression was increased in the same samples. As a control, MC4100 was transformed with the OmpN overexpression plasmid (pSD04) and the corresponding empty vector (pTrc99A). Cultures were induced with IPTG to allow OmpN expression; OM extracts were prepared and tested for OmpN expression by WB. For this, we generated antibodies against a peptide in loop 7 present in OmpN, but absent in OmpF and OmpC. A single protein of about 39 kDa was detected in the OM extracts of MC4100 (pSD04), but not in that of MC4100 (pTrc99A), suggesting that the detected band is OmpN without cross-reactivity to other porins, and that OmpN production from the chromosome is undetectable (Figure 2b). However, OmpN production was also undetectable in OM extracts prepared from cells grown in the presence of sub-inhibitory concentrations of *micC* inducing compounds (Figure 2b).

These results suggest that transient exposure of the cells to sub-inhibitory concentrations of *micC–lacZ* inducing compounds was not sufficient to yield high levels of MicC and concomitant changes in the porin expression profile. Moreover, it is worth to note that Western blot analysis only provides steady-state levels of OmpC and OmpN. Additional reverse transcription PCR and pulse-chase experiments are needed to conclude the effects of *micC* and *ompN* inducing conditions on the expression of OmpC and OmpN at the transcriptional and post-transcriptional levels, respectively.

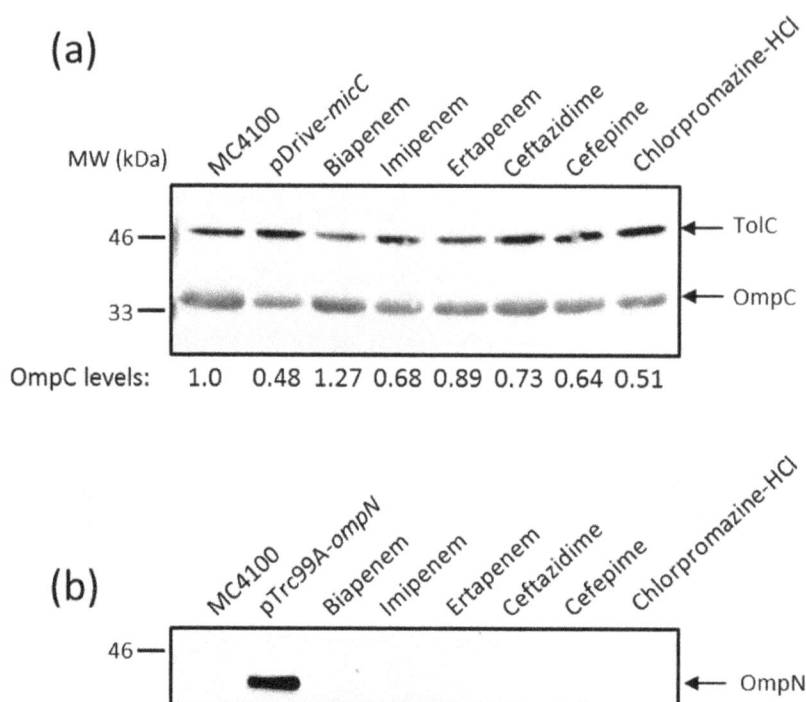

Figure 2. Western blot (WB) analysis of outer membrane (OM) proteins. Cells were grown, and OM extracts were prepared as described in the Materials and Methods. OM proteins equivalent to 0.2 OD_{600} units of cultures were separated by SDS-PAGE, electrotransferred on nitrocellulose membranes, and blotted with the appropriate anti-sera. Data show the production of OmpC (**a**) and OmpN (**b**). Both the positive controls pDrive-*micC* and pTrc99A-*ompN* were induced by 0.4 mM IPTG for 3 h. TolC expression was used for normalizing sample loading, and the expression of normalized OmpC has been expressed in mean values from three independent experiments.

2.3. Identification of Genetic Factors That Impact on MicC and OmpN Expression

micC–lacZ and *ompN–lacZ* transcriptional fusions were transformed into MC4100 derivatives carrying either chromosomal null mutations or overexpression plasmids of several regulatory factors, in order to identify putative repressors or activators, respectively. In *Enterobacteriaceae*, global regulators MarA and RamA have been reported to induce MDR associated with an increase in efflux pump production and a decrease in OmpF expression levels [31,32]. We detected no induction of the reporter fusions, either when these factors were overexpressed from multicopy plasmids or when the corresponding genes were inactivated (data not shown). This observation suggests that the *micC–ompN* operon is not part of the MarA and RamA regulatory pathways, or is strongly silenced by an upstream repressor.

Previous Northern blotting analysis showed that the expression of MicF (repressor of OmpF) was opposite to that of MicC (repressor of OmpC) under most of the tested conditions [24]. Because the osmoregulator OmpR is known to modulate MicF and control the opposite expression of OmpF and OmpC, we tested the impact of an *ompR* mutation on *micC* and *ompN* expression. Here, the activity of the *micC–lacZ*, but not that of the *ompN-lacZ* fusion, was slightly increased in the *ompR* null mutant, thus confirming that OmpR represses MicC (Figure 3a). Whether this regulation is direct or indirect is still unknown.

The last decade has been marked by the identification of several sRNAs. These are differentially expressed, and have been assigned to various important regulons of *E. coli* and *Salmonella*. Examples include the RyhB sRNA as a member of the iron-responsive Fur regulon [33]; MicA and RybB, which are activated by the envelope stress sigma factor, σ^E [26,34,35]; CyaR, whose transcription is governed by the cAMP-CRP complex [36,37]; ArcZ and FnrS, which respond to oxygen availability via the

ArcA/B or Fnr systems [38,39]; MgrR, which is a member of the Mg^{2+}-responsive PhoP/Q regulon [40]; SdsR, which is selectively transcribed by the major stationary phase and stress sigma factor, σ^S [41]; and CpxQ, which responds to the CpxA/R two-component envelope stress system [42,43]. Focusing on envelope stress responses and expression of OM proteins, we examined the impact of CpxA/R and σ^E on *micC* and *ompN* induction. Constitutive activation of the Cpx stress response, by multicopy plasmids expressing an autoactivated CpxA [15] or the signaling lipoprotein NlpE [44], did not increase the activity of the reporter fusion (data not shown). In the opposing scenario, when cells were depleted of σ^E upon the overexpression of its cognate anti-sigma RseA, the activity of both the *micC*– and *ompN*–*lacZ* fusions resulted in a 3–4-fold increase (Figure 3a). Additionally, OmpN was detected in OM extracts of cells grown under the same conditions (Figure 3b). We suggest this regulation is most likely indirect, as the *micC*–*ompN* intergenic region does not contain a σ^E core promoter motif [45]. Because RybB is one of the most abundant sRNA, represses OmpC as well as other OM proteins, and is part of the σ^E regulon in *E. coli* [46], we hypothesized that OmpN could be silenced by RybB. However, the activity of the *ompN*–*lacZ* fusion did not increase in *rybB* and *hfq* mutants, suggesting that the *ompN* mRNA is not targeted by RybB or any other Hfq-dependent sRNA (Figure 3a,b).

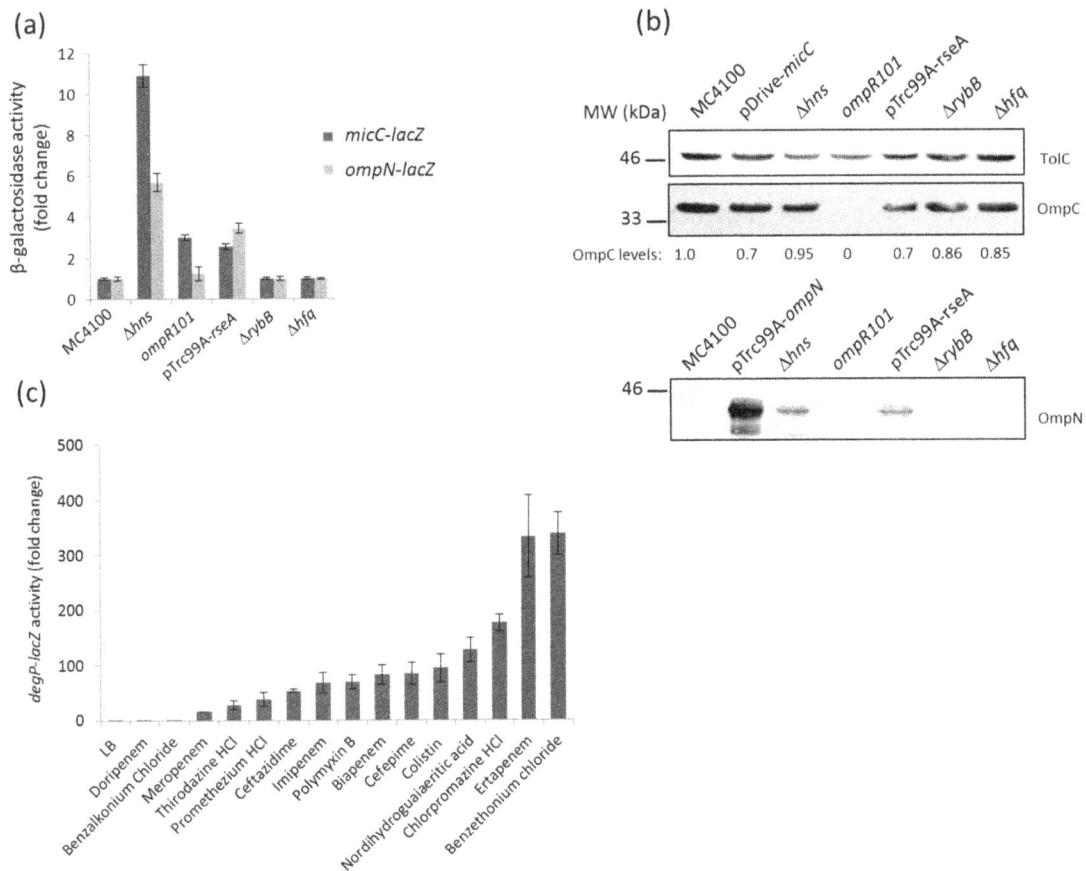

Figure 3. (a) β-Galactosidase activity of the *micC*– and *ompN*–*lacZ* fusions in different genetic backgrounds. Envelope stress sigma factor σ^E is essential in *Escherichia coli*. Therefore, cells were temporarily depleted of σ^E by the overexpression of the anti-sigma factor RseA with 0.4 mM IPTG under heat shock conditions at 42 °C; (b) WB analysis of OM proteins. Cells were grown, and OM extracts were prepared as described in the Materials and Methods. OM proteins equivalent to 0.2 ODU of cultures were separated by SDS-PAGE, electrotransferred on nitrocellulose membranes, and blotted with the appropriate anti-sera. Data show the production of OmpC (upper panel) and OmpN (lower panel). TolC expression was evaluated for normalizing sample loading and the expression of normalized OmpC has been expressed in numerical values below the bands; (c) β-galactosidase activity of a *degP*–*lacZ* chromosomal fusion in response to various external stresses.

In order to explore the connection between σ^E and the MicC/OmpN inducing compounds, we examined the effect of the latter on the expression of DegP, a periplasmic protease/chaperone member of the σ^E regulon, by using a *degP–lacZ* fusion [47]. Interestingly, all the compounds that had been identified as inducers of *micC–* and *ompN–lacZ* also activated *degP–lacZ* (Figure 3c). These results suggest a strong link between toxic compounds that target the bacterial envelope, the envelope stress σ^E pathway, and MicC/OmpN expression [48].

Previous studies on porin regulation reported that the H-NS nucleoid protein binds to the *micF–ompC* intergenic region. Expression of the major OM proteins, OmpF and OmpC, is affected by *hns* mutations, such that OmpC expression increases via direct effect at the transcriptional level, while OmpF expression decreases via indirect regulation by the MicF sRNA at the post-transcriptional level [49,50]. Comparative transcriptomic and proteomic studies further confirmed the influence of H-NS on the expression of OmpF and OmpC, but also indicated that *ompN* was upregulated in an *hns* mutant [51]. Here, the activity of both the *micC–* and *ompN–lacZ* fusions was significantly increased (approximately by 11- and 6-fold, respectively) in an *hns* mutant (Figure 3a). The OM profile of this mutant is shown and indicates that the expression level of both OmpC and OmpN is increased by 2–3-fold (Figure 3b). Considering that MicC functions as a repressor of OmpC, negative regulation of non-identified OmpC repressors by H-NS could explain upregulation of OmpC in the *hns* mutant.

2.4. Role of OmpN in Antibiotic Translocation

OmpF and OmpC porins represent the preferred route for the uptake of β-lactam antibiotics across the OM of *E. coli* [6,8,9]. Although OmpN is quiescent porin in *E. coli* [25], the orthologous OmpK37 of *Klebsiella pneumoniae* has been shown to be expressed at low levels under standard laboratory growth conditions, but highly expressed in β-lactam-resistant clinical isolates [52]. As a first step to investigate the role of MicC/OmpN in antibiotic susceptibility profile, we examined the expression levels of OmpF, OmpC, and OmpN in a collection of *E. coli* β-lactam-resistant clinical isolates by WB analysis. None of these isolates produced detectable OmpF, OmpC, or OmpN (Supplementary Data 3). Here, it should be noted that the anti-OmpN antibodies are directed against amino acid residues of the extracellular loop 7, which are specific of *E. coli* OmpN, but also submitted to variability between strains of this species. The impact of MicC in the downregulation of OmpC in these isolates is not known, and should be further investigated by Northern blot analysis. Second, we used a whole cell-based assay to compare the role of OmpN to that of OmpF and OmpC in the uptake of β-lactam antibiotics. To do this, the metabolic activity of *E. coli* W3100Δ*ompF*(pTrc99A) (OmpF⁻ OmpC⁺), W3100Δ*ompC*(pTrc99A) (OmpF⁺ OmpC⁻), W3100Δ*ompF*Δ*ompC*(pTrc99A) (OmpF⁻ OmpC⁻) and W3100Δ*ompF*Δ*ompC*(pSD04) (OmpF⁺ OmpC⁻ OmpN⁺) was monitored in the absence and in presence of representative β-lactams added at inhibitory concentrations, with regards to their capacity to inhibit the reduction of the viability dye resazurin [6]. The results showed that the metabolic activity of *E. coli* expressing either OmpF or OmpC, but not OmpN, was significantly inhibited upon exposure to β-lactams, suggesting that OmpN is not competent for translocation of this class of antibiotics (Figure 4). However, other approaches, such as liposome swelling assays with reconstituted OmpN, are necessary to conclude on this point.

OmpF and OmpC channels are also used for the translocation of various colicins across the OM of *E. coli* [53]. We examined the sensitivity of *E. coli* strains expressing OmpF, OmpC, or OmpN to colicins E2 and E3, by spotting serial 2-fold dilutions onto cell lawns. Interestingly, the expression of any of the three porins yields similar sensitivity (titers of 2×10^{-7}), suggesting that OmpN channels are able to bind and transport porin-dependent group A colicins across the OM of *E. coli* (data not shown). This also points to the different mechanism of antibiotic versus colicin translocation through OM porin channels.

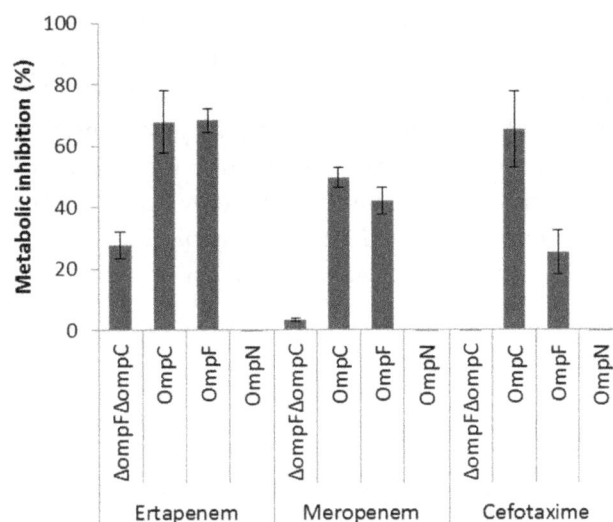

Figure 4. Metabolic inhibition of intact cells expressing OmpF, OmpC, or OmpN in the presence of selected β-lactam antibiotics using a resazurin-reduction-based assay. Actively metabolizing bacterial cells are able to reduce blue resazurin into red resofurin, which emits fluorescence at 590 nm. The experiment was performed in a microtiter plate, and fluorescence was measured every 10 min with an excitation wavelength of 530 nm and an emission wavelength of 590 nm. Inhibition of resazurin reduction in the presence of appropriate concentrations of each antibiotic was translated into % metabolic inhibition.

3. Discussion

sRNAs have become important players in bacterial gene regulation. To date, systematic genome-wide searches have led to the identification of approximately 80 sRNAs in *E. coli*, the majority of which are conserved in *Salmonella* and other closely related species. About one-third of the reported sRNAs repress synthesis of OM proteins. Evidence for important roles of sRNAs in this post-transcriptional regulation was previously established by the fact that the loss of Hfq, the sRNA chaperone [54], results in the overproduction of OM proteins [24,26,27,36,37,41].

In *E. coli*, the conserved Hfq-associated sRNA, MicC, was identified as a repressor of the synthesis of OmpC [24,54]. MicC inhibits the 30S ribosome binding through a conserved 22 bp RNA duplex near the start codon of the *ompC* mRNA [24]. Many parallels have been drawn between the MicC and MicF sRNAs. Both repress the expression of abundant porins by base pairing near the RBS, thereby blocking translation. Both are encoded opposite to another porin gene. Both are also conserved, together with their *omp* target sequences in *Salmonella*, *K. pneumoniae*, and *Enterobacter* spp. However, major questions such as (i) environmental conditions and/or intracellular regulatory pathways that promote maximal expression of MicC; (ii) the co-regulation of MicC and OmpN; (iii) the impact of such regulation on antibiotic susceptibility; and (iv) the prevalence of MicC/OmpN in MDR clinical isolates remain unanswered. In this work, we used *lacZ* transcriptional fusions and β-galactosidase assays to show that the expression of *micC* and *ompN* is co-regulated in response to antibiotic stress. In particular, β-lactam antibiotics are among the most potent inducers of both *micC* and *ompN*. Interestingly, we found that expression of OmpN from a plasmid could not restore the susceptibility of an *E. coli* porin-less strain to β-lactams. In addition, other studies have demonstrated that strains expressing OmpN, but not OmpF or OmpC, were less susceptible to β-lactams [52,55].

Our results also identified that envelop stress sigma factor σ^E and H-NS are two major negative regulators of MicC/OmpN. σ^E is widespread among pathogenic and non-pathogenic bacteria, and becomes activated when bacterial envelope homeostasis is perturbed due to misfolding of OM proteins in the periplasm, or severe OM damage by external stresses [56]. In both cases, the bacteria must decrease the synthesis of major OM proteins. It has been shown that MicA and RybB are the two most abundant sRNAs responsible for the rapid decay of *omp* mRNAs upon activation of the σ^E envelope stress response [46,57]. Although β-lactams were found to be potent inducers of the σ^E envelope stress response, RybB nor any other Hfq-dependent sRNA could be responsible for *ompN* silencing. This suggests that *ompN* is not subjected to sRNA post-transcriptional regulation. On the other hand, H-NS is a major component of the bacterial nucleoid, and has pleiotropic effects on gene expression, genome stability, and DNA recombination. Previous work has shown that H-NS was required for full expression of OmpF, and that this involves a role for H-NS in repressing the expression of MicF sRNA [48]. Our results also showed that H-NS had a role in repressing the expression of MicC and OmpN.

4. Materials and Methods

4.1. Plasmids and Bacterial Strains

All the *E. coli* strains and plasmids used in this study are listed in Table 1. *E. coli* MC4100 and derivatives were used for *lacZ* reporter gene assays and protein expression analysis. Knockout mutants were generated by P1 transduction from different sources and cured by using the FLP helper plasmid pCP20 to remove the kanamycin resistance cassette [58]. Strains were routinely grown in Luria Bertani (LB) broth (Sigma, Saint Quentin Fallavier, France), supplemented with the following antibiotics when necessary: ampicillin, 100 μg/mL (Amp); kanamycin, 50 μg/mL (Kan); chloramphenicol (Cam), 30 μg/mL; streptomycin 50 μg/mL (Str). *E. coli* W3110 and derivatives were used for translocation assays.

4.2. Plasmid Construction

Genomic DNA was extracted from MC4100 by using the Wizard® Genomic purification kit (Promega, Charbonnières-les-Bains, France) according to the manufacturer's instructions, and used as a template for all PCR-amplifications. *micC*– and *ompN–lacZ* transcriptional fusions were constructed in the promoter-less *lacZ* containing vector pFus2K [59]. A 184 nt fragment containing the MicC promoter was amplified by using the primer pair SD1 (5′-*TTACGTATC*GGATCC TCGGGGAGTGAAAACATCCT-3′) and SD2 (5′-GC*GGATCC*CCGCGCAGAATAACGTAT-3′), which contain BamHI restriction sites (underlined) for classic restriction/ligation cloning into BamHI restricted pFus2K (Supplementary data 4) in the orientation of *micC–lacZ* (pSD02). Because the transcription start of *ompN* is only based on promoter prediction, the entire intergenic region between MicC and OmpN was PCR-amplified by using the primer pair SD3 (5′-*GAGCTCGCATGC* GGATCCTGAATAAATCCTTTAGTTATT-3′) and SD4 (5′-*CAGGACTCTAGA*GGATCCCCGCGC AGAATAACGTAT-3′). This generated a 227 nt fragment, which contained BamHI restriction sites (underlined) and extension homologous to BamHI restricted pFus2K for cloning using the In-Fusion ™ cloning kit (Clontech, Saint Germaine n Laye, France), in the orientation of *ompN–lacZ* (pSD03) (Supplementary Data 4). For overexpression of the MicC sRNA, a 410 nt PCR fragment was generated by using the primer pair SD1 and SD5 (5′-*AGGCTCGAG*AAGCTT AGATGCTGCAGCTGAATTTG-3′) inserted into the pDrive vector restricted with BamHI and HindIII under the control of an IPTG inducible promoter by using the In-Fusion ™ cloning kit (pSD01) (Supplementary Data 1). Recombinant plasmids pSD04 and pSD05 were obtained by InFusion cloning of fragments into the pTrc99A vector after digestion with appropriate restriction enzymes. pSD04 contains ompN, which was PCR-amplified by using the primer set SD6 (5′-*CATG*GAATTCATGAAAAGCAAAGTACTGGCAC-3′) and SD7 (5′-*CGACTCAGA*GGATCCTTAGAACTGATAAACCAGACCTAAAGCG-3′) that contain the EcoRI and BamHI restriction sites respectively. pSD05 contains rseA, which was PCR-amplified by using the primer pair SD8 (5′-*GGTATTAG*CCATGGAGAAAG-3′) and SD9 (5′-*CTGTGCCGC* CCCGGGTACTTTCTG-3′) that contain the NcoI and SmaI restriction sites, respectively. All the plasmid constructs were confirmed by sequencing.

Table 1. Strains and plasmids used in this study.

Strain or Plasmid	Description	Source or Reference
E. coli strains		
MC4100	F⁻ [araD139]_{B/r} Δ(argF-lac)169 λ⁻ e14 flhD5301 Δ(fruK-yeiR)725(fruA25) relA1 rpsL150(Str^R) rbsR22 Δ(fimB-fimE)632(::IS1) deoC1	[60]
MH1160	MC4100 ompR101	[61]
TR49	MC4100 λRS88[degP-lacZ]	[47]
W3110	F⁻ λ⁻ IN(rrnD-rrnE)1 rph-1	[62]
SR8265	W3110 rybB< >aph, Kan^R, source for P1 transduction	[63]
PS2209	W3110 ΔlacZ169	[64]
PS2652	ΔlacZ169 zch-506::TnlO hns-1001::Tnseq1, Kan^R, source for P1 transduction	[64]
AG100	F⁻ glnX44(AS) galK2(Oc) rpsL704(Str^R) xylA5 mtl-1 argE3(Oc) thiE1 tfr-3	[65]
CH164	AG100 marA zdd-230::Tn9, Cam^R, source for P1 transduction	[66]
BW25113	F⁻ Δ(araD–araB)567 ΔlacZ4787(::rrnB-3) λ⁻ rph-1 Δ(rhaD–rhaB)568 hsdR514	[67]
JW4130	BW25113 hfq::kan, Kan^R, source for P1 transduction	GE Healthcare
SD01	MC4100 ΔrybB	This study
SD02	MC4100 marA zdd-230::Tn9, Cam^R,	This study
SD03	MC4100 Δhfq	This study
SD04	MC4100 Δhns	This study
SD05	MC4100 ΔrpoS	This study
W3110ΔompF	W3110 ompF::kan	M.G. Page
W3110ΔompC	W3110 ompC::kan	M.G. Page
W3110ΔompFΔompC	W3110 ΔompFΔompC	M.G. Page
Plasmids		
pDrive	PCR cloning vector; Amp^R, Kan^R	Qiagen
pRC1	pDrive containing *Enterobacter aerogenes* MarA	[31]
pRC2	pDrive containing *Enterobacter aerogenes* RamA	[32]
pSD01	pDrive encoding MicC sRNA	This study
pFus2K	Cloning vector with promoter-less *lacZ*, Kan^R	[59]
pSD02	pFus2K containing the *micC–lacZ* fusion	This study
pSD03	pFus2K containing the *ompN–lacZ* fusion	This study
pTrc99A	Expression vector with the inducible P_{TRC} promoter, Amp^R	Pharmacia
pSD04	pTrc99A containing OmpN	This study
pSD05	pTrc99A containing RseA	This study
pBAD24	Expression vector with the inducible P_{BAD} promoter, Amp^R	[68]
pBAD24-NlpE	pBAD24 containing NlpE	M. Masi
pBAD33	Expression vector with the inducible P_{BAD} promoter, Cam^R	[68]
pBAD33-CpxA*	pBAD33 containing an autoactivated (*) CpxA	M. Masi

4.3. β-Galactosidase Assays

β-Galactosidase activity was routinely assayed on log-phase bacterial cultures, as described by Miller [69].

4.4. Determination of Minimal Inhibitory Concentrations (MIC)

MIC values of antibiotics were determined by the microdilution method in Mueller Hinton II broth (MHIIB) (Sigma). Susceptibilities were determined in 96-well microtiter plates with an inoculum of 2×10^5 cfu in 200 µL containing two-fold serial dilutions of each compound. The MIC was defined as the lowest concentration of each compound for which no visible growth was observed after 18 h of incubation at 37 °C. Each assay was systematically performed in triplicate. The average of three independent assays was considered in µg/mL.

4.5. Preparation of the Microtiter Plates for β-Galactosidase Assays

The standard β-galactosidase assay was adapted for compound screening by using 96-well microtiter plates and a SUNRISE™ Tecan for absorbance readings. Briefly, strains were grown to an OD_{600} of 0.6. Cultures were diluted to an OD_{600} of 0.2, and added (200 μL) to the Phenotype MicroArrays ™ test plates (Biolog plates PM11 to PM19) (Supplementary Data 2). After overnight incubation at 37 °C, cells were centrifuged, washed, and treated with ONPG (2-nitrophenyl β-D-galactoside, Sigma) (4 mg/mL). Curves of OD_{420} were plotted over the time (30 min) to identify optimal inducers (Supplementary data 2). Similar experiments were repeated in 96-well microtiter plates preloaded with a chosen concentration range for each compound: each well was loaded with 20 μL of ONPG (4 mg/mL) and 10 μL of compound dilutions (Supplementary Data 3), then cells (170 μL at an OD_{600} of 0.2) were added. The plates were incubated at 37 °C inside the reader, and curves of OD_{420} were plotted over the time (6 h). The obtained readings in presence of ONPG were used to calculate Miller units and for determining the fold change in *lacZ* activity, relatively to standard growth conditions. Experiments were independently repeated at least three times.

4.6. Preparation of OM Extracts

Bacterial cultures (50 mL), grown in the presence or absence of stress, were incubated according to the optimum *micC/ompN* induction conditions determined by the β-galactosidase assay. The cells were washed and concentrated 12.5 fold in 20 mM sodium phosphate buffer (pH 7.4), and lysed by one passage through a cell disruptor (Constant Systems) at 2 kbar. After removal of cell debris by centrifugation ($7000 \times$ g, 20 min, 4 °C) the supernatant was ultracentrifuged ($100,000 \times$ g, 60 min, 4 °C) to collect the whole cell envelopes. These were resuspended in 0.3% N-laurylsarcosinate, and incubated for 30 min at room temperature to solubilize the IM. The insoluble OM extracts were pelleted by centrifugation ($100,000 \times$ g, 60 min, 4 °C).

4.7. SDS-PAGE and Western Blot Analysis

OM were prepared as described above, resuspended in 20 mM sodium phosphate buffer (pH 7.4), and kept at −20 °C until use. All samples were diluted in Laemmli buffer (2×: 4% SDS, 20% glycerol, 10% 2-mercaptoethanol, 0.004% bromophenol blue, 125 mM Tris-HCl, pH 6.8) and heated for 5 min at 100 °C before loading. Samples corresponding to 0.2 OD units were separated on 10% SDS-PAGE. To better resolve OmpF and OmpC, 4 M urea was added to the running gel. Proteins were either visualized after straining with Coomassie Brilliant Blue R250 or transferred onto nitrocellulose blotting membranes (GE Healthcare, Aulnay-sous-Bois, France). Primary rabbit antibodies and dilutions were: TolC (1:5000), OmpFd (1:5000), OmpC1 (1:5000), and OmpN (1:1000). Goat anti-rabbit HRP-conjugated secondary antibodies and Clarity Max™ Western ECL Blotting substrates (Bio-Rad, Marnes-la-Coquette, France) were used for detection. Protein bands were visualized with a molecular imager Chemidoc-XRS System (Bio-Rad) and quantified using the Image Lab software (Bio-Rad) by using the TolC band as a standard. Peptide-specific antibodies were used to avoid cross-detection of OmpC and OmpN: OmpC1 antibodies are directed against KNGNPSGEGTSGVTNNG amino acid sequence present in loop 4 [70], and OmpN1 antibodies are directed against the GGADNPAGVDDKDLVKYAD amino acid sequence found in loop 7 (Thermo Scientific Pierce custom antibody service, Villebon-sur-Yvette, France).

4.8. Whole Cell-Based Viability Assay

Resazurin-based CellTiter-Blue® Cell Viability Assay (Promega) was used to determine the metabolic inhibition of cells expressing single porins in the presence of clinically relevant antibiotics as an indicator of porin permeation properties [6]. These assays were performed on W3110 derivatives, i.e., W3110ΔF (expressing OmpC), W3110ΔC (expressing OmpF), and W3110ΔFC transformed with pTrc99A-*ompN* (expressing OmpN). Overnight cultures were diluted to 1:100 and grown until mid-log phase in MHIIB. Strain containing pTrc99A-*ompN* was grown in the presence of Amp, and OmpN expression was induced with 0.1 mM IPTG for 1 h at 37 °C. When tested for β-lactam permeation, cultures were diluted to 10^7 cells/mL in fresh MHIIB containing 10% of CellTiter Viability Reagent. For strains containing pTrc99A-*ompN*, MHIIB was supplemented with 0.1 mM IPTG, and β-lactamase inhibitors tazobactam and clavulanic acid (4 μg/mL each), to inhibit the activity of the plasmidic AmpC, but not Amp. Microtiter plates (96 well) with black sides and a clear bottom were preloaded with 10 μL of $20\times$ concentrated antibiotic solutions. For each antibiotic, the final concentration in the wells was defined as the maximal concentration that did not alter the metabolism of the porin-less strain, i.e., ertapenem, 0.125 μg/mL; meropenem, 0.125 μg/mL; cefotaxime, 0.0625 μg/mL. Cells (190 μL) were then added to separate wells. Control wells also contained cells with resazurin, but no antibiotic, and resaruzin with antibiotics without cells. Fluorescent signals of resorufin were measured with a TECAN Infinite Pro M200 spectrofluorometer (excitation wavelength 530 nm and emission wavelength 590 nm). Kinetic readings were taken at 37 °C every 10 min for 300 min. The % of metabolic inhibition for each strain exposed to each antibiotic was calculated from the measured difference of relative fluorescence units (RFUs) in the presence (RFU_{ATB}) as compared to in the absence (RFU_{MAX}) of antibiotic. All experiments were performed at least four times.

4.9. Colicin Killing Assays

LB agar plates were overlaid with 4 mL of soft agar (with a final agar concentration of 0.75%) containing 100 μL of *E. coli* overnight cultures. Serial two-fold dilutions of ColE2 or ColE3 (laboratory collection), were spotted in 5 μL drops onto the lawns, and the plates were incubated overnight at 37 °C. Efficiencies of killing were taken as the reciprocal of the highest dilution that gave complete clearing of the lawn.

5. Conclusions

Altogether, these data suggest that exposure to β-lactams induce a complex stress response to reduce the translocation of these antibiotics across the OM in *Enterobacteriaceae*. Further work will analyze how external stresses, such as β-lactams, interact with the σ^E envelope stress response and H-NS in laboratory strains, as well as in MDR clinical isolates.

Supplementary Materials: The following are available online at www.mdpi.com/2079-6382/6/4/33/s1, Supplementary Data 1: Screening of *micC* expression by β-galactosidase assay using preloaded 96-well Phenotype MicroArrays™ plates (Biolog PM11 to PM19) for bacterial chemical susceptibility, Supplementary Data 2: Fifteen compounds were selected to investigate their effects on MicC and OmpN, Supplementary Data 3: The expression of OmpN was evaluated in laboratory and clinical strains of *E. coli* by Western blot analysis, Supplementary Data 4: Partial *pfo(ybdK)-micC-ompN* genetic region.

Acknowledgments: We thank E. Dumont, J. Vergalli and members of the laboratory for helpful discussions throughout this work. The research leading to the discussions presented here was conducted as part of the Marie Curie Initial Training Network TRANSLOCATION consortium and has received support from the ITN-2013-607694-Translocation (SD). This work was also supported by Aix-Marseille Univ and Service de Santé des Armées.

Author Contributions: Jean-Marie Pagès and Muriel Masi conceived and designed the experiments; Sushovan Dam performed the experiments; Sushovan Dam, Jean-Marie Pagès and Muriel Masi analyzed the data; Sushovan Dam, Jean-Marie Pagès and Muriel Masi wrote the paper.

References

1.   The Review on Antimicrobial Resistance Chaired by Jim O'Neill. Tackling Drug-Resistant Infections Globally: Final Report and Recommandations. Available online: https://amr-review.org/sites/default/files/160525_Final%20paper_with%20cover.pdf (accessed on 3 March 2016).

2.   World Health Organization (WHO). Antimicrobial Resistance: Global Report on Surveillance. Available online: http://apps.who.int/iris/bitstream/10665/112642/1/9789241564748_eng.pdf (accessed on 3 March 2016).

3.   National Institute of Allergy and Infectious Diseases (NIAID). NIAID's Antibacterial Resistance Program: Currtent Status and Future Directions. Available online: https://www.niaid.nih.gov/sites/default/files/arstrategicplan2014.pdf (accessed on 3 March 2016).

4.   Stavenger, R.A.; Winterhalter, M. Translocation project: How to get good drugs into bad bugs. *Sci. Transl. Med.* **2014**, *6*, 228ed7. [CrossRef] [PubMed]

5.   Laxminarayan, R.; Duse, A.; Wattal, C.; Zaidi, A.K.; Wertheim, H.F.; Sumpradit, N.; Vlieghe, E.; Hara, G.L.; Gould, I.M.; Goossens, H.; et al. Antibiotic resistance-the need for global solutions. *Lancet Infect. Dis.* **2013**, *13*, 1057–1098. [CrossRef]

6.   Masi, M.; Réfregiers, M.; Pos, K.M.; Pagès, J.-M. Mechanisms of envelope permeability and antibiotic influx and efflux in Gram-negative bacteria. *Nat. Microbiol.* **2017**, *2*, 17001. [CrossRef] [PubMed]

7.   Silhavy, T.J.; Kahne, D.; Walker, S. The bacterial cell envelope. *Cold Spring Harb. Perspect. Biol.* **2010**, *2*, a000414. [CrossRef] [PubMed]

8.   Nikaido, H. Molecular basis of bacterial outer membrane permeability revisited. *Microbiol. Mol. Biol. Rev.* **2003**, *67*, 593–656. [CrossRef] [PubMed]

9.   Pagès, J.-M.; James, C.E.; Winterhalter, M. The porin and the permeating antibiotic: A selective diffusion barrier in Gram-negative bacteria. *Nat. Rev. Microbiol.* **2008**, *6*, 893–903. [CrossRef] [PubMed]

10. Nikaido, H.; Pagès, J.-M. Broad-specificity efflux pumps and their role in multidrug resistance of Gram-negative bacteria. *FEMS Microbiol. Rev.* **2012**, *36*, 340–363. [CrossRef] [PubMed]

11. Davin-Regli, A.; Bolla, J.-M.; James, C.E.; Lavigne, J.-P.; Chevalier, J.; Garnotel, E.; Molitor, A. Membrane permeability and regulation of drug "influx and efflux" in enterobacterial pathogens. *Curr. Drug Targets* **2008**, *9*, 750–759. [CrossRef] [PubMed]

12. Pratt, L.A.; Hsing, W.; Gibson, K.E.; Silhavy, T.J. From acids to *osmZ*: Multiple factors influence synthesis of the OmpF and OmpC porins in *Escherichia coli*. *Mol. Microbiol.* **1996**, *20*, 911–917. [CrossRef] [PubMed]

13. Guest, R.L.; Raivio, T.L. Role of the Gram-negative envelope stress response in the presence of antimicrobial agents. *Trends Microbiol.* **2016**, *24*, 377–390. [CrossRef] [PubMed]

14. Gerken, H.; Charlson, E.S.; Cicirelli, E.M.; Kenney, L.J.; Misra, R. MzrA: A novel modulator of the EnvZ/OmpR two-component regulon. *Mol. Microbiol.* **2009**, *72*, 1408–1422. [CrossRef] [PubMed]

15. Philippe, N.; Maigre, L.; Santini, S.; Pinet, E.; Claverie, J.-M.; Davin-Régli, A.V.; Pagès, J.-M.; Masi, M. In vivo evolution of bacterial resistance in two cases of *Enterobacter aerogenes* infections during treatment with imipenem. *PLoS ONE* **2015**, *10*, e0138828. [CrossRef] [PubMed]

16. Mizuno, T.; Chou, M.Y.; Inouye, M. A unique mechanism regulating gene expression: Translational inhibition by a complementary RNA transcript (micRNA). *Proc. Natl. Acad. Sci. USA* **1984**, *81*, 1966–1970. [CrossRef] [PubMed]

17. Delihas, N. Discovery and characterization of the first non-coding RNA that regulates gene expression, *micF* RNA: A historical perspective. *World J. Biol. Chem.* **2015**, *6*, 272–280. [CrossRef] [PubMed]

18. Inouye, M. The first demonstration of RNA interference to inhibit mRNA function. *Gene* **2016**, *592*, 332–333. [CrossRef] [PubMed]

19. Andersen, J.; Delihas, N. *micF* RNA binds to the 5' end of *ompF* mRNA and to a protein from *Escherichia coli*. *Biochemistry* **1990**, *29*, 9249–9256. [CrossRef] [PubMed]

20. Delihas, N.; Forst, S. *MicF*: An antisense RNA gene involved in response of *Escherichia coli* to global stress factors. *J. Mol. Biol.* **2001**, *313*, 1–12. [CrossRef] [PubMed]

21. Ramani, N.; Hedeshian, M.; Freundlich, M. *micF* antisense RNA has a major role in osmoregulation of OmpF in *Escherichia coli*. *J. Bacteriol.* **1994**, *176*, 5005–5010. [CrossRef] [PubMed]

22. Chou, J.H.; Greenberg, J.T.; Demple, B. Posttranscriptional repression of *Escherichia coli* OmpF protein in response to redox stress: Positive control of the *micF* antisense RNA by the *soxRS* locus. *J. Bacteriol.* **1993**, *175*, 1026–1031. [CrossRef] [PubMed]

23. Cohen, S.P.; McMurry, L.M.; Levy, S.B. MarA locus causes decreased expression of OmpF porin in multiple-antibiotic-resistant (Mar) mutants of *Escherichia coli*. *J. Bacteriol.* **1988**, *170*, 5416–5422. [CrossRef] [PubMed]

24. Chen, S.; Zhang, A.; Blyn, L.B.; Storz, G. MicC, a second small-RNA regulator of Omp protein expression in *Escherichia coli*. *J. Bacteriol.* **2004**, *186*, 6689–6697. [CrossRef] [PubMed]

25. Prilipov, A.; Phale, P.S.; Koebnik, R.; Widmer, C.; Rosenbusch, J.-P. Identification and characterization of two quiescent porin genes, *nmpC* and *ompN*, in *Escherichia coli* B[E]. *J. Bacteriol.* **1998**, *180*, 3388–3392. [PubMed]

26. Johansen, J.; Rasmussen, A.A.; Overgaard, M.; Valentin-Hansen, P. Conserved small non-coding RNAs that belong to the sigma[E] regulon: Role in down-regulation of outer membrane proteins. *J. Mol. Biol.* **2006**, *364*, 1–8. [CrossRef] [PubMed]

27. Douchin, V.; Bohn, C.; Bouloc, P. Down-regulation of porins by a small RNA bypasses the essentiality of the regulated intramembrane proteolysis protease RseP in *Escherichia coli*. *J. Biol. Chem.* **2006**, *281*, 12253–12259. [CrossRef] [PubMed]

28. Castillo-Keller, M.; Vuong, P.; Misra, R. Novel mechanism of *Escherichia coli* porin regulation. *J. Bacteriol.* **2006**, *188*, 576–586. [CrossRef] [PubMed]

29. Vogel, J.; Papenfort, K. Small non-coding RNAs and the bacterial outer membrane. *Curr. Opin. Microbiol.* **2006**, *9*, 605–611. [CrossRef] [PubMed]

30. Guillier, M.; Gottesman, S.; Storz, G. Modulating the outer membrane with small RNAs. *Genes Dev.* **2006**, *20*, 2338–2348. [CrossRef] [PubMed]

31. Chollet, R.; Bollet, C.; Chevalier, J.; Malléa, M.; Pagès, J.-M.; Davin-Regli, A. *mar* operon involved in multidrug resistance of *Enterobacter aerogenes*. *Antimicrob. Agents Chemother.* **2002**, *46*, 1093–1097. [CrossRef] [PubMed]

32. Chollet, R.; Chevalier, J.; Bollet, C.; Pages, J.-M.; Davin-Regli, A. RamA is an alternate activator of the multidrug resistance cascade in *Enterobacter aerogenes*. *Antimicrob. Agents Chemother.* **2004**, *48*, 2518–2523. [CrossRef] [PubMed]

33. Massé, E.; Gottesman, S. A small RNA regulates the expression of genes involved in iron metabolism in *Escherichia coli*. *Proc. Natl. Acad. Sci. USA* **2002**, *99*, 4620–4625. [CrossRef] [PubMed]

34. Thompson, K.M.; Rhodius, V.A.; Gottesman, S. Sigma[E] regulates and is regulated by a small RNA in *Escherichia coli*. *J. Bacteriol.* **2007**, *189*, 4243–4256. [CrossRef] [PubMed]

35. Skovierova, H.; Rowley, G.; Rezuchova, B.; Homerova, D.; Lewis, C.; Roberts, M.; Kormanec, J. Identification of the sigma[E] regulon of *Salmonella enterica* serovar Typhimurium. *Microbiology* **2006**, *152*, 1347–1359. [CrossRef] [PubMed]

36. Johansen, J.; Eriksen, M.; Kallipolitis, B.; Valentin-Hansen, P. Down-regulation of outer membrane proteins by noncoding RNAs: Unraveling the cAMP-CRP- and sigma[E]-dependent CyaR-OmpX regulatory case. *J. Mol. Biol.* **2008**, *383*, 1–9. [CrossRef] [PubMed]

37. Papenfort, K.; Pfeiffer, V.; Lucchini, S.; Sonawane, A.; Hinton, J.C.; Vogel, J. Systematic deletion of *Salmonella* small RNA genes identifies CyaR, a conserved CRP-dependent riboregulator of OmpX synthesis. *Mol. Microbiol.* **2008**, *68*, 890–906. [CrossRef] [PubMed]

38. Mandin, P.; Gottesman, S. Integrating anaerobic/aerobic sensing and the general stress response through the ArcZ small RNA. *EMBO J.* **2010**, *29*, 3094–3107. [CrossRef] [PubMed]

39. Durand, S.; Storz, G. Reprogramming of anaerobic metabolism by the FnrS small RNA. *Mol. Microbiol.* **2010**, *75*, 1215–1231. [CrossRef] [PubMed]

40. Moon, K.; Six, D.A.; Lee, H.J.; Raetz, C.R.; Gottesman, S. Complex transcriptional and post-transcriptional regulation of an enzyme for lipopolysaccharide modification. *Mol. Microbiol.* **2013**, *89*, 52–64. [CrossRef] [PubMed]

41. Fröhlich, K.S.; Papenfort, K.; Berger, A.A.; Vogel, J. A conserved RpoS-dependent small RNA controls the synthesis of major porin OmpD. *Nucleic Acids Res.* **2012**, *40*, 3623–3640. [CrossRef] [PubMed]

42. Grabowicz, M.; Koren, D.; Silhavy, T.J. The CpxQ sRNA negatively regulates Skp to prevent mistargeting of β-barrel outer membrane proteins into the cytoplasmic membrane. *mBio* **2016**, *7*, e00312-16. [CrossRef] [PubMed]

43. Chao, Y.; Vogel, J. A 3′ UTR-derived small RNA provides the regulatory noncoding arm of the inner membrane stress response. *Mol. Cell* **2016**, *61*, 352–363. [CrossRef] [PubMed]

44. Snyder, W.B.; Davis, L.J.; Danese, P.N.; Cosma, C.L.; Silhavy, T.J. Overproduction of NlpE, a new outer membrane lipoprotein, suppresses the toxicity of periplasmic LacZ by activation of the Cpx signal transduction pathway. *J. Bacteriol.* **1995**, *177*, 4216–4223. [CrossRef] [PubMed]

45. Nonaka, G.; Blankschien, M.; Herman, C.; Gross, C.A.; Rhodius, V.A. Regulon and promoter analysis of the *E. coli* heat-shock factor, sigma32, reveals a multifaceted cellular response to heat stress. *Genes Dev.* **2006**, *20*, 1776–1789. [CrossRef] [PubMed]

46. Gogol, E.B.; Rhodius, V.A.; Papenfort, K.; Vogel, J.; Gross, C.A. Small RNAs endow a transcriptional activator with essential repressor functions for single-tier control of a global stress regulon. *Proc. Natl. Acad. Sci. USA* **2011**, *108*, 12875–12880. [CrossRef] [PubMed]

47. Raivio, T.L.; Silhavy, T.J. Transduction of envelope stress in *Escherichia coli* by the Cpx two-component system. *J. Bacteriol.* **1997**, *179*, 7724–7733. [CrossRef] [PubMed]

48. Viveiros, M.; Dupont, M.; Rodrigues, L.; Couto, I.; Davin-Regli, A.; Martins, M.; Pagès, J.-M.; Amaral, L. Antibiotic stress, genetic response and altered permeability of *E. coli*. *PLoS ONE* **2007**, *2*, e365. [CrossRef] [PubMed]

49. Deighan, P.; Free, A.; Dorman, C.J. A role for the *Escherichia coli* H-NS-like protein StpA in OmpF porin expression through modulation of *micF* RNA stability. *Mol. Microbiol.* **2000**, *38*, 126–139. [CrossRef] [PubMed]

50. Suzuki, T.; Ueguchi, C.; Mizuno, T. H-NS regulates OmpF expression through *micF* antisense RNA in *Escherichia coli*. *J. Bacteriol.* **1996**, *178*, 3650–3653. [CrossRef] [PubMed]

51. Hommais, F.; Krin, E.; Laurent-Winter, C.; Soutourina, O.; Malpertuy, A.; Le Caer, J.P.; Danchin, A.; Bertin, P. Large-scale monitoring of pleiotropic regulation of gene expression by the prokaryotic nucleoid-associated protein, H-NS. *Mol. Microbiol.* **2001**, *40*, 20–36. [CrossRef] [PubMed]

52. Doménech-Sánchez, A.; Hernández-Allés, S.; Martínez-Martínez, L.; Benedí, V.J.; Albertí, S. Identification and characterization of a new porin gene of *Klebsiella pneumoniae*: Its role in beta-lactam antibiotic resistance. *J. Bacteriol.* **1999**, *181*, 2726–2732. [PubMed]

53. Housden, N.G.; Kleanthous, C. Colicin translocation across the *Escherichia coli* outer membrane. *Biochem. Soc. Trans.* **2012**, *40*, 1475–1479. [CrossRef] [PubMed]

54. Zhang, A.; Wassarman, K.M.; Rosenow, C.; Tjaden, B.C.; Storz, G.; Gottesman, S. Global analysis of small RNA and mRNA targets of Hfq. *Mol. Microbiol.* **2003**, *50*, 1111–1124. [CrossRef] [PubMed]

55. Fàbrega, A.; Rosner, J.L.; Martin, R.G.; Solé, M.; Vila, J. SoxS-dependent coregulation of *ompN* and *ydbK* in a multidrug-resistant *Escherichia coli* strain. *FEMS Microbiol. Lett.* **2012**, *332*, 61–67. [CrossRef] [PubMed]

56. Raivio, T.L.; Silhavy, T.J. Periplasmic stress and ECF sigma factors. *Annu. Rev. Microbiol.* **2001**, *55*, 591–624. [CrossRef] [PubMed]

57. Papenfort, K.; Pfeiffer, V.; Mika, F.; Lucchini, S.; Hinton, J.C.; Vogel, J. Sigma^E-dependent small RNAs of *Salmonella* respond to membrane stress by accelerating global *omp* mRNA decay. *Mol. Microbiol.* **2006**, *62*, 1674–1688. [CrossRef] [PubMed]

58. Datsenko, K.A.; Wanner, B.L. One-step inactivation of chromosomal genes in *Escherichia coli* K-12 using PCR products. *Proc. Natl. Acad. Sci. USA* **2000**, *97*, 6640–6645. [CrossRef] [PubMed]

59. Masi, M.; Pagès, J.-M.; Villard, C.; Pradel, E. The *eefABC* multidrug efflux pump operon is repressed by H-NS in *Enterobacter aerogenes*. *J. Bacteriol.* **2005**, *187*, 3894–3897. [CrossRef] [PubMed]

60. Casadaban, M.J. Transposition and fusion of the *lac* genes to selected promoters in *Escherichia coli* using bacteriophage lambda and Mu. *J. Mol. Biol.* **1976**, *104*, 541–555. [CrossRef]

61. Sarma, V.; Reeves, P. Genetic locus (*ompB*) affecting a major outer-membrane protein in *Escherichia coli* K-12. *J. Bacteriol.* **1977**, *132*, 23–27. [PubMed]

62. Bachmann, B.J. Pedigrees of some mutant strains of *Escherichia coli* K-12. *Bacteriol. Rev.* **1972**, *36*, 525–557. [PubMed]

63. Klein, G.; Lindner, B.; Brade, H.; Raina, S. Molecular basis of lipopolysaccharide heterogeneity in *Escherichia coli*: Envelope stress-responsive regulators control the incorporation of glycoforms with a third 3-deoxy-α-D-manno-oct-2-ulosonic acid and rhamnose. *J. Biol. Chem.* **2011**, *286*, 42787–42807. [CrossRef] [PubMed]

64. Bertin, P.; Terao, E.; Lee, E.H.; Lejeune, P.; Colson, C.; Danchin, A.; Collatz, E. The H-NS protein is involved in the biogenesis of flagella in *Escherichia coli*. *J. Bacteriol.* **1994**, *176*, 5537–5540. [CrossRef] [PubMed]

65. George, A.M.; Levy, S.B. Amplifiable resistance to tetracycline, chloramphenicol, and other antibiotics in *Escherichia coli*: Involvement of a non-plasmid-determined efflux of tetracycline. *J. Bacteriol.* **1983**, *155*, 531–540. [PubMed]

66. Rosner, J.L.; Slonczewski, J.L. Dual regulation of *inaA* by the multiple antibiotic resistance (*mar*) and superoxide (*soxRS*) stress response systems of *Escherichia coli*. *J. Bacteriol.* **1994**, *176*, 6262–6269. [CrossRef] [PubMed]

67. Baba, T.; Ara, T.; Hasegawa, M.; Takai, Y.; Okumura, Y.; Baba, M.; Datsenko, K.A.; Tomita, M.; Wanner, B.L.; Mori, H. Construction of *Escherichia coli* K12 in-frame, single-gene knockout mutants: The Keio collection. *Mol. Syst. Biol.* **2006**. [CrossRef] [PubMed]

68. Guzman, L.M.; Belin, D.; Carson, M.J.; Beckwith, J. Tight regulation, modulation, and high-level expression by vectors containing the arabinose PBAD promoter. *J. Bacteriol.* **1995**, *177*, 4121–4130. [CrossRef] [PubMed]

69. Miller, J.H. *Experiments in Molecular Genetics*; Cold Spring Harbor Laboratory: Cold Spring Harbor, NY, USA, 1972.

70. Simonet, V.; Malle, M.; Fourel, D.; Bolla, J.-M.; Pages, J.-M. Crucial domains are conserved in Enterobacteriaceae porins. *FEMS Microbiol. Lett.* **1996**, *136*, 91–97. [CrossRef] [PubMed]

5

High-Throughput Sequencing Analysis of the Actinobacterial Spatial Diversity in Moonmilk Deposits

Marta Maciejewska [1], Magdalena Całusińska [2] (iD), Luc Cornet [3], Delphine Adam [1], Igor S. Pessi [1], Sandrine Malchair [4], Philippe Delfosse [2], Denis Baurain [3], Hazel A. Barton [5], Monique Carnol [4] and Sébastien Rigali [1,* (iD)

[1]   InBioS—Centre for Protein Engineering, Institut de Chimie B6a, University of Liège, B-4000 Liège, Belgium; maciejewska.m@wp.pl (M.M.); delphine.adam@doct.ulg.ac.be (D.A.); ispessi@alumni.ulg.ac.be (I.S.P.)
[2]   Environmental Research and Innovation Department, Luxembourg Institute of Science and Technology, Belvaux, Luxembourg; magdalena.calusinska@list.lu (M.C.); philippe.delfosse@list.lu (P.D.)
[3]   InBioS—PhytoSYSTEMS, Eukaryotic Phylogenomics, University of Liège, B-4000 Liège, Belgium; luc.cornet@uliege.be (L.C.); Denis.Baurain@uliege.be (D.B.)
[4]   InBioS—Plant and Microbial Ecology, Botany B22, University of Liège, B-4000 Liège, Belgium; S.Malchair@uliege.be (S.M.); S.Malchair@uliege.be (M.C.)
[5]   Department of Biology, University of Akron, Akron, OH 44325, USA; bartonh@uakron.edu
*   Correspondence: srigali@uliege.be

Abstract: Moonmilk are cave carbonate deposits that host a rich microbiome, including antibiotic-producing Actinobacteria, making these speleothems appealing for bioprospecting. Here, we investigated the taxonomic profile of the actinobacterial community of three moonmilk deposits of the cave "Grotte des Collemboles" via high-throughput sequencing of 16S rRNA amplicons. Actinobacteria was the most common phylum after Proteobacteria, ranging from 9% to 23% of the total bacterial population. Next to actinobacterial operational taxonomic units (OTUs) attributed to uncultured organisms at the genus level (~44%), we identified 47 actinobacterial genera with *Rhodoccocus* (4 OTUs, 17%) and *Pseudonocardia* (9 OTUs, ~16%) as the most abundant in terms of the absolute number of sequences. Streptomycetes presented the highest diversity (19 OTUs, 3%), with most of the OTUs unlinked to the culturable *Streptomyces* strains that were previously isolated from the same deposits. Furthermore, 43% of the OTUs were shared between the three studied collection points, while 34% were exclusive to one deposit, indicating that distinct speleothems host their own population, despite their nearby localization. This important spatial diversity suggests that prospecting within different moonmilk deposits should result in the isolation of unique and novel Actinobacteria. These speleothems also host a wide range of non-streptomycetes antibiotic-producing genera, and should therefore be subjected to methodologies for isolating rare Actinobacteria.

Keywords: antibiotics; geomicrobiology; Illumina sequencing; microbiome diversity; *Streptomyces*; Actinobacteria

1. Introduction

Molecular approaches evaluating microbial communities in caves have revealed a level of diversity greater than initially expected [1]. Microorganisms have been found to inhabit virtually all subterranean niches, including cave walls, ceilings, speleothems, soils, sediments, pools, and aquifers [2]. Cave bacteria often represent novel taxonomic groups [3–7], which are frequently more closely related to other cave-derived bacterial lineages than to the microbiota of other environments [8–10].

Among cave speleothems, moonmilk draws a particular scientific attention due to its distinctive crystal morphology. The origins of various moonmilk crystalline habits, including monocrystalline rods, polycrystalline chains, and nanofibers, are tentatively attributed to the moonmilk indigenous microbial population [11]. Among a moonmilk microbiome comprising Archaea, Fungi, and Bacteria [9,10,12–19], the indigenous filamentous Fungi [20] and Actinobacteria [11,21] are believed to mediate moonmilk genesis with cell surfaces promoting $CaCO_3$ deposition [11,20,21]. Actinobacteria were additionally reported to be metabolically capable of inducing favorable conditions for $CaCO_3$ precipitation, or even directly precipitating carbonate minerals [12,21]. Members of the phylum Actinobacteria are routinely found in this speleothem [9,10,12–14,18,19], as well as in the other subterranean deposits within limestone caves [3,8,22,23], volcanic caves [24–26], and ice caves [27]. The broad distribution of Actinobacteria in the subsurface systems stimulates investigation in order to understand the factors driving their existence in mainly inorganic and highly oligotrophic environments, and the processes that enable them to mediate speleogenesis. The successful adaptation of Actinobacteria to a wide range of environments could probably be a consequence of their broad-spectrum metabolism, which includes prolific secreted hydrolytic systems that are capable of generating nutrient sources from various substrates, along with their extraordinary faculty to produce specialized metabolites (metal chelators, antimicrobials, hormones, etc.) [28].

As recently reported, moonmilk Actinobacteria represent novel microorganisms, which is a discovery that opens great avenues for the bioprospecting of novel drugs [6,10,18]. Rooney et al. (2010) [13] showed that spatially separated moonmilk speleothems in Ballynamintra Cave are inhabited by taxonomically distinct fungal and bacterial communities. Instead, in our attempt to isolate moonmilk-dwelling Actinobacteria for assessing their potential for participating in the genesis of these speleothems [21] and producing antimicrobial compounds [10], we only recovered members of the genus *Streptomyces*. Such a dominance of streptomycetes was rather unexpected, according to other moonmilk microbial diversity studies performed through culture-dependent [10,12,13,18] and culture-independent approaches using clone libraries [9], denaturing gradient gel electrophoresis (DGGE) fingerprinting [14,16,17], automated ribosomal intergenic spacer analysis (ARISA) [13], and, more recently, high-throughput sequencing (HTS) [19]. The actinobacterial genera identified in those studies included *Rhodococcus, Pseudonocardia, Propionibacterium, Nocardia, Amycolatopsis, Saccharothrix, Geodermatophilus, Mycobacterium, Aeromicrobium, Kribella, Nocardioides, Actinomycetospora, Nonomuraea, Euzebya, Rubrobacter,* and *Arthrobacter*, in addition to *Streptomyces*. Nonetheless, the diversity of the moonmilk actinobacterial microbiome still remains largely unknown and, beyond evaluating *"what and how much have we missed in our culture-dependent bioprospecting approach"* [10], a major important question that arises is: *to what extent are moonmilk-dwelling Actinobacteria different between the moonmilk deposits within a single cave, or in different caves?*

In this work, we carried out a comparative (HTS) of 16S small subunit (SSU) rRNA gene from DNA extracted from spatially separated moonmilk deposits within the same cave, "Grotte des Collemboles" (Springtails' Cave) in Comblain-au-Pont, Belgium (Figure S1), in order to draw a detailed taxonomic picture of the intra-phylum diversity. Identifying the presence of rare Actinobacteria and unveiling to which degree they exhibit a spatial variability would help determining whether it is worth prospecting from different moonmilk deposits to isolate unique and novel natural compound producers.

2. Results

2.1. Actinobacterial Abundance within the Whole Moonmilk Bacterial Microbiome

Libraries spanning the V4–V6 variable regions of the 16S rRNA gene using universal bacterial primers were used to assess the proportion of Actinobacteria in comparison to the whole bacterial community of three moonmilk deposits of the cave "Grotte des Collemboles" (Table S1a). The observed bacterial communities differed in species richness, evenness, and diversity between the three sampling points (Table 1). Phylotype richness (total number of operational taxonomic units (OTUs) per site) was the highest in COL4 (1863 OTUs), followed by COL1 and COL3, with 1332 and 1161 OTUs, respectively (Table 1, Figure 1a). Across the three sampling points, we found a total of 2301 different OTUs, amongst which 710 (31%) were common to all of the deposits (Figure 1a). Interestingly, pairwise comparison revealed highly similar percentages (~31.7 ± 0.53%) of shared bacterial OTUs between moonmilk deposits (Table 2, Figure 1a). A total of 956 OTUs (42%) were found to be exclusive to one sampling site, with COL4 having the highest number of unique bacterial phylotypes (584 OTUs), along with the most diverse bacterial population, as reflected by the highest diversity indices (Table 1, Figure 1a).

Table 1. Richness, specificity, diversity, and evenness of the bacterial and actinobacterial communities in the three moonmilk deposits of the "Grotte des Collemboles". OTUs: operational taxonomic units.

Target Group	Site	Total OTUs (Richness)	Unique OTUs (Specificity)	Inverse Simpson Index (Diversity)	Simpson Index (Evenness)
Bacteria	COL1	1332	238 (17.9%)	13.23	0.01
	COL3	1161	134 (11.6%)	58.94	0.05
	COL4	1863	584 (31.3%)	155.31	0.08
Actinobacteria	COL1	150	14 (9.3%)	6.21	0.04
	COL3	147	15 (10.2%)	7.74	0.05
	COL4	211	54 (25.6%)	24.13	0.11

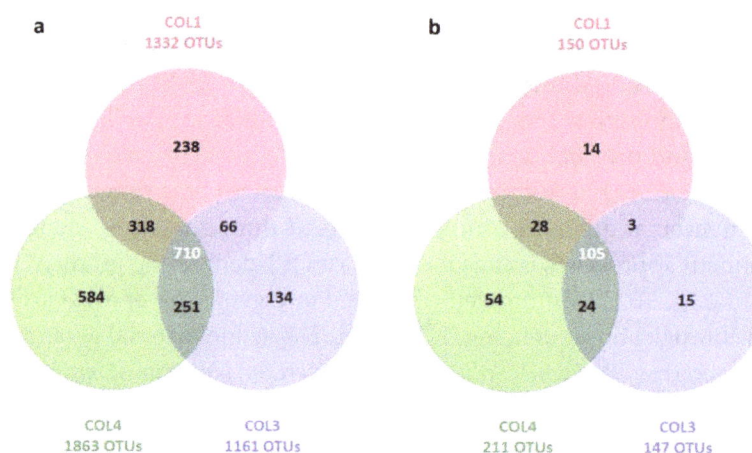

Figure 1. Venn diagrams showing the numbers of shared and unique bacterial (**a**) and actinobacterial (**b**) OTUs between the three moonmilk sampling points (COL1, COL3, COL4).

Table 2. Pairwise comparisons of shared OTUs between the moonmilk deposits.

Target Group	COL1 and COL3	COL1 and COL4	COL4 and COL3
Bacteria	776/2493 (31.1%)	1028/3195 (32.2%)	961/3024 (31.8%)
Actinobacteria	108/297 (36.4%)	133/361 (36.9%)	129/358 (36.0%)

Bacterial OTUs were grouped into 21 phyla and 18 candidate phyla (Table S2, Figure 2). Actinobacteria represented 9%, 23%, and 10% of the total bacterial population in COL1, COL3, and COL4, respectively (Table S2, Figure 2a). In terms of abundance, they were the most common phylum after Proteobacteria, which accounted for 52%, 34%, and 30% of the total community in COL1, COL3, and COL4, respectively (Table S2, Figure 2a). The other major phyla of the moonmilk microbiome included Acidobacteria, Nitrospirae, Chloroflexi, Gemmatimonadetes, Planctomycetes, Latescibacteria, Verrucomicrobia, Zixibacteria, Armatimonadetes, Bacteroidetes, and Parcubacteria (Table S2, Figure 2a). Together, these phyla constituted 93.4%, 94.7%, and 91.5% of the total community in COL1, COL3, and COL4, respectively (Table S2, Figure 2a). The remaining phyla (with a relative abundance of <1%) were pooled as 'other' (Figure 2a), and included most of the candidate divisions identified in this study (Figure 2b). Sequences that could not be affiliated to any bacterial phylum accounted for 4%, 3%, and 5% of the sequences in COL1, COL3, and COL4, respectively (Table S2). Some fraction of the moonmilk microbial diversity still remains to be discovered for all of the three sampling sites, as the rarefaction curves did not reach a plateau (Figure S2a).

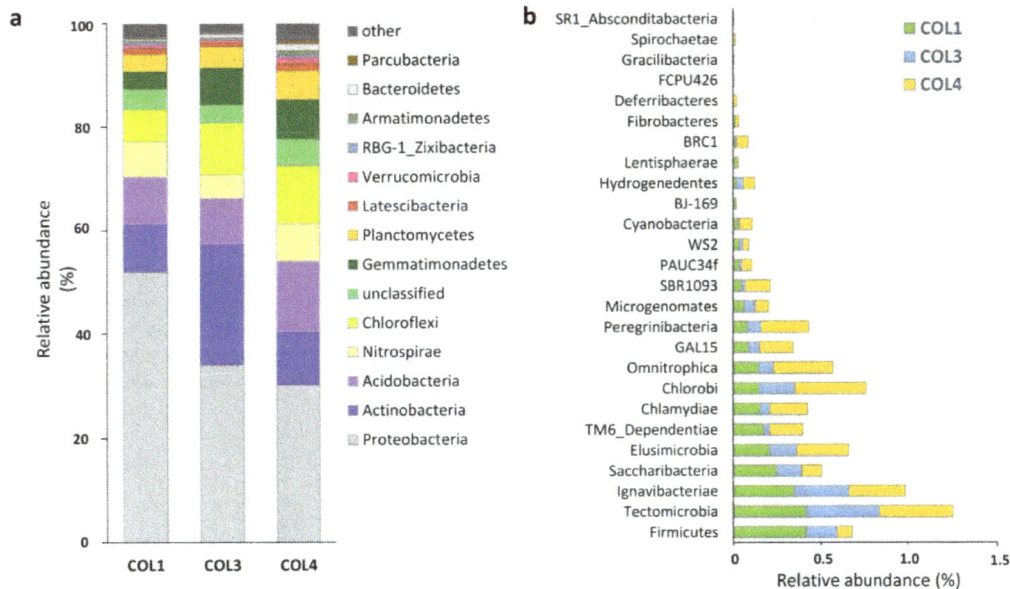

Figure 2. Taxonomic profiles of the moonmilk-associated microbiome at the phylum level across the three moonmilk sampling points (COL1, COL3, COL4). The main phyla of the microbiome are presented on the left (**a**), while the pattern of low-abundance taxa, named as 'other' (with a relative abundance of <1%) is displayed on the right (**b**).

2.2. Actinobacterial Diversity in Moonmilk Deposits

Evaluation of the actinobacterial profile was performed with libraries spanning the V6–V7 variable regions of 16S rRNA gene, and using modified Actinobacteria-specific primers (Table S1a). The specificity of the primers was confirmed by the detection of only 1%, 0.2%, and 2% of non-actinobacterial sequences in COL1, COL3, and COL4, respectively (Figure S3). In contrast to the bacterial dataset, the diversity of Actinobacteria appeared to be exhaustively sampled with the phylum-specific primers (Figure S2b).

The diversity indices for Actinobacteria showed the same trends as the ones observed for the whole Bacteria domain, i.e., evenness and diversity were the highest in COL4, followed by COL3, and COL1 (Table 1). Phylotype richness was the highest in COL4 with 211 OTUs, followed by COL1 and COL3 with 150 OTUs and 147 OTUs, respectively (Figure 1b and Table 1). Among the 243 different OTUs, 105 OTUs (43%) were found in all three of the studied moonmilk deposits (Figure 1b). Hence, the moonmilk-associated actinobacterial community appeared to be more conservative than the moonmilk-associated bacterial population (31%, Figure 1a). If we also include OTUs shared between at least two sampling points, the level of conservation rises to 66% of OTUs for Actinobacteria, and 58% for Bacteria. Still, 34% of the 243 OTUs (14, 15, and 54 OTUs in COL1, COL3, and COL4, respectively) remained specific to a moonmilk deposit, despite the close localization of collection points within the studied cave (Figure 1b). COL4 was characterized not only with the highest number of unique phylotypes (54 OTUs) (Figure 1b), but also with the most diverse population, as revealed by diversity indices (Table 1). As observed for the bacterial dataset, pairwise comparisons showed highly similar percentages (~36.4% ± 0.41%) of shared actinobacterial OTUs between moonmilk deposits (Table 2).

A taxonomic assignment of actinobacterial OTUs revealed the presence of two major classes—Acidimicrobiia and Actinobacteria, next to the low-abundant Thermoleophilia class (Table S3, Figure 3a). Acidimicrobiia was represented by one single order, the Acidimicrobiales, which dominated sample COL4, constituting 55.3% of the population (Table S3, Figure 3a). The Acidimicrobiales order consisted of two families, i.e., Acidimicrobiaceae and Iamiaceae (Table S3). The Actinobacteria class was represented by 15 orders, with Corynebacteriales dominating in COL1, and Pseudonocardiales in COL3 and COL4 (Table S3, Figure 3b). The most abundant families among the Actinobacteria class were Pseudonocardiaceae, Nocardiaceae, and Streptomycetaceae (Table S3). The proportion of unclassified and uncultured sequences at the family level ranged from 9% in COL3, to 25% in COL1, and 53% in COL4 (Table S3).

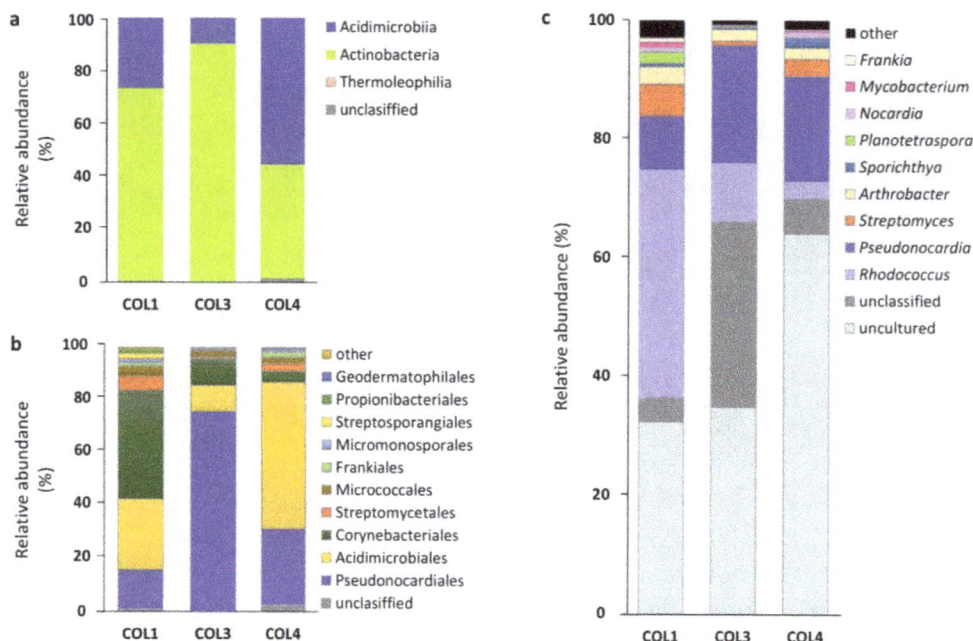

Figure 3. Taxonomic profiles of moonmilk-associated Actinobacteria at different taxonomic levels—(**a**) class; (**b**) order; (**c**) family—observed across the three moonmilk-sampling points (COL1, COL3, COL4). 'Other' includes orders and families with a relative abundance of <1%.

Among 28 families, a total of 47 genera were identified across the investigated samples (Table S3 and Table 3), with 35 genera identified for the first time in moonmilk (Table 3). COL1 was dominated by *Rhodococcus* (38.37%), while uncultured and unclassified Actinobacteria were the most abundant in COL3 and COL4 (Table 3). When only known genera were taken into account, *Pseudonocardia* prevailed in those samples, accounting for 20% and 18% of the population in COL3 and COL4, respectively (Table 3). Other genera, which constituted more than 1% of the population in at least one moonmilk deposit, included *Streptomyces, Arthrobacter, Sporichthya, Planotetraspora, Nocardia, Mycobacterium,* and *Frankia* (Table 3). While accounting in average for only 3% of the actinobacterial community, streptomycetes displayed the highest diversity, with 19 OTUs identified across the three moonmilk deposits (Table 3).

Some taxa showed important differences in their relative abundance between investigated samples, particularly *Rhodococcus*, which was approximately four and 14 times more abundant in COL1 than in COL3 and COL4, respectively (Table 3). The *Streptomyces* genus represented only 0.8% of the population in COL3, while it was detected at the level of 5.3% and 3% in the COL1 and COL4, respectively (Table 3). An important discrepancy in the relative abundance between speleothems was also observed for the genera *Planotetraspora, Mycobacterium,* and *Frankia*, whereas some taxa (e.g., *Pseudoclavibacter, Lentzea, Propionibacterium*) were exclusively found in a single sampling site (Table 3).

Table 3. Actinobacterial genera pattern in moonmilk deposits of the "Grotte des Collemboles" based on 16S rRNA amplicon libraries.

Genus	COL1			COL3			COL4			TOTAL		
	Seq.	%	OTUs	Seq.	%	OTUs	Seq.	%	OTUs	Seq.	Av. %	Diff. OTUs
Uncultured	46,346	32.38	65	58,903	34.80	63	92,444	63.98	90	197,693	43.7	96
Rhodococcus	54,920	38.37	3	16,636	9.83	3	4102	2.84	3	75,658	17.0	4
Pseudonocardia †	12,913	9.02	7	33,640	19.87	8	25,545	17.68	9	72,098	15.5	9
Unclassified	5762	4.03	18	52,908	31.26	20	8668	6.00	26	67,338	13.8	32
Streptomyces †	7628	5.33	10	1292	0.76	11	4347	3.01	18	13,267	3.0	19
Arthrobacter	4323	3.02	4	3214	1.90	4	2649	1.83	5	10,186	2.3	5
Sporichthya *	771	0.54	1	556	0.33	2	2515	1.74	2	3842	0.9	2
Planotetraspora *	2769	1.93	1	294	0.17	1	113	0.08	1	3176	0.7	1
Nocardia	1023	0.71	2	157	0.09	2	1212	0.84	2	2392	0.5	2
Mycobacterium †	1299	0.91	2	127	0.08	2	440	0.30	3	1866	0.4	3
Frankia *	1067	0.75	2	77	0.05	1	126	0.09	3	1270	0.3	3
Luedemannella *	555	0.39	2	212	0.13	2	276	0.19	2	1043	0.2	2
Longispora *	371	0.26	1	374	0.22	1	110	0.08	1	855	0.2	1
Agromyces *	310	0.22	2	136	0.08	2	355	0.25	2	801	0.2	2
Actinoplanes *	591	0.41	2	85	0.05	2	111	0.08	2	787	0.2	2
Nakamurella *	416	0.29	1	114	0.07	1	101	0.07	1	631	0.1	1
Nocardioides †	360	0.25	4	52	0.03	3	158	0.11	8	570	0.1	9
Geodermatophilus †	78	0.05	1	70	0.04	2	374	0.26	2	522	0.1	2
Catellatospora *	95	0.07	3	70	0.04	2	141	0.10	4	306	0.07	4
Kribbella †	120	0.08	1	36	0.02	1	135	0.09	2	291	0.07	2
Kocuria *	261	0.18	1	23	0.01	1	-	-	-	284	0.1	2
Actinomyces *	247	0.17	5	1	0.001	1	6	0.004	1	254	0.06	5
Corynebacterium *	151	0.11	1	32	0.02	3	10	0.01	2	193	0.04	5
Rhizocola *	-	-	-	27	0.02	1	145	0.10	1	172	0.06	1
Microbacterium *	108	0.08	1	48	0.03	1	5	0.003	1	161	0.04	1
Iamia *	107	0.07	1	-	-	-	31	0.02	1	138	0.05	1
Pseudoclavibacter *	138	0.10	1	-	-	-	-	-	-	138	0.1	1
Lentzea *	-	-	-	-	-	-	111	0.08	1	111	0.08	1
Aeromicrobium †	73	0.05	1	-	-	-	28	0.02	2	101	0.04	2
Amycolatopsis	86	0.06	1	-	-	-	5	0.003	1	91	0.03	2
Cryptosporangium *	-	-	-	71	0.04	1	10	0.01	1	81	0.02	1
Glycomyces *	35	0.02	1	-	-	-	45	0.03	1	80	0.03	1
Streptosporangium *	61	0.04	1	-	-	-	19	0.01	1	80	0.03	1
Smaragdicoccus *	43	0.03	1	-	-	-	34	0.02	1	77	0.03	1
Propionibacterium	57	0.04	1	-	-	-	-	-	0	57	0.04	1
Kineosporia *	44	0.03	1	-	-	-	8	0.01	1	52	0.02	1
Jatrophihabitans *	-	-	-	21	0.01	1	24	0.02	1	45	0.01	1
Promicromonospora *	-	-	-	22	0.01	1	21	0.01	1	43	0.01	2
Millisia *	-	-	-	22	0.01	1	6	0.004	1	28	0.01	1
Rothia *	2	0.001	1	13	0.01	1	7	0.005	1	22	0.005	1
Tessaracoccus *	-	-	-	17	0.01	1	-	-	-	17	0.01	1
Acidothermus *	-	-	-	-	-	-	16	0.01	1	16	0.01	1
Marmoricola *	-	-	-	-	-	-	14	0.01	2	14	0.01	2
Dermacoccus *	-	-	-	-	-	-	11	0.008	1	11	0.01	1
Ponticoccus *	-	-	-	8	0.005	1	-	-	-	8	0.005	1
Stackebrandtia *	-	-	-	-	-	-	8	0.006	1	8	0.01	1
Umezawaea *	-	-	-	-	-	-	2	0.001	1	2	0.001	1
Actinospica *	-	-	-	-	-	-	1	0.001	1	1	0.001	1
Propionimicrobium *	-	-	-	-	-	-	1	0.001	1	1	0.001	1

For each taxon, the number of obtained sequences (Seq.) and their relative abundance (%), together with the number of OTUs, are given. The total number of sequences, average relative abundance, and total number of different OTUs obtained per genus are shown in the last three columns. Taxa marked with an asterisk (*) were reported for the first time in moonmilk deposits in this study Taxa marked with a cross (†) were detected in moonmilk deposits in this work, and in the high-throughput sequencing (HTS)-based study of Dhami et al. [19]. Taxa underlined represent the ones that were also detected in other moonmilk microbial diversity studies [12–15,18]. Cases filled in grey highlight the most abundant genera in each studied sampling point. Abbreviations: Seq.—number of sequences identified.

2.3. Analysis of the Most Abundant Actinobacterial OTUs

In order to obtain more information about the most dominant moonmilk-dwelling Actinobacteria, a detailed analysis was conducted for the 41 most abundant OTUs (~17% of all of the OTUs) accounting together for 90% (413,739 out of 456,878) of the sequences obtained via our HTS approach (Table 4). Out of the subset of 41 OTUs, 16 phylotypes belonged to the class Acidimicrobiia, with most of them being uncultured at the family level, and the remaining 25 OTUs belonged to the class Actinobacteria (Table 4). In the latter case, all of the OTUs were associated with major families previously identified in moonmilk deposits, including Pseudonocardiaceae, Propionibacteriaceae, Micrococcaceae, Nocardiaceae, Streptomycetaceae, and Streptosporangiaceae (Table 4). Only 16

OTUs could be classified at the genus level and were affiliated to genera *Rhodococcus*, *Pseudonocardia*, *Arthrobacter*, *Sporichthya*, *Streptomyces*, *Planotetraspora*, and *Nocardia* (Table 4).

Table 4. The relative abundance (%) and taxonomy assignment of the most abundant actinobacterial OTUs found across moonmilk samples within the "Grotte des Collemboles".

OTU	COL1	COL3	COL4	Av. %	Class	Family	Genus
OTU1	38.28	9.68	2.74	16.90	Actinobacteria	Nocardiaceae	*Rhodococcus*
OTU2	0.31	28.89	2.13	10.44	Actinobacteria	Pseudonocardiaceae	unclassified
OTU8	0.75	13.96	0.58	5.10	Actinobacteria	Pseudonocardiaceae	uncultured
OTU4	3.35	1.13	11.47	5.32	Acidimicrobiia	uncultured	uncultured
OTU3	0.52	7.80	4.87	4.40	Actinobacteria	Pseudonocardiaceae	*Pseudonocardia*
OTU262	3.45	4.12	5.89	4.49	Actinobacteria	Pseudonocardiaceae	*Pseudonocardia*
OTU6	7.53	1.00	3.98	4.17	Acidimicrobiia	uncultured	uncultured
OTU12	2.97	6.61	1.82	3.80	Actinobacteria	Pseudonocardiaceae	uncultured
OTU5	3.53	1.70	5.87	3.70	Acidimicrobiia	uncultured	uncultured
OTU13	0.46	4.91	3.65	3.01	Actinobacteria	Pseudonocardiaceae	*Pseudonocardia*
OTU98	0.99	1.07	6.94	3.00	Acidimicrobiia	uncultured	uncultured
OTU203	1.73	0.31	5.92	2.66	Acidimicrobiia	uncultured	uncultured
OTU432	3.68	1.40	1.66	2.25	Actinobacteria	Pseudonocardiaceae	*Pseudonocardia*
OTU142	0.72	1.91	2.35	1.66	Actinobacteria	Pseudonocardiaceae	unclassified
OTU7	0	1.70	3.31	1.67	Actinobacteria	Pseudonocardiaceae	uncultured
OTU19	2.06	0.52	1.65	1.41	Actinobacteria	Micrococcaceae	*Arthrobacter*
OTU190	0.46	0.31	2.84	1.20	Acidimicrobiia	uncultured	uncultured
OTU10	0.81	0.29	1.68	0.93	Acidimicrobiia	Acidimicrobiaceae	uncultured
OTU9	0.24	0.15	2.39	0.93	Acidimicrobiia	uncultured	uncultured
OTU251	0.77	0.65	1.12	0.85	Actinobacteria	Pseudonocardiaceae	*Pseudonocardia*
OTU14	0.54	0.31	1.73	0.86	Actinobacteria	Sporichthyaceae	*Sporichthya*
OTU30	2.11	0.13	0.31	0.85	Actinobacteria	Streptomycetaceae	*Streptomyces*
OTU360	0.40	0.17	1.68	0.75	Acidimicrobiia	uncultured	uncultured
OTU24	1.93	0.17	0.08	0.73	Actinobacteria	Streptosporangiaceae	*Planotetraspora*
OTU11	0.38	0.03	1.72	0.71	Acidimicrobiia	uncultured	uncultured
OTU20	0.71	0.47	0.81	0.67	Acidimicrobiia	Iamiaceae	uncultured
OTU47	0.75	0.26	0.98	0.66	Acidimicrobiia	uncultured	uncultured
OTU15	0.30	0.17	1.48	0.65	Actinobacteria	Streptomycetaceae	*Streptomyces*
OTU192	0.01	1.65	0.01	0.56	Actinobacteria	Pseudonocardiaceae	uncultured
OTU16	0.24	0.51	1.11	0.62	Acidimicrobiia	uncultured	uncultured
OTU50	0.88	0.54	0.37	0.60	Actinobacteria	Pseudonocardiaceae	uncultured
OTU22	1.61	0.16	0.06	0.61	Actinobacteria	Propionibacteriaceae	unclassified
OTU23	0.27	1.19	0.10	0.52	Actinobacteria	Micrococcaceae	*Arthrobacter*
OTU54	0.13	0.92	0.46	0.50	Actinobacteria	Pseudonocardiaceae	*Pseudonocardia*
OTU18	0.48	0.12	1.04	0.54	Acidimicrobiia	uncultured	uncultured
OTU25	0.56	0.09	0.83	0.49	Actinobacteria	Nocardiaceae	*Nocardia*
OTU21	0.80	0.19	0.34	0.45	Actinobacteria	Streptomycetaceae	*Streptomyces*
OTU99	1.05	0.09	0.17	0.44	Actinobacteria	Streptomycetaceae	*Streptomyces*
OTU36	0.22	0.04	0.96	0.41	Acidimicrobiia	uncultured	uncultured
OTU44	0.80	0.14	0.26	0.40	Acidimicrobiia	uncultured	uncultured
OTU32	0.22	0.03	0.92	0.39	Actinobacteria	unclassified	unclassified

Taking into account the spatial differences in terms of the most abundant taxa across the cave, COL1 was highly dominated by OTU1, affiliated to the genus *Rhodococcus*, and accounting for 38% of the total population in this speleothem (Table 4). This phylotype highly outnumbered other two *Rhodococcus* OTUs detected in COL1 (Table 3), which together constituted only 0.1% (data not shown). The predominant phylotypes identified in speleothems COL3 and COL4 were OTU2, representing an unclassified Pseudonocardiaceae in COL3 (29%), and OTU4, representing uncultured bacterium from Acidimicrobiia class in COL4 (11%) (Table 4). Among the known genera, *Rhodococcus* (OTU1, 10%) was also prevailing in COL3, while *Pseudonocardia* (OTU262, 6%) was found to be the most abundant in COL4 (Table 4).

In total, 40 out of 41 OTUs were present in all the three studied moonmilk deposits, often with an extreme variation in terms of their relative abundance across the different collection points. This is well demonstrated by OTU2 (Pseudonocardiaceae, unclassified at the genus level), which largely dominated the actinobacterial community in COL3 (29%), while only representing 0.3% of the actinobacterial microbiome in COL1 (Table 4).

2.4. Comparison of Moonmilk Streptomyces OTUs and Streptomyces Strains Isolated via the Culture-Dependent Approach

The true diversity of microbial communities is known to be strongly biased by cultivation-based methods in comparison to molecular techniques; therefore, we wanted to assess how much of the *Streptomyces* moonmilk-dwelling community we managed to isolate in our previous bioprospection work [10]. For this purpose, we compared the 16S rRNA sequences of the 19 *Streptomyces* OTUs retrieved from the HTS approach with the sequences of the 31 previously isolated *Streptomyces* phylotypes (MM strains), which were trimmed to the corresponding V6–V7 variable regions of HTS amplicons. Figure 4 presents the phylogenetic tree generated by maximum likelihood with all the 252 nt 16S rRNA sequences from the *Streptomyces* phylotypes (MM strains) and OTUs. The identity threshold for clustering sequences in the same branch of the tree was fixed to 97%, i.e., the same threshold as the one used to define OTUs in our HTS approach (see methods for details). As deduced from the generated phylogenetic tree, the 31 isolated *Streptomyces* strains matched with only five of the 19 *Streptomyces* OTUs, suggesting that the isolated strains represent a minor fraction of the *Streptomyces* species dwelling in the moonmilk deposits of the studied cave. Expectedly, Figure 4 further shows that we isolated *Streptomyces* species that are associated with the most abundant *Streptomyces* OTUs, e.g., OTU15, OTU21, OTU30, and OTU99 (Table 4), which together represent 79% of the *Streptomyces* sequences retrieved by our HTS approach. Moreover, 21 out of the 31 phylotype strains (68%) clustered together with OTU21 (Figure 4). Finally, two *Streptomyces* isolates, i.e., MM24 and MM106, did not cluster with any of the identified *Streptomyces* OTUs (Figure 4).

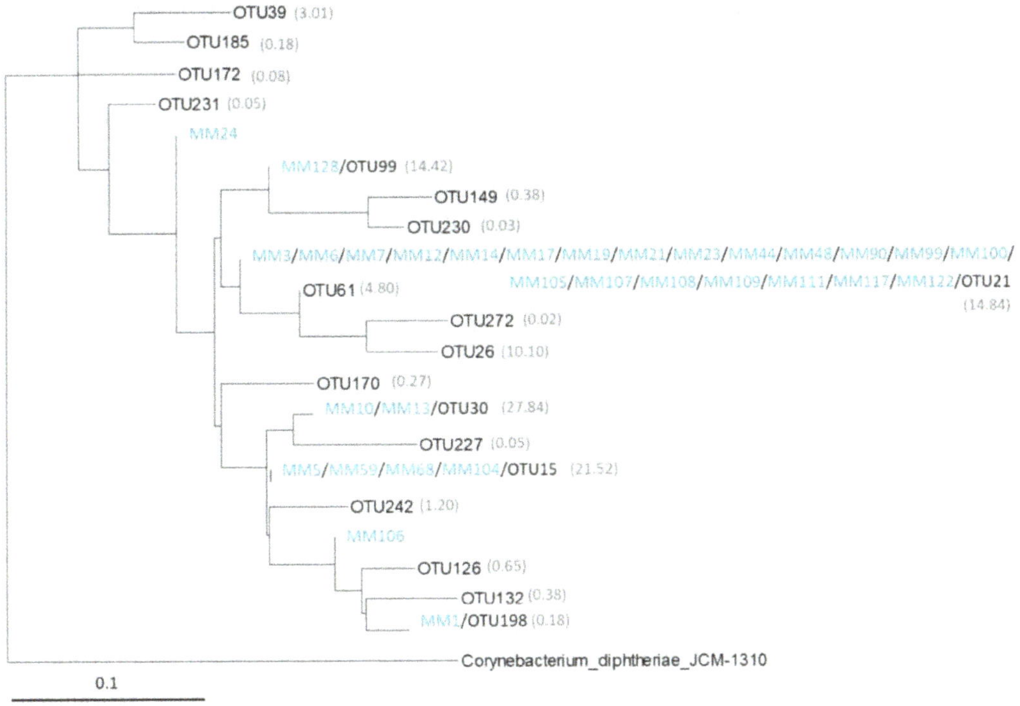

Figure 4. Phylogenetic relationships between culturable and non-culturable *Streptomyces* originating from moonmilk of "Grotte des Collemboles". The tree was inferred by maximum likelihood. Scale bar is in substitution per site. Numbers between brackets reflect the predicted mean abundance of *Streptomyces* OTUs in the studied deposits based on the percentage of sequences retrieved from the HTS analysis. *Streptomyces* phylotypes isolated in our previous bioprospection study (MM strains) are marked in blue.

3. Discussion

3.1. New Insights into Moonmilk Bacterial Diversity Revealed by High-Throughput Sequencing

Previous investigations on the moonmilk microbiome revealed a very diverse microbial community in these deposits [9,13–17,19]. The high-throughput sequencing approach used in this work complemented previous findings by providing an in-depth picture of the bacterial population, together with a detailed taxonomic fingerprint of the phylum Actinobacteria.

Comparison of the bacterial diversity in moonmilk between earlier investigations and the present work is limited to some extent by the differences in experimental procedures, such as DNA isolation and PCR-based approaches, and the sensitivity of the sequencing techniques. Nonetheless, the profile of the major taxonomic groups found in this work is consistent with that observed for the moonmilk communities in the caves "Grotta della Foos" and "Bus della Genziana" in Italy, which were obtained from 16S rRNA clone libraries [9]. All of the phyla detected in the above-mentioned caves, including Bacteroidetes, Acidobacteria, Chloroflexi, Planctomycetes, Verrucomicrobia, Actinobacteria, Firmicutes, Nitrospirae, Chlorobi, Proteobacteria, and WS3 (now Latescibacteria), were also identified in the cave "Grotte des Collemboles", although their relative abundance varied between the studies. While Proteobacteria were found to be the most abundant phylum in both cases, the second most abundant population identified in Italian caves was the phylum Bacteroidetes, which constituted a minor part of the bacterial community in the present study. The Actinobacteria population was found to be an important part of the moonmilk microbiome in the "Grotte des Collemboles" (from 9% to 23%), but instead represented only a minor fraction (<2%) of the bacterial population in the two Italian caves investigated by Engel et al. (2013). Very recently, a study by Dhami et al. has reported the moonmilk microbiome profile in the Australian "Lake Cave" using an HTS approach [19], as in this work. The presence of Proteobacteria, Actinobacteria, Acidobacteria, Chloroflexi, Nitrospirae, Gemmatimonadetes, Firmicutes, and Bacteroidetes were detected in the moonmilk deposit of the "Lake Cave", similarly to the "Grotte des Collemboles". However, many of the low-abundance taxa identified in the Belgian cave were not reported, possibly because their phylogenetic profiles were based on different regions of 16S rRNA gene—V3/V4 for the "Lake Cave", and V6–V7 for the "Grotte des Collemboles". Interestingly, unlike in Italian and Belgian caves, the "Lake Cave" moonmilk deposit was strongly dominated by Actinobacteria, which were more than twice as abundant as the Proteobacteria [19]. The highly sensitive HTS amplicon sequencing approach employed in this work revealed the presence of 26 phyla within the moonmilk microbiome that had not been previously described in this speleothem. These included Zixibacteria (formerly RBG-1), Armatimonadetes (formerly OP10), and Parcubacteria (formerly OD1) among the main phyla of moonmilk microbiome (Figure 2a), which have been previously reported from other subterranean environments [24,29–33], and 23 low-abundant taxa that were found below the level of 1%, and included many candidate divisions (Figure 2b).

This new study uncovered a surprisingly diverse Actinobacteria taxonomic profile that demonstrates the limitations of our previous cultivation-based screening, in which only the *Streptomyces* species could be isolated from the three moonmilk deposits [10]. Here, a total of 47 actinobacterial genera from 28 families were identified across the investigated samples. Beyond the previously reported members of the Actinomycetales family—including *Nocardia* and *Rhodococcus* (Nocardiaceae) [15,18], *Pseudonocardia, Amycolatopsis* and *Saccharothrix* (not identified in our study) (Pseudonocardiaceae) [12,14,19], *Propionibacterium* (Propionibacteriaceae) [14], *Streptomyces* (Streptomycetaceae) [10,12,18,19], *Arthrobacter* (Micrococcaceae) [13], *Mycobacterium* (Mycobacteriaceae) [19], *Nocardioides, Aeromicrobium,* and *Kribbella* (Nocardioidaceae) [19], and *Geodermatophilus* (Geodermatophilaceae) [19]—35 other genera were identified in the moonmilk deposits of the "Grotte des Collemboles". The population of each investigated sample was also found to include representatives of the Acidimicrobiia class, which were not previously reported in moonmilk. Their presence in all the three sampling sites, with an abundance up to 55% in COL4, and the dominance of the unclassified Acidimicrobiia phylotype (OTU 4) within the community of COL4, suggest that the chemical composition of the investigated moonmilk would be particularly suitable for the development of the representatives of this class of Actinobacteria, of which the ecology and metabolism are still largely unknown.

3.2. Moonmilk Deposits as Appealing Source of Novel Producers of Bioactive Compounds

Extreme environmental niches have recently become the main targets for intense bioprospecting, as they are expected to host diverse yet-unknown microorganisms, which could offer unexplored chemical diversity. While *Streptomyces* are reported as the most prolific "antibiotic makers", advances in the cultivation and characterization of rare Actinobacteria revealed similarly promising capabilities for the production of bioactive natural compounds [34–36]. The results obtained in this work suggest a significant biodiversity of the moonmilk-dwelling actinobacterial population, with a wide spectrum of rare genera. Next to *Streptomyces*, other members of Actinobacteria with valuable secondary metabolism were detected at a high proportion, such as *Pseudonocardia*, *Amycolatopsis*, *Streptosporangium*, *Nocardia*, *Nocardioides*, and *Rhodococcus*. Such findings clearly prompt to apply appropriate selective cultivation methods to isolate rare Actinobacteria from moonmilk deposits.

Moreover, particular importance should be also focused on Acidimicrobiia, which constituted an important part of the community in the studied deposits. Members of this class are a recently identified taxonomic unit [37] that is considered to represent an early-branching lineage within the phylum [38]. Due to their phylogenetic isolation and novelty, they are likely to hide a yet-uncovered valuable bioactive arsenal.

The great potential of moonmilk as a source of diverse and metabolically beneficial Actinobacteria is illustrated by the comparison of *Streptomyces* isolated in our previous study and the *Streptomyces* OTUs identified in this work (Figure 4). Most *Streptomyces* OTUs are phylogenetically distinct from culturable representatives (Figure 4), indicating that a great number of species still remain to be isolated. On the other hand, our culture-dependent study identified *Streptomyces* strains (MM24 and MM106, Figure 4) that were not associated with OTUs deduced from the HTS approach, confirming that both strategies are complementary, and should be used in parallel for microbial diversity assessment [39,40]. In addition, next to the identification methods themselves, our data suggests that the diversity level can be also biased by the identity threshold that is used for OTU definition. The tree revealed that a single OTU (OTU21, Figure 4) clustered together with most of the phylotypes deduced from MLSA (multilocus sequence analysis), each most likely representing a distinct species [10]. This indicates that the 97% sequence homology threshold applied to the comparative analysis of the V6–V7 regions of the 16S RNA gene largely underestimated the number of *Streptomyces* species dwelling in a studied environmental niche.

4. Materials and Methods

4.1. Site description and Sampling

The cave "Grotte des Collemboles" (Springtails' Cave), located in Comblain-au-Pont (GPS coordinates 50°28′41″ N, 5°36′35″ E), Belgium (Figure S1, Maciejewska et al. 2017 for full description), was formed in Visean limestone and has the shape of a 70-m long meander. White to brown–orange moonmilk deposits are found on the walls in the first narrow chamber located at the entrance of the cave, as well as in the narrow passages leading deeper into the cave (Figure S1). Moonmilk samples used for total DNA extractions were aseptically collected in January 2012 from three spatially separated locations along about a 20-m transect in the cave. Soft moonmilk speleothems were scratched with sterile scalpels into sterile Falcon tubes from the wall in the first chamber, adjacent to the cave entrance (COL4), and from the walls in a narrow passage after the first chamber (COL1, COL3) (Figure S1). COL4 was located approximately 6 m from COL1, and 20 m from COL3 (Figure S1).

Samples were immediately transferred to the laboratory, freeze-dried on a VirTis Benchtop SLC Lyophilizer (SP Scientific, Warminster, PA, USA), and stored at −20 °C.

4.2. Total DNA Extraction and 16S rRNA Gene Amplicon High-Throughput Sequencing

The metagenetic approach applied in this work was performed on DNA extracted from three moonmilk deposits (COL1, COL3, and COL4) originating from the "Grotte des Collemboles". Environmental genomic DNA isolation was carried out from 200 mg of the freeze-dried moonmilk samples COL1, COL3, and COL4 (Figure S1), using the PowerClean Soil DNA kit (MoBio, Carlsbad, CA, USA), according to manufacturer's instructions. The integrity of purified DNA was assessed by agarose gel electrophoresis (1% w/v), and the dsDNA concentration was evaluated by Qubit fluorometer (Invitrogen, Carlsbad, CA, USA).

The 16S rRNA gene amplicon libraries were generated using bacterial (S-D-Bact-0517-a-S-17/S-D-Bact-1061-a-A-17 spanning V4–V6 region [41]) and actinobacterial (Com2xf/Ac1186r, spanning V6–V7 region [42]) specific primer pairs. The Illumina platform-compatible dual index paired-end approach was designed as previously described [43] (detailed description provided in the Table S1a). Each forward and reverse primer consisted of an Illumina-compatible forward/reverse primer overhang attached to the $5'$ end. Additionally, a heterogeneity spacer of four degenerate nucleotides (Ns) was added to the forward primer, between the primer overhang and the locus-specific sequence. The Illumina barcodes and sequencing adapters were added during the subsequent cycle-limited amplification step using Nextera XT Index kit (Illumina, San Diego, CA, USA). Triplicated PCR reactions were performed for each sample in 25 μL of volume containing 2.5 μL of total DNA, 5 μL of each primer (1 μM), and 12.5 μL of 2× Q5 High-Fidelity Master Mix (New England Biolabs, Ipswich, MA, USA). Amplification conditions for each set of primers are listed in Table S1b. The triplicated amplicons were visualized on 3% agarose gel, pulled, purified with Agencourt AMPure XP beads (Beckman Coulter, Brea, CA, USA), and quantified with the Qubit HS dsDNA assay kit (Invitrogen, Carlsbad, CA,) before being processed for index ligation, using the Nextera XT Index kit (Illumina, San Diego, CA, USA). The PCR amplifications were performed with the same enzyme and cycling conditions as described above [43], with the total number of cycles reduced to eight, and an annealing temperature of 55 °C. The resulting amplicons were purified with the Agencourt AMPure XP magnetic beads (Beckman Coulter, CA, USA), quantified, and pooled in equimolar concentrations. The library concentration was quantified by qPCR using a Kappa SYBR FAST kit (Kapa Biosystems, Wilmington, MA, USA), and subsequently, the library was normalized to 4 nM, denatured, and diluted to the final concentration of 8 p.m. The resulting pool was mixed with the PhiX control and subjected to 2 × 300 bp paired-end sequencing on Illumina MiSeq platform (Illumina, San Diego, CA, USA). Raw sequences were deposited in the NCBI Sequence Read Archive (SRA) database under the Bioproject PRJNA428798 with accession numbers SRX3540524–SRX3540529.

4.3. 16S rRNA Amplicon Analysis

16S rRNA amplicon analysis was based for both Bacteria and Actinobacteria on forward reads only, owing to the poor quality of reverse reads. Quality trimming (prohibiting mismatches and ambiguities, ensuring a minimum quality score of 20 and removing the four degenerate nucleotides from the $5'$ end) was carried out using CLC Genomic Workbench (Qiagen, Hilden, Germany). USEARCH [44] was applied for length trimming (minimum length = 240 nt) and dereplication. Operational taxonomic units (OTUs) for both bacterial and actinobacterial datasets were defined using a 97% identity threshold on 16S rRNA sequences. OTUs were clustered using the UPARSE algorithm [45], and their taxonomic position was assigned by MOTHUR [46] with SILVA v128 database [47]. OTUs were further classified using BLASTN [48] analyses against a local mirror of NCBI nt database (downloaded on 9 August 2017), through manual and automatic analyses. For the automatic approach, a last common ancestor (LCA) classification was performed with a custom parser mimicking the MEGAN algorithm [49], which we developed for analyses of genome contamination (Cornet et al., 2017, under review). A maximum number of 100 hits per OTU were taken into account. To consider a BLASTN hit, the E-value threshold was set at 1e-15, the minimum identity threshold was set at 95.5%, the minimum bit score was set at 200, and the bit score percentage threshold was set at 99% of the best hit. These thresholds were defined through preliminary analyses (data not shown). When the BLASTN hits are too numerous, the MEGAN-like algorithm frequently yields high-ranking LCAs (e.g., Bacteria) that are not informative in practice. In order to minimize this effect, we decided to skip uncultured/unclassified hits whenever other, more informative, hits also passed the thresholds. Moreover, when computing LCAs, we only considered the most frequent taxa, provided that they represented $\geq$95% of the (up to 100) accumulated BLASTN hits, so as to avoid uninformative classifications due to a few (possibly aberrant) outliers.

Normalized OTU abundance data was used to calculate α-diversity and β-diversity estimators using MOTHUR [46]. Community richness, evenness, diversity, and differential OTU abundance between samples were calculated using sobs, the Simpson index, the inverse Simpson index and Venn diagrams, respectively.

The 19 OTUs identified as *Streptomyces* were combined to 31 sequences (16S rRNA region V6–V7) from previously isolated *Streptomyces* phylotypes (MM strains) and dereplicated with the UCLUST algorithm [44] using an identity threshold of 97%. This yielded 21 clusters, to which we added the homologous region of *Corynebacterium diphtheriae* JCM-1310 as an outgroup. A multiple sequence alignment was built with MUSCLE [50] (default parameters), and then analyzed with PhyML [51] under a K80 + Γ_4 model. Due to the limited amount of phylogenetic signal (short sequences from very related organisms), the resolution of the tree was low (bootstrap proportions <50 for nearly all nodes; data not shown).

5. Conclusions

Before the advent of metagenomics, bioprospecting was carried out blindly, with poor knowledge on the real potential of an ecological niche mined for novel organisms, enzymes, or bioactive compounds. The results of the metagenetic study presented here confirmed that different moonmilk deposits host their own indigenous microbial population, and thus each individual speleothem can be a source of a great biodiversity. Consequently, the observed important differences in the spatial diversity of Actinobacteria imply that bioprospecting within different moonmilk deposits—from different caves or within the same cave—could result in the isolation of unique and novel natural compound producers. Our study also revealed how many and which actinobacterial genera have been missed in our first attempt to isolate antibiotic producers. We now know that the *Streptomyces* strains of our collection isolated from the moonmilk deposits of the cave 'Grotte des Collemboles' [10] are just the tip of the iceberg. These results prompted us to apply a series of *'tips and tricks'* to isolate other *Streptomyces* and representatives of other antibiotic-producing Actinobacteria that are present in different proportions in each moonmilk deposit. The results of our adapted protocols for the isolation of rare Actinobacteria are presented in the article *'Isolation, Characterization, and Antibacterial Activity of Hard-to-Culture Actinobacteria from Cave Moonmilk Deposits'*, which is published in the same special issue [52].

Supplementary Materials: The following are available online at http://www.mdpi.com/2079-6382/7/2/27/s1, Figure S1: Localization of the "Grotte des Collemboles" (Springtails' Cave) together with the cave map and visualization of the moonmilk deposit sampling points, Figure S2: Rarefaction curves of OTUs clustered at 97% sequence identity across the three moonmilk-sampling points for Bacteria (a) and Actinobacteria (b), Figure S3: Taxonomic profile of bacterial phyla generated with Actinobacteria-specific primers. Note the high specificity of Actinobacteria primers, Table S1: Details of the PCR primers used for community profiling of moonmilk samples (a) and—PCR conditions used for 16S rRNA amplification from moonmilk samples (b), Table S2: Relative abundance (%) of bacterial phyla identified in the three moonmilk deposits in "Grotte des Collemboles". Low-abundant taxa with relative abundance <1% are marked in red, Table S3: Relative abundance (%) of the phylum Actinobacteria at different taxonomic levels identified in the three moonmilk deposits in the "Grotte des Collemboles".

Acknowledgments: The authors are grateful to Luc Willems for the introduction to the subject and help with sampling. MM, DA, and LC work was supported by a Research Foundation for Industry and Agriculture (FRIA) grant. MC and PD were supported by the Luxembourg National Research Fund (FNR CORE 2011 project

GASPOP; C11/SR/1280949: Influence of the Reactor Design and the Operational Parameters on the Dynamics of the Microbial Consortia Involved in the Biomethanation Process). Computational resources ("durandal" grid computer) were funded by three grants from the University of Liège, "Fonds spéciaux pour la recherche", "Crédit de démarrage 2012" (SFRD-12/03 and SFRD-12/04) and "Crédit classique 2014" (C-14/73) and by a grant from the F.R.S.-FNRS "Crédit de recherche 2014" (CDR J.0080.15). This work is supported in part by the Belgian program of Interuniversity Attraction Poles initiated by the Federal Office for Scientific Technical and Cultural Affairs (PAI No. P7/44). SR is a Research Associate at Belgian Fund for Scientific Research (F.R.S-FNRS). The authors declare no conflict of interest. We dedicate the work to the memory of Leonard Maculewicz (1936–2017) who always supported our work with great enthusiasm.

Author Contributions: M.M., Ma.C., S.M., Mo.C., P.D., and S.R. designed and performed experiments. Bioinformatic analyses were performed by M.M., Mo.C., Ma.C., L.C., D.B., and S.R. Data were analyzed by all authors. The manuscript was written and/or corrected by all authors.

References

1. Engel, A.S. Microbial diversity of cave ecosystems. In *Geomicrobiology: Molecular and Environmental Perspective*; Springer: Berlin, Germany, 2010, ISBN 9789048192038.

2. Barton, H.A.; Northup, D.E. Geomicrobiology in cave environments: Past, current and future perspectives. *J. Cave Karst Stud.* **2007**, *69*, 163–178.

3. Groth, I.; Vettermann, R.; Schuetze, B.; Schumann, P.; Saiz-Jimenez, C. Actinomycetes in Karstic caves of northern Spain (Altamira and Tito Bustillo). *J. Microbiol. Methods* **1999**, *36*, 115–122. [CrossRef]

4. Jurado, V.; Kroppenstedt, R.M.; Saiz-Jimenez, C.; Klenk, H.P.; Mouniée, D.; Laiz, L.; Couble, A.; Pötter, G.; Boiron, P.; Rodríguez-Nava, V. Hoyosella altamirensis gen. nov., sp. nov., a new member of the order Actinomycetales isolated from a cave biofilm. *Int. J. Syst. Evol. Microbiol.* **2009**, *59*, 3105–3110. [CrossRef] [PubMed]

5. Jurado, V.; Groth, I.; Gonzalez, J.M.; Laiz, L.; Saiz-Jimenez, C. Agromyces salentinus sp. nov. and Agromyces neolithicus sp. nov. *Int. J. Syst. Evol. Microbiol.* **2005**, *55*, 153–157. [CrossRef] [PubMed]

6. Maciejewska, M.; Pessi, I.S.; Arguelles-Arias, A.; Noirfalise, P.; Luis, G.; Ongena, M.; Barton, H.; Carnol, M.; Rigali, S. *Streptomyces lunaelactis* sp. nov., a novel ferroverdin A-producing *Streptomyces* species isolated from a moonmilk speleothem. *Antonie van Leeuwenhoek Int. J. Gen. Mol. Microbiol.* **2015**, *107*, 519–531. [CrossRef] [PubMed]

7. Lee, S.D.; Kang, S.O.; Hah, Y.C. Hongia gen, nov., a new genus of the order Actinomycetales. *Int. J. Syst. Evol. Microbiol.* **2000**, *50*, 191–199. [CrossRef] [PubMed]

8. Ortiz, M.; Neilson, J.W.; Nelson, W.M.; Legatzki, A.; Byrne, A.; Yu, Y.; Wing, R.A.; Soderlund, C.A.; Pryor, B.M.; Pierson, L.S.; et al. Profiling Bacterial Diversity and Taxonomic Composition on Speleothem Surfaces in Kartchner Caverns, AZ. *Microb. Ecol.* **2013**, *65*, 371–383. [CrossRef] [PubMed]

9. Engel, A.S.; Paoletti, M.G.; Beggio, M.; Dorigo, L.; Pamio, A.; Gomiero, T.; Furlan, C.; Brilli, M.; Dreon, A.L.; Bertoni, R.; et al. Comparative microbial community composition from secondary carbonate (moonmilk) deposits: Implications for the Cansiliella servadeii cave hygropetric food web. *Int. J. Speleol.* **2013**, *42*, 181–192. [CrossRef]

10. Maciejewska, M.; Adam, D.; Martinet, L.; Naômé, A.; Calusinska, M.; Smargiasso, N.; De Pauw, E.; Barton, H.; Carnol, M.; Hanikenne, M.; et al. A Phenotypic and Genotypic Analysis of the Antimicrobial Potential of Cultivable *Streptomyces* isolated from Cave Moonmilk Deposits. *Front. Microbiol.* **2016**. [CrossRef] [PubMed]

11. Cañaveras, J.C.; Cuezva, S.; Sanchez-Moral, S.; Lario, J.; Laiz, L.; Gonzalez, J.M.; Saiz-Jimenez, C. On the origin of fiber calcite crystals in moonmilk deposits. *Naturwissenschaften* **2006**, *93*, 27–32. [CrossRef] [PubMed]

12. Cañaveras, J.C.; Hoyos Gómez, M.; Sánchez-Moral, S.; Sanz Rubio, E.; Bedoya, J.; Hoyos, V.; Groth, I.; Schumann, P.; Laiz Trobajo, L. Microbial Communities Associated with Hydromagnesite and Needle-Fiber Aragonite Deposits in a Karstic Cave (Altamira, Northern Spain). *Geomicrobiol. J.* **1999**, *16*, 9–25.

13. Rooney, D.C.; Hutchens, E.; Clipson, N.; Baldini, J.; McDermott, F. Microbial Community Diversity of Moonmilk Deposits at Ballynamintra Cave, Co. Waterford, Ireland. *Microb. Ecol.* **2010**, *60*, 753–761. [CrossRef] [PubMed]

14. Portillo, M.C.; Gonzalez, J.M. Moonmilk Deposits Originate from Specific Bacterial Communities in Altamira Cave (Spain). *Microb. Ecol.* **2011**, *61*, 182–189. [CrossRef] [PubMed]

15. Reitschuler, C.; Lins, P.; Schwarzenauer, T.; Spotl, C.; Wagner, A.O.; Illmer, P. New Undescribed Lineages of Non-extremophilic Archaea Form a Homogeneous and Dominant Element within Alpine Moonmilk Microbiomes. *Geomicrobiol. J.* **2015**, *32*. [CrossRef]

16. Reitschuler, C.; Spötl, C.; Hofmann, K.; Wagner, A.O.; Illmer, P. Archaeal Distribution in Moonmilk Deposits from Alpine Caves and Their Ecophysiological Potential. *Microb. Ecol.* **2016**, *71*, 686–699. [CrossRef] [PubMed]

17. Reitschuler, C.; Lins, P.; Wagner, A.O.; Illmer, P. Cultivation of moonmilk-born non-extremophilic Thaum and Euryarchaeota in mixed culture. *Anaerobe* **2014**, *29*, 73–79. [CrossRef] [PubMed]

18. Axenov-Gibanov, D.V.; Voytsekhovskaya, I.V.; Tokovenko, B.T.; Protasov, E.S.; Gamaiunov, S.V.; Rebets, Y.V.; Luzhetskyy, A.N.; Timofeyev, M.A. Actinobacteria isolated from an underground lake and moonmilk speleothem from the biggest conglomeratic karstic cave in Siberia as sources of novel biologically active compounds. *PLoS ONE* **2016**, *11*. [CrossRef] [PubMed]

19. Dhami, N.K.; Mukherjee, A.; Watkin, E. Characterisation of Mineralogical-Mechanical-Microbial properties of calcitic speleothems and the in vitro biomineralization potential of associated microbial communities. *Front. Microbiol.* **2018**, *9*, 40. [CrossRef] [PubMed]

20. Bindschedler, S.; Milliere, L.; Cailleau, G.; Job, D.; Verrecchia, E.P. Calcitic nanofibres in soils and caves: A putative fungal contribution to carbonatogenesis. *Geol. Soc. Lond. Spec. Publ.* **2010**, *336*, 225–238. [CrossRef]

21. Maciejewska, M.; Adam, D.; Naômé, A.; Martinet, L.; Tenconi, E.; Calusinska, M.; Delfosse, P.; Hanikenne, M.; Baurain, D.; Compère, P.; et al. Assessment of the potential role of *Streptomyces* in cave moonmilk formation. *Front. Microbiol.* **2017**, *8*. [CrossRef] [PubMed]

22. Nimaichand, S.; Devi, A.M.; Tamreihao, K.; Ningthoujam, D.S.; Li, W.J. Actinobacterial diversity in limestone deposit sites in Hundung, Manipur (India) and their antimicrobial activities. *Front. Microbiol.* **2015**, *6*. [CrossRef] [PubMed]

23. Wu, Y.; Tan, L.; Liu, W.; Wang, B.; Wang, J.; Cai, Y.; Lin, X. Profiling bacterial diversity in a limestone cave of the western Loess Plateau of China. *Front. Microbiol.* **2015**, *6*. [CrossRef] [PubMed]

24. Northup, D.E.; Melim, L.A.; Spilde, M.N.; Hathaway, J.J.M.; Garcia, M.G.; Moya, M.; Stone, F.D.; Boston, P.J.; Dapkevicius, M.L.N.E.; Riquelme, C. Lava Cave Microbial Communities within Mats and Secondary Mineral Deposits: Implications for Life Detection on Other Planets. *Astrobiology* **2011**, *11*, 601–618. [CrossRef] [PubMed]

25. Riquelme, C.; Hathaway, J.J.M.; Dapkevicius, M.d.L.N.E.; Miller, A.Z.; Kooser, A.; Northup, D.E.; Jurado, V.; Fernandez, O.; Saiz-Jimenez, C.; Cheeptham, N. Actinobacterial diversity in volcanic caves and associated geomicrobiological interactions. *Front. Microbiol.* **2015**, *6*. [CrossRef] [PubMed]

26. Cheeptham, N.; Sadoway, T.; Rule, D.; Watson, K.; Moote, P.; Soliman, L.C.; Azad, N.; Donkor, K.K.; Horne, D. Cure from the cave: Volcanic cave actinomycetes and their potential in drug discovery. *Int. J. Speleol.* **2013**, *42*, 35–47. [CrossRef]

27. Tebo, B.M.; Davis, R.E.; Anitori, R.P.; Connell, L.B.; Schiffman, P.; Staudigel, H. Microbial communities in dark oligotrophic volcanic ice cave ecosystems of Mt. Erebus, Antarctica. *Front. Microbiol.* **2015**, *6*. [CrossRef] [PubMed]

28. Chater, K.F.; Biró, S.; Lee, K.J.; Palmer, T.; Schrempf, H. The complex extracellular biology of *Streptomyces*. *FEMS Microbiol. Rev.* **2010**, *34*, 171–198. [CrossRef] [PubMed]

29. Castelle, C.J.; Hug, L.A.; Wrighton, K.C.; Thomas, B.C.; Williams, K.H.; Wu, D.; Tringe, S.G.; Singer, S.W.; Eisen, J.A.; Banfield, J.F. Extraordinary phylogenetic diversity and metabolic versatility in aquifer sediment. *Nat. Commun.* **2013**, *4*. [CrossRef] [PubMed]

30. Schabereiter-Gurtner, C.; Saiz-Jimenez, C.; Pinar, G.; Lubitz, W.; Rolleke, S. Phylogenetic diversity of bacteria associated with Paleolithic paintings and surrounding rock walls in two Spanish caves (Llonin and La Garma). *FEMS Microbiol. Ecol.* **2004**, *47*, 235–247. [CrossRef]

31. Pedersen, K.; Arlinger, J.; Ekendahl, S.; Hallbeck, L. 16S rRNA gene diversity of attached and unattached bacteria in boreholes along the access tunnel to the Äspö hard rock laboratory, Sweden. *FEMS Microbiol. Ecol.* **1996**, *19*, 249–262. [CrossRef]

32. Zhou, J.; Gu, Y.; Zou, C.; Mo, M. Phylogenetic diversity of bacteria in an earth-cave in Guizhou Province, Southwest of China. *J. Microbiol.* **2007**, *45*, 105–112. [PubMed]

33. De Mandal, S.; Chatterjee, R.; Kumar, N.S. Dominant bacterial phyla in caves and their predicted functional roles in C and N cycle. *BMC Microbiol.* **2017**, *17*, 90. [CrossRef] [PubMed]

34. Tiwari, K.; Gupta, R.K. Rare actinomycetes: A potential storehouse for novel antibiotics. *Crit. Rev. Biotechnol.* **2012**, *32*, 108–132. [CrossRef] [PubMed]

35. Choi, S.S.; Kim, H.J.; Lee, H.S.; Kim, P.; Kim, E.S. Genome mining of rare actinomycetes and cryptic pathway awakening. *Process Biochem.* **2015**, *50*, 1184–1193. [CrossRef]

36. Rigali, S.; Anderssen, S.; Naômé, A.; van Wezel, G.P. Cracking the regulatory code of biosynthetic gene clusters as a strategy for natural product discovery. *Biochem. Pharmacol.* **2018**. [CrossRef] [PubMed]

37. Norris, P. Class II. Acidimicrobiia class. nov. In *Bergey's Manual of Systematic Bacteriology*; Whitman, W., Goodfellow, M., Kämpfer, P., Busse, H.-J., Trujillo, M., Ludwig, W., Suzuki, K.-I., Parte, A., Eds.; Springer: New York, NY, USA, 2012; Volume 5, p. 1968.

38. Bull, A.T. Actinobacteria of the extremobiosphere. In *Extremophiles Handbook*; Springer: Tokyo, Japan, 2011; pp. 1203–1240, ISBN 9784431538981.

39. Stefani, F.O.P.; Bell, T.H.; Marchand, C.; de la Providencia, I.E.; El Yassimi, A.; St-Arnaud, M.; Hijri, M. Culture-Dependent and -Independent Methods Capture Different Microbial Community Fractions in Hydrocarbon-Contaminated Soils. *PLoS ONE* **2015**, *10*, e0128272. [CrossRef] [PubMed]

40. Vaz-Moreira, I.; Egas, C.; Nunes, O.C.; Manaia, C.M. Culture-dependent and culture-independent diversity surveys target different bacteria: A case study in a freshwater sample. *Antonie van Leeuwenhoek, Int. J. Gen. Mol. Microbiol.* **2011**, *100*, 245–257. [CrossRef] [PubMed]

41. Klindworth, A.; Pruesse, E.; Schweer, T.; Peplies, J.; Quast, C.; Horn, M.; Glöckner, F.O. Evaluation of general 16S ribosomal RNA gene PCR primers for classical and next-generation sequencing-based diversity studies. *Nucleic Acids Res.* **2013**, *41*. [CrossRef] [PubMed]

42. Schäfer, J.; Jäckel, U.; Kämpfer, P. Development of a new PCR primer system for selective amplification of Actinobacteria. *FEMS Microbiol. Lett.* **2010**, *311*, 103–112. [CrossRef] [PubMed]

43. Goux, X.; Calusinska, M.; Fossépré, M.; Benizri, E.; Delfosse, P. Start-up phase of an anaerobic full-scale farm reactor—Appearance of mesophilic anaerobic conditions and establishment of the methanogenic microbial community. *Bioresour. Technol.* **2016**, *212*, 217–226. [CrossRef] [PubMed]

44. Edgar, R.C. Search and clustering orders of magnitude faster than BLAST. *Bioinformatics* **2010**, *26*, 2460–2461. [CrossRef] [PubMed]

45. Edgar, R.C. UPARSE: Highly accurate OTU sequences from microbial amplicon reads. *Nat. Methods* **2013**, *10*, 996–998. [CrossRef] [PubMed]

46. Schloss, P.D.; Westcott, S.L.; Ryabin, T.; Hall, J.R.; Hartmann, M.; Hollister, E.B.; Lesniewski, R.A.; Oakley, B.B.; Parks, D.H.; Robinson, C.J.; et al. Introducing mothur: Open-source, platform-independent, community-supported software for describing and comparing microbial communities. *Appl. Environ. Microbiol.* **2009**, *75*, 7537–7541. [CrossRef] [PubMed]

47. Pruesse, E.; Peplies, J.; Glöckner, F.O. SINA: Accurate high-throughput multiple sequence alignment of ribosomal RNA genes. *Bioinformatics* **2012**, *28*, 1823–1829. [CrossRef] [PubMed]

48. Boratyn, G.M.; Schäffer, A.A.; Agarwala, R.; Altschul, S.F.; Lipman, D.J.; Madden, T.L. Domain enhanced lookup time accelerated BLAST. *Biol. Direct* **2012**, *7*. [CrossRef] [PubMed]

49. Huson, D.H.; Auch, A.F.; Qi, J.; Schuster, S.C. MEGAN analysis of metagenomic data. *Genome Res.* **2007**, *17*, 377–386. [CrossRef] [PubMed]

50. Edgar, R.C. MUSCLE: Multiple sequence alignment with high accuracy and high throughput. *Nucleic Acids Res.* **2004**, *32*, 1792–1797. [CrossRef] [PubMed]

51. Guindon, S.; Dufayard, J.F.; Lefort, V.; Anisimova, M.; Hordijk, W.; Gascuel, O. New algorithms and methods to estimate maximum-likelihood phylogenies: Assessing the performance of PhyML 3.0. *Syst. Biol.* **2010**, *59*, 307–321. [CrossRef] [PubMed]

52. Adam, D.; Maciejewska, M.; Naômé, A.; Martinet, L.; Coppieters, W.; Karim, L.; Baurain, D.; Rigali, S. Isolation, Characterization, and Antibacterial Activity of Hard-to-Culture Actinobacteria from Cave Moonmilk Deposits. *Antibiotics* **2018**, in press. [CrossRef]

6

The Peptidoglycan Pattern of *Staphylococcus carnosus* TM300—Detailed Analysis and Variations Due to Genetic and Metabolic Influences

Julia Deibert [1,†], Daniel Kühner [1,2,‡], Mark Stahl [3], Elif Koeksoy [1,§] and Ute Bertsche [1,2,*]

[1]   Interfaculty Institute of Microbiology and Infection Medicine Tübingen (IMIT) — Microbial Genetics, University of Tuebingen, Auf der Morgenstelle 28 E, 72076 Tuebingen, Germany; antibiotics@mdpi.com (J.D.); antibiotics@mdpi.com (D.K.); elif.koeksoy@uni-tuebingen.de (E.K.)

[2]   Interfaculty Institute of Microbiology and Infection Medicine Tübingen (IMIT) — Infection Biology, University of Tuebingen, Auf der Morgenstelle 28 E, 72076 Tuebingen, Germany

[3]   Center for Plant Molecular Biology (ZMBP), University of Tuebingen, Auf der Morgenstelle 32, 72076 Tuebingen, Germany; mark.stahl@zmbp.uni-tuebingen.de

*   Correspondence: ute.bertsche@uni-tuebingen.de

†   Present address: CureVac AG, Paul-Ehrlich-Strasse 15, 72076 Tübingen, Germany.

‡   Present address: Agilent Technologies, Hewlett-Packard-Strasse 8, 76337 Waldbronn, Germany.

§   Present address: University of Tuebingen, Center for Applied Geoscience—Geomicrobiology, Sigwartstr. 10, 72076 Tuebingen, Germany.

Academic Editor: Waldemar Vollmer

Abstract: The Gram-positive bacterium *Staphylococcus carnosus* (*S. carnosus*) TM300 is an apathogenic staphylococcal species commonly used in meat starter cultures. As with all Gram-positive bacteria, its cytoplasmic membrane is surrounded by a thick peptidoglycan (PGN) or murein sacculus consisting of several layers of glycan strands cross-linked by peptides. In contrast to pathogenic staphylococci, mainly *Staphylococcus aureus* (*S. aureus*), the chemical composition of *S. carnosus* PGN is not well studied so far. UPLC/MS analysis of enzymatically digested *S. carnosus* TM300 PGN revealed substantial differences in its composition compared to the known pattern of *S. aureus*. While in *S. aureus* the uncross-linked stem peptide consists of a pentapeptide, in *S. carnosus*, this part of the PGN is shortened to tripeptides. Furthermore, we found the PGN composition to vary when cells were incubated under certain conditions. The collective overproduction of HlyD, FtsE and FtsX—a putative protein complex interacting with penicillin-binding protein 2 (PBP2)—caused the reappearance of classical penta stem peptides. In addition, under high sugar conditions, tetra stem peptides occur due to overflow metabolism. This indicates that *S. carnosus* TM300 cells adapt to various conditions by modification of their PGN.

Keywords: *S. carnosus*; peptidoglycan; muropeptides; UPLC/MS; FtsEX; CcpA; carboxypeptidases

1. Introduction

Staphylococcus carnosus (*S. carnosus*, *S. c.*) TM300 is an apathogenic, coagulase-negative, "food grade" staphylococcal species [1] commonly used as meat starter culture for raw sausages [2]. Its 2.56 Mbp genome has the highest GC content of all staphylococcal species sequenced so far. While virulence and toxicity factors are almost completely missing from the genome, most of the metabolic pathways are present. As typical for starter cultures, it harbors various sugar degradation pathways [3,4]. The general features of the peptidoglycan (PGN) of *S. carnosus* TM300 are already known. Like *Staphylococcus aureus* (*S. aureus*, *S. a.*) it belongs to the A3α-type with a penta glycine interpeptide bridge [1,5]. *N*-acetylmuramic acid (MurNAc) residues in the glycan backbone are not O-acetylated at position six, therefore rendering S. carnosus sensitive against lysozymes like all apathogenic Staphylococcus species [6,7].

PGN biosynthesis starts in the cytoplasm where the precursor UDP-MurNAc-pentapeptide is synthesized by the sequential addition of the stem peptide to UDP-MurNAc. At the cytoplasmic membrane, this precursor is attached to the lipid carrier undecaprenol leading to lipid I. Addition of the second sugar moiety UDP-N-acetylglucosamine (UDP-GlcNAc) results in lipid II formation, which is flipped across the cytoplasmic membrane by an enzyme, that is still highly debated in its identity, as there are two possible candidates [8]: either FtsW [9,10] or MurJ [11,12]. The S. aureus stem peptide consists of L-Ala-D-iGlu-L-Lys-D-Ala-D-Ala [5] with the D-iGlu being modified at the stage of lipid II to D-iGln [13,14]. The murein synthesizing enzymes—called penicillin-binding proteins (PBPs)—need at least one amidated stem peptide for their transpeptidase activity during cross-linking [15]. In general, PBPs are divided into high molecular weight (HMW) PBPs, that perform PGN synthesis, and low molecular weight (LMW) PBPs, which are PGN hydrolases [16]. S. aureus contains four native synthesizing PBPs and homologues of all of these can be found in the genome of S. carnosus TM300. PBP2 is considered to be the main enzyme for cell wall biosynthesis in staphylococci and is localized to the division septum by binding to its transpeptidation substrate lipid II [17]. PBP2 is the only bifunctional PBP in S. aureus and S. carnosus. It catalyzes the polymerization of the glycan moieties of lipid II by its transglycosylase activity resulting in glycan chains of alternating β-1,4-linked GlcNAc-MurNAc residues. In addition PBP2 is able to cross-link adjacent stem peptides by its transpeptidase activity [18,19]. Transpeptidation occurs between the D-Ala on position four of the donor stem peptide and the N-terminal Gly of the interpeptide bridge of the acceptor stem peptide by the expense of the last D-Ala of the donor stem peptide. The resulting tetra stem peptide can serve as an acceptor for further cross-linking reactions (Supplementary Materials Figure S1). The penta stem peptide of the first acceptor or of free acceptors in S. aureus however has never been reported to be modified in any way.

In S. aureus there are three additional monofunctional PBPs: (1) the essential enzyme PBP1, which is crucial for the cell division mechanism [20]; (2) the non-essential PBP3, which is involved in autolysis [21] and (3) the non-essential PBP4, which belongs to the low molecular weight PBPs and normally is considered to be a murein hydrolase. In S. aureus however, PBP4 is responsible for the high degree of cross-linking [22] and for the resistance against β-lactams in community-acquired methicillin-resistant S. aureus strains (caMRSA) [23]. There are two possible candidates for PBP4 in S. carnosus TM300 found in KEGG [24]: SCA_0291 with 64.7% or SCA_2445 with 37.6% sequence identity to S. aureus COL, respectively. While PBPs are generally considered to contain a non-cleavable signal peptide functioning as a single N-terminal transmembrane anchor [16], these three proteins are all predicted to contain a second transmembrane domain on the C-terminus [25].

The concerted actions of transglycosylase and transpeptidase reactions of the PBPs build a mesh-like macromolecule that surrounds the whole cell. During cell division this PGN sacculus has to be divided into two parts without compromising integrity. S. aureus is a spherical bacterium that divides along three orthogonal planes over the course of three division cycles [26]. While it was long believed that spheres like staphylococci grow by PGN synthesis at the cell division site only, recent investigations by super-resolution microscopy revealed additional peripheral PGN biosynthesis catalyzed by PBP4 [27]. Cell division in all bacteria depends on formation of the FtsZ-ring and the sequential recruitment of various proteins such as FtsE and FtsX to the divisome [28,29]. FtsEX is similar to an ABC transporter on a structural and sequence level [30] with FtsE being the ATP binding subunit and FtsX being the integral membrane part. Rather than being transporters, these two proteins are proposed to regulate the activity of murein hydrolases like PcsB in Streptococcus pneumoniae [31–33] and the amidases AmiA and AmiB—both via EnvC—in E. coli [34]. In Bacillus subtilis, FtsX interacts with the endopeptidase CwlO [35]. Genes encoding for FtsE and FtsX can also be found in S. carnosus TM300. However, the resulting proteins do not possess sequence similarity but only structural similarity. The role of FtsE and FtsX during synthesis of the PGN sacculus has not been investigated in staphylococci so far.

The PGN sacculus can be isolated and digested by a muraminidase such as mutanolysin into fragments called muropeptides. Muropeptides are disaccharide units with peptide moieties that can be cross-linked to other stem peptides and disaccharides thereby resulting in oligomeric structures [36]. During the analyses of *S. carnosus* TM300 muropeptides, we observed degradation of the first acceptor stem peptides from five (pentapeptide) to three (tripeptide) amino acids, which is in contrast to the known muropeptide pattern of *S. aureus* [37,38]. This gave us reason to perform a detailed Ultra Performance Liquid Chromatography (UPLC) and UPLC mass spectrometry (UPLC/MS) analysis of the *S. carnosus* TM300 muropeptide pattern. Our results show that almost all stem peptides that were not part of a cross-link contain only three amino acids (L-Ala-D-iGln-L-Lys) under standard conditions. However, overexpression of HlyD-FtsE-FtsX, a putative protein complex interacting with PBP2, partly inhibited this degradation process. A similar effect was observed for high glucose and fructose concentrations.

2. Results

2.1. Peptidoglycan Analysis

We analyzed the PGN of *S. carnosus* TM300 by UPLC (Figure 1) and observed that it differed substantially from the known pattern of *S. aureus* [37,38]. The whole muropeptide pattern of *S. carnosus* was shifted to shorter retention times compared to *S. aureus*. We performed UPLC-MS analysis to determine the chemical composition of the muropeptide peaks (Table 1). All main peaks in the monomeric as well as in the cross-linked fractions (dimer to pentamer fraction) contained muropeptides with stem peptides only consisting of three amino acids: L-Ala-D-iGln-L-Lys, explaining the shift in retention time. In *S. aureus*, the non-cross-linked stem peptides of monomeric muropeptides as well as the acceptor stem peptide of multimeric muropeptides harbor the complete penta stem peptide. These penta muropeptides are also present in *S. carnosus*, but in small amounts compared to the respective tri muropeptide. The cross-linked stem peptides are still tetra peptides and do not get degraded into tri peptides, leading to Tri-Tetra$_n$ muropeptides (Table 1). During the course of our experiments, we realized that the amount of different muropeptides varied and was influenced by genetic factors as well as composition of the medium.

Table 1. Muropeptides of *S. carnosus* TM300 analyzed by UPLC-MS. Each muropeptide contains one to five stem-peptides and each consists of the three to five amino acids L-Ala-D-iGln-L-Lys(-D-Ala)(-D-Ala). The interpeptide bridges are built of Gly molecules. The sum of all Gly residues present in each muropeptide is given. Muropeptide peaks 4, 7 and 10 (highlighted in bold) are strongly elevated by *hlyD-ftsE-ftsX* overexpression. Muropeptide peaks 3, 6 and 9 (highlighted in italics) are strongly elevated by high glucose and fructose concentrations.

Peak	Retention Time (min)	M + H⁺ (Da)	Proposed Molecular Formula	Lengths of the Stem Peptides	Inter-Peptide Bridges
					Gly
1	7.5	1111.5192	$C_{43}H_{75}N_{12}O_{22}{}^+$	Tri	5
2	8.6	1036.4937	$C_{40}H_{70}N_{13}O_{19}{}^+$	Tetra w/o GlcNAc	6
		1093.5164	$C_{42}H_{73}N_{14}O_{20}{}^+$		7
		1150.5417	$C_{44}H_{76}N_{15}O_{21}{}^+$		8
		1207.5699	$C_{46}H_{79}N_{16}O_{22}{}^+$		9
		1239.5699	$\mathbf{C_{48}H_{83}N_{14}O_{24}{}^+}$	Tetra	**6**
		1296.5939	$C_{50}H_{86}N_{15}O_{25}{}^+$		7
		1353.6135	$C_{52}H_{89}N_{16}O_{26}{}^+$		8
		1410.6370	$C_{54}H_{92}N_{17}O_{27}{}^+$		9
3	*10.2*	*979.4691*	$C_{38}H_{67}N_{12}O_{18}{}^+$	*Tetra w/o GlcNAc*	*5*
		1182.5502	$C_{46}H_{80}N_{13}O_{23}{}^+$	*Tetra*	*5*
4	**11.1**	**1253.5856**	$\mathbf{C_{49}H_{85}N_{14}O_{24}{}^+}$	**Penta**	**5**
5	19.2	2275.0595	$C_{89}H_{152}N_{25}O_{44}{}^+$	Tri-Tetra	10

Table 1. *Cont.*

Peak	Retention Time (min)	M + H⁺ (Da)	Proposed Molecular Formula	Lengths of the Stem Peptides	Inter-Peptide Bridges Gly
6	21.5	2346.0815	$C_{92}H_{157}N_{26}O_{45}^{+}$	Tetra$_2$	10
7	**21.9**	**2417.1143**	$\mathbf{C_{95}H_{162}N_{27}O_{46}^{+}}$	**Penta-Tetra**	**10**
8	25.4	3438.5927	$C_{135}H_{229}N_{38}O_{66}^{+}$	Tri-Tetra$_2$	15
9	27.2	3509.6465	$C_{138}H_{234}N_{39}O_{67}^{+}$	Tetra$_3$	15
10	**27.5**	**3580.6553**	$\mathbf{C_{141}H_{239}N_{40}O_{68}^{+}}$	**Penta-Tetra$_2$**	**15**
11	29.1	4602.0920	$C_{181}H_{306}N_{51}O_{88}^{+}$	Tri-Tetra$_3$	20
12	31.6	5765.6142	$C_{227}H_{383}N_{64}O_{110}^{+}$	Tri-Tetra$_4$	25

Note: w/o—without.

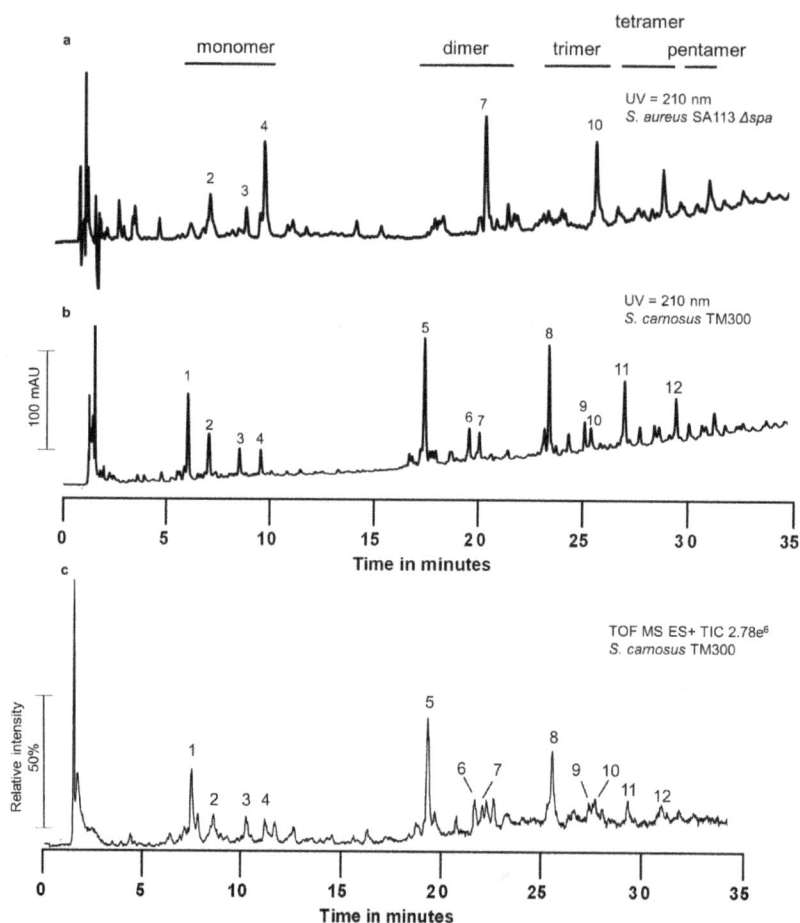

Figure 1. Muropeptide profile of *S. carnosus* TM300 by UPLC and UPLC/MS. Peptidoglycan was isolated, digested into muropeptides and analyzed by reversed phase UPLC and UPLC/MS. (**a**) Muropeptide profile of *S. aureus* SA113 Δspa obtained by UPLC. Muropeptide peaks that are identical with the ones of *S. carnosus* TM300 are numbered; (**b**) Muropeptide profile of *S. carnosus* TM300 as obtained by UPLC; (**c**) TIC of UPLC/MS analysis of *S. carnosus* TM300 peptidoglycan. Muropeptides of *S. carnosus* TM300 exhibit shorter retention times compared to *S. aureus* SA113 Δspa. UPLC/MS analysis revealed the presence of stem peptides containing only three amino acids instead of five. Masses of indicated peaks are shown in Table 1 including molecule composition and proposed molecular formula. Retention time of peaks in the UPLC (quaternary pumping system) was about 1 min longer than in the binary UPLC/MS system. Therefore, in Table 1 only TIC retention times are given (TIC: Total Ion current, recorded in positive mode).

2.2. Search for New Proteins Involved in PGN Biosynthesis

We performed a Bacterial-Two-Hybrid (BTH) screen using a genomic library of *S. carnosus* TM300 to search for new interaction partners of PBP2. This bifunctional transglycosylase/transpeptidase is considered to be one of the main players of PGN biosynthesis in *S. aureus* [16–19,39,40]. Among others, we found the so far uncharacterized protein SCA_1997, a conserved hypothetical protein that belongs to the HlyD family of secretion proteins (K02005). Therefore, we refer to this gene as *hlyD*. Bioinformatical analyses using the Kyoto Encyclopedia of Genes and Genomes (KEGG) [24] showed that if *hlyD* is present in *Bacillus spec.* and *Staphylococcus spec.* it is always located in an operon with two other genes. Each of them possesses its own start codon but they share one Shine-Dalgarno sequence and one promotor region. The first gene (SCA_1996) encodes for a putative ABC transport system ATP-binding protein (K02003) with structural similarity to FtsE of *E. coli*. The second gene (SCA_1995) is predicted to produce an ABC transport system permease protein (K02004) with structural similarity to *E. coli* FtsX [30,41]. So far, there is no function described for the staphylococcal HlyD, FtsE and FtsX proteins.

We cloned the genes of each of these proteins into the two vectors of the BTH system and performed interaction studies with all possible pairs (Table 2). PBP2 interacted with itself as well as with HlyD and FtsX. HlyD also interacted with FtsX. In addition, FtsX interacted with itself and with FtsE. There was no self-interaction of FtsE detected, and FtsE did not directly interact with HlyD (Figure 2). The interactions of the full length proteins confirmed our genetic screen results, and suggest that HlyD, FtsX and FtsE are involved in the same or in closely related biosynthetic pathways, most likely in cell wall biosynthesis and/or cell division.

Table 2. BTH interaction of proteins related to PGN biosynthesis. Interactions between proteins putatively involved in PGN biosynthesis were tested by BTH experiments. The mean values of three independent experiments are given in Miller Units per mg dry weight bacteria. (Gray: <460; orange: 1500–3000; red: >3000)

		pUT18C				
	Units/mg	*pbp2*	*ftsX*	*ftsE*	*hlyD*	*zip*
pKT25	*pbp2*			136 ± 13		164 ± 28
	ftsX		2502 ± 491	2008 ± 289	2842 ± 287	165 ± 25
	ftsE	109 ± 21		354 ± 138	132 ± 27	201 ± 103
	hlyD		2280 ± 456	205 ± 29		156 ± 36
	zip	113 ± 20	155 ± 4	126 ± 7	157 ± 59	

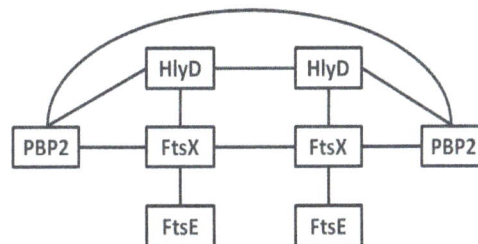

Figure 2. Protein-Protein interactions. BTH analyses revealed that PBP2 interacted with itself as well as with HlyD and FtsX. HlyD also interacted with FtsX. In addition, FtsX interacted with itself and with FtsE. There was no self-interaction of FtsE determined, and FtsE did not interact with HlyD or PBP2.

Therefore, we deleted the whole operon and examined the resulting mutant strain *S. carnosus* TM300 Δ*hlyD-ftsEX*. We did not observe any difference in growth behavior under standard BM conditions (Supplementary Materials Figure S2A), in minimal M9 medium (Supplementary Materials Figure S2B), or when the amount of NaCl in the medium was varied (Figure S2C). In addition, deletion of this operon did not have any effect on the muropeptide composition (Figure S3A). However, when the three genes were overexpressed from a plasmid harboring a xylose inducible promoter, all peaks with muropeptides containing a penta stem peptide were highly elevated while the tri muropeptides were still present in comparable amounts. Muropeptides with tetra stem peptides were slightly elevated as well. As 25 mM xylose itself had no effect on the wild type strain, the observed effect is due to overexpression of the *hlyD-ftsEX* operon (Figure 3) while overexpression of *hlyD* or *ftsEX* had no effect on muropeptide composition (Supplementary Materials Figure S3B). Astonishingly, we also observed elevated tetra and—to a lower extent—penta muropeptides when we repressed plasmid gene expression with 25 mM glucose, indicating that the PGN of *S. carnosus* is influenced by genetic as well as metabolic factors.

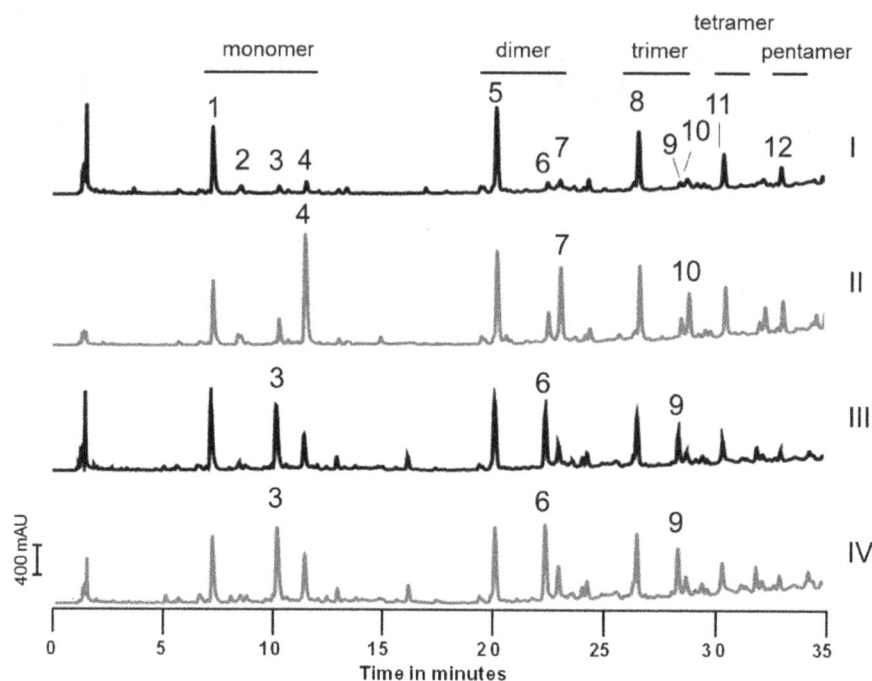

Figure 3. Variations in muropeptide profile caused by genetic and metabolic factors. PGN from different *S. carnosus* TM300 variants was isolated, digested into muropeptides and analyzed by UPLC. (**I**) *S. carnosus* TM300 grown in the presence of 25 mM xylose; (**II**) *S. carnosus* TM300 pPTX-*hlyD-ftsEX* induced with 25 mM xylose; (**III**) *S. carnosus* TM300 pPTX-*hlyD-ftsEX* repressed with 25 mM glucose; (**IV**) *S. carnosus* TM300 grown in the presence of 25 mM glucose. Overexpression of *hlyD-ftsEX* led to an accumulation of penta muropeptides (peak 4, 7 and 10 in panel **II**) which was not observed when the wild type strain was grown in the presence of 25 mM xylose. Addition of 25 mM glucose in the medium lead to an increase in tetra muropeptides independent of the plasmid pPTX-*hlyD-ftsEX* (peaks 3, 6 and 9 in panel **III** and **IV**, respectively).

2.3. Precursor Analysis

To examine if *S. carnosus* TM300 synthesizes already shortened variants of the classical PGN precursor UDP-MurNAc-pentapeptide, we accumulated and analyzed the PGN precursor of the wild type strain *S. carnosus* TM300 and of the overexpression strain *S. carnosus* TM300 pPTX-*hlyD-ftsEX* (Figure 4). In *S. aureus*, the PGN precursor is the UDP-MurNAc-pentapeptide with a mass of 1149.37 g/mol. In both tested *S. carnosus* strains, this mass was only found in a broad peak group at about 11 min in the TIC of the UPLC-MS. None of the other masses obtained correlated with the UDP-MurNAc-tripeptide (1007.2774 g/mol) or UDP-MurNAc-tetrapeptide (1078.3145 g/mol). This shows that *S. carnosus* TM300 only synthesizes the classical precursor UDP-MurNAc-pentapeptide and truncation to the tetra and tri stem peptide must occur at a later time point.

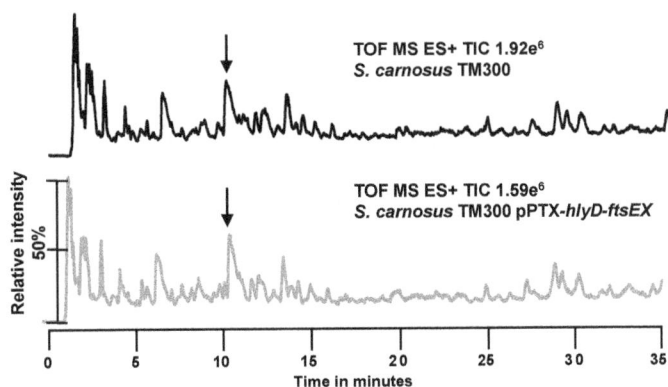

Figure 4. UPLC/MS analysis of the PGN precursor. *S. carnosus* TM300 wild type and *S. c.* TM300 pPTX-*hlyD-ftsEX* were grown in B medium supplemented with 25 mM xylose. Precursors were concentrated, isolated and analyzed by UPLC/MS. Peaks highlighted by arrows were identified to harbor the same masses including the mass for the classical precursor UDP-MurNAc-pentapeptide (1149.37 g/mol). Masses for UDP-MurNAc-tripeptide (1007.2774 g/mol) or UDP-MurNAc-tetrapeptide (1078.3145 g/mol) were not detected in any of the analyses.

2.4. Investigation of a Putative L,D-Carboxypeptidase

A logical explanation for the observed truncation of the penta stem peptide to a tri stem peptide would be an L,D-carboxypeptidase (LD-CP) activity. Even though such an activity has never been described for staphylococci, we found one potential candidate in the genome of *S. carnosus* TM300: SCA_0214 is annotated as a cytoplasmic muramoyl-tetrapeptide carboxypeptidase that hydrolyses the bond between a di-basic amino acid and the C-terminal D-alanine in the tetra peptide moiety of PGN. An orthologous gene was not found in *S. aureus* and no paralog was annotated in *S. carnosus* TM300. Therefore, a deletion mutant of SCA_0214 was created in *S. carnosus* TM300. However, deletion of this gene did not alter the PGN pattern compared to the wild type strain (Supplementary Materials Figure S4A). When we overexpressed this gene, we found the resulting protein to accumulate in the cytoplasm and not be transported to the supernatant (Supplementary Materials Figure S4B). As truncation of the stem peptide most likely occurs outside the cell, we exclude SCA_0214 as the sought-after LD-CP.

2.5. Influence of Sugars on PGN Composition

As we had observed that high concentrations of glucose (25 mM) led to an increase in muropeptides with tetra stem peptides, we tested other C-sources in this concentration as well. While fructose had the same effect, the muropeptide pattern in the presence of glycerol or ribose was unchanged. PGN of cells grown in B0 medium (B medium without an additional C-source) was also unaffected (Supplementary Materials Figure S5A). Therefore, we examined whether this observation was due to overflow metabolism and deleted the gene for the catabolite control protein A (*ccpA*). CcpA mainly functions as a gene repressor, but it is also involved in the transcription activation of genes involved in fermentation and overflow metabolism [42,43]. It is itself activated by glucose intermediates like glucose-6-phosphate and fructose-1,6-bisphosphate [44]. Indeed, the effect of high amounts of glucose on PGN composition was lost in the ΔccpA mutant (Figure 5). In the complemented mutant, the *ccpA* gene was constitutively expressed from a plasmid, and addition of 25 mM glucose to the medium again caused the appearance of muropeptides with tetra stem peptides in addition to tri stem peptides. Alterations in the PGN pattern of *S. carnosus* TM300 were not solely reduced to high glucose concentrations and were lost in a *ccpA* deletion mutant. Therefore, this effect can be explained by an overflow metabolism when an abundance of nutrients is present in the medium rather than solely by a glucose effect. In *S. aureus*, SA113 an increased glucose concentration showed no effect on the muropeptide pattern (Supplementary Materials Figure S6).

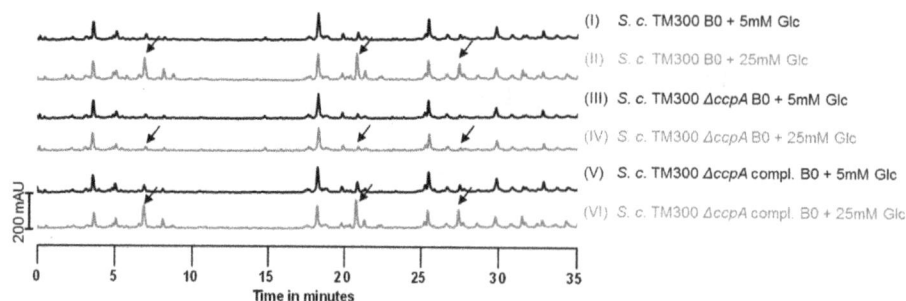

Figure 5. Deletion of *ccpA* prevents the effect of high sugar concentrations. The catabolite repressor gene *ccpA* was deleted in *S. carnosus* TM300. PGN of the wild type, the mutant and the complemented strain grown with 5 or 25 mM glucose was isolated and analyzed by UPLC. In the *ccpA* deletion mutant, 25 mM glucose did not cause accumulation of tetra muropeptides (arrows in panel 4), while complementation with a constitutively expressed *ccpA* gene completely restored this effect (panel 6).

2.6. Deletion of ccpA Causes a Decrease in Colony Size and Growth Rate

While the observed variation in PGN composition was lost in the *ccpA* deletion mutant, this strain was influenced in its growth behavior. There was a decrease in colony size (Figure 6 and Table 3) of the *S. carnosus* TM300 Δ*ccpA* mutant of ~60% compared to the wild type strain. Complementation restored the mutant phenotype completely. In liquid culture, the *S. carnosus* TM300 Δ*ccpA* mutant showed a growth defect during log phase compared to the wild type strain that was restored again by complementation (Figure 6). Growth rate of the mutant was reduced to 60% in low glucose concentration and to 68% in high glucose concentrations compared to the wild type. This effect was restored by complementation (Table 4). Therefore, in these experiments, the glucose concentration itself had only minor influence, indicating observed effects on the PGN are specific.

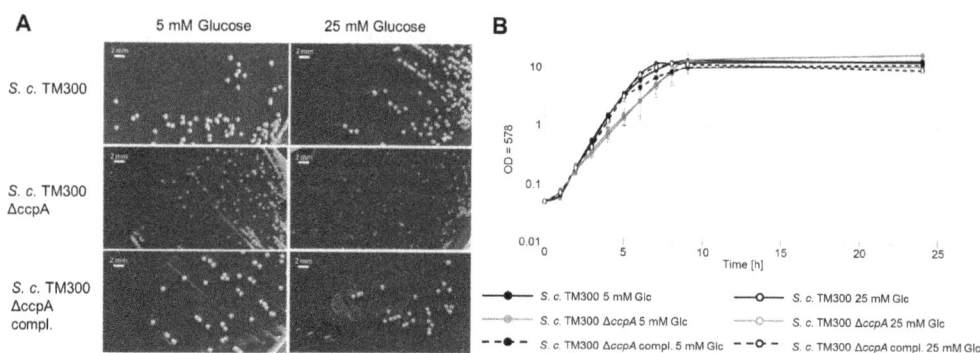

Figure 6. The Δ*ccpA* mutant showed a decrease in colony size and a reduction in growth rate. (**A**) On solid media colonies, the deletion mutant appeared clearly smaller than the parental strains. The glucose concentration seemed to have only a minor influence on colony size; (**B**) In liquid media, *S. carnosus* TM300 Δ*ccpA* also showed a growth defect compared to the wild type strain. In both cases, the effect could be complemented. The influence of the glucose concentration in both experiments was negligible. (Bar size: 2 mm; Glc: glucose).

Table 3. Determination of colony size. The size of ten individual grown colonies was measured digitally. The *ccpA* mutant showed a 57% decrease in cell size that could be complemented again. The influence of glucose was only minor. The mean values of three independent experiments are given.

Strain	5 mM Glucose (mm)	25 mM Glucose (mm)
S. carnosus TM300	0.91 ± 0.07	0.83 ± 0.09
S. carnosus TM300 Δ*ccpA*	0.39 ± 0.07	0.33 ± 0.06
S. carnosus TM300 Δ*ccpA* compl.	0.92 ± 0.04	0.89 ± 0.07

Table 4. Calculation of growth rate. Growth rate for each strain was calculated for the mid exponential phase between time point 4 and 5 h and is given as doubling time per hour (t_d/h). *S. carnosus* TM300 Δ*ccpA* showed a decreased doubling time compared to its parental strain. The influence of high glucose concentrations was only minor. The mean values of three independent experiments are given.

Strain	5 mM Glucose (t_d/h)	25 mM Glucose (t_d/h)
S. carnosus TM300	1.82 ± 0.16	2.10 ± 0.35
S. carnosus TM300 Δ*ccpA*	0.71 ± 0.31	0.67 ± 0.19
S. carnosus TM300 Δ*ccpA* compl.	1.90 ± 0.40	2.00 ± 0.38

3. Discussion

3.1. The Peptidoglycan Composition of S. carnosus TM300

UPLC/MS analysis of the PGN of *S. carnosus* TM300 revealed a muropeptide pattern different from the one known of *S. aureus*. Instead of stem peptides containing the classical five amino acids L-Ala-D-iGln-L-Lys-D-Ala-D-Ala) typical for *S. aureus*, most stem peptides were degraded to tri peptides missing the two D-Ala. This is the case for monomeric muropeptides (Figure 1a, peak 1) as well as for all cross-linked muropeptides, in which the acceptor stem peptide was also degraded, while the former donor stem peptides are still classical tetra peptides (Figure 1a, peaks 5, 8, 11 and 12). We were able to identify the cross-linked muropeptides up to the pentamer (Tri-Tetra$_4$). Acceptor stem peptides with penta peptides were also found (Figure 1a, peaks 4, 7 and 10), but in small amounts only. We also found tetra muropeptides containing five (Figure 1a, peak 3) or six to nine glycine residues in the interpeptide bridge (Figure 1a, peak 2). The latter indicates that these muropeptides had been released again from mature PGN. This peak was not influenced by the genetic and metabolic factors tested.

In *S. aureus* PGN—the best studied PGN in staphylococci—this degradation was never observed [37,38,45]. Tri stem peptides are a classical feature of *E. coli* [36] but also of other firmicutes like *Bacillus subtilis*, where the PGN is modified after cross-linking has occurred. Interestingly, we observed the length of the *S. carnosus* TM300 stem peptide not only to be influenced by genetic factors (in our study *hlyD-ftsE-ftsX*) but also by the composition of the growth medium (see below). Especially 25 mM glucose, a concentration frequently used for plasmid repression, caused an increase in muropeptides with tetra stem peptides. Changes in stem peptide composition due to medium ingredients have been reported for example for *Caulobacter crescentus*. It incorporates glycine at position five, even if only traces of free glycine are present in the growth medium [46]. When glycine is depleted in the medium, *S. aureus* PGN is directly cross-linked and lacks the interpeptide bridge [47]. Cells then enter the stationary phase, indicating this to be a protection mechanism.

3.2. The hlyD-ftsE-ftsX Operon

A gene for HlyD (hemolysin D) is present in e.g., *Escherichia coli* (*E. coli*) but the orthologue could not be found in staphylococci. The database KEGG and a Blast search for orthologous genes did not lead to any positive results. However, SCA_1997, which was identified in the BTH screen with a genomic library of *S. carnosus* TM300 as a putative interaction partner for PBP2, was annotated as a conserved hypothetical protein belonging to the HlyD family of secretion proteins. The nomenclature was maintained as SCA_1997 and orthologous genes possess a short HlyD motif that is eponymous for these proteins.

Like the *E. coli* HlyD, the staphylococcal HlyD is highly similar to the membrane fusion component of the RND family of transporters (RND: Resistance, Nodulation, Cell Division). As the proposed function is to facilitate and enable transport (e.g., resistance through efflux) by bringing the inner and outer membrane together, most members of this family are found in Gram-negative bacteria [48]. Nevertheless, also in Gram-positive bacteria, there are a few representatives of this family. But *hlyD* is not omnipresent in *Staphylococcus*. Only about 47% (34 out of 73) of all annotated staphylococci harbor a copy of *hlyD*. In contrast, in *Bacillus*, 98% of strains (112 out of 114 strains sequenced) possess this gene. There is also no correlation between *hlyD* and pathogenicity, as it can be found throughout the whole genus of staphylococci.

While the *S. carnosus* TM300 FtsEX complex has no sequence similarity to FtsEX of *E. coli*, the predicted structures of the respective proteins are very similar. An *ftsEX* depletion mutant in *E. coli* forms filaments, and growth in LB medium was shown to be salt dependent as the septal ring does not properly assemble in the absence of FtsEX and salt [30]. However, growth of the *S. carnosus* TM300 *hlyD-ftsEX* mutant was not affected by the absence or presence of NaCl nor by the use of minimal medium M9 (Supplementary Materials Figure S2) and we did not observe any obvious changes in cell appearance. This indicates the septal ring in staphylococci does not necessarily need *ftsEX* for stabilization.

Our BTH results are in accordance with known results for PBP2 of *S. aureus* which was also shown to self-interact [49]. In our experiments, FtsX also interacted with HlyD, with itself and with FtsE (Figure 2 and Table 2). We could not detect homodimerization of FtsE as was published for the *Streptococcus pneumoniae* orthologue. In this organism, both FtsE and FtsX formed homodimers and interacted with each other [31]. In various species, FtsE and FtsX have been shown to interact with each other and thereby activate murein hydrolases. This includes PcsB of *Streptocccus pneumoniae* [31–33], the endopeptidase CwlO of *Bacillus subtilis* [35] and an amidase of *E. coli* that was activated by FtsEX via EnvC [34]. Our results from *S. carnosus* point to a role for HlyD-FtsEX in the regulation of a carboxypeptidase, as the overexpression of the *hlyD-ftsEX* operon led to an increase in muropeptides containing penta stem peptides. To a minor extent, tetra stem peptides were also observed (Figure 3). Penta stem peptides of *S. carnosus* are normally degraded into tri stem peptides by a so far unknown enzyme(s). We propose that HlyD-FtsEX must have an inhibitory effect on this/these enzyme/s, as deletion of the whole operon did not alter the muropeptide pattern and therefore did not influence degradation activity. In addition, only overproduction of all three proteins caused an increase in penta and tetra muropeptides, indicating a necessity for complex formation for activity. As tri muropeptides are present in similar amounts to pentas, inhibition of the degradation enzymes is not complete and other factors might contribute to their regulation. This is corroborated by the notion that the *hlyD-ftsEX* operon is not essential and its deletion had no effect on bacterial growth under various conditions tested.

3.3. Investigation of a Putative L,D-Carboxypeptidase (SCA_0214)

The PGN of *S. carnosus* TM300 mainly consists of tri and tetra peptide structures (Table 1) suggesting L,D-carboxypeptidase (LD-CP) activity. Bioinformatical analysis led to only one possible candidate in *S. carnosus* TM300: SCA_0214, which is located between SCA_0213 (an NAD dependent epimerase/dehydratase family protein) and SCA_0215 (*ilvE*, a branched chain amino acid aminotransferase). In contrast to *S. carnosus* TM300, a gene for an LD-CP is missing from the genome of *S. aureus*. For instance, the genome of *S. a.* USA300 does not contain a homologous gene for SCA_0214. Instead, the two genes SCA_0213 and SCA_0215 are located directly next to each other. The absence of a putative LD-CP is in accordance with the presence of only penta and tetra stem peptides in *S. aureus* PGN [37]. However, deletion of SCA_0214 in *S. carnosus* TM300 had no effect at all on the muropeptide pattern. It still harbored mainly tri stem peptides (Figure S4A). Even if SCA_0214 was only able to cleave off D-Ala from a tetrapeptide but not from a pentapeptide, as could be expected from a carboxypeptidase, its deletion should have resulted in an accumulation of tetrapeptides. As this is not the case, we exclude SCA_0214 as being responsible for the occurrence of tripeptides in *S. carnosus* TM300.

But what could be the role of SCA_0214? Overproduction resulted in protein accumulation in the cytoplasm. This is in accordance with the LD-CP sequence analysis that revealed neither a TAT (Twin Arginine Translocation) nor a Sec (Secretion) sequence. This could point to a role in the cytoplasm, but could also be a mere side effect of protein overproduction.

But which enzyme(s) could cause the reduction from penta to tri stem peptides? As trimming of the stem-peptides during PGN maturation is widely seen in eubacteria, *S. carnosus* might be "normal", while actually *S. aureus* is an exception by keeping its pentapeptide intact. Another bioinformatical search in KEGG revealed three annotated DD-CPs in *S. carnosus*: (1) SCA_0291, the homologue of *S. aureus* PBP4, which is actually a PGN synthase responsible for secondary cross-linking of PGN [22]; (2) SCA_2445, which is also assigned as an *S. aureus* PBP4 homologue, but with less homology; and (3) SCA_1643 that is orthologous to LdcB of *Streptococcus pneumoniae* and *B. subtilis* but has no orthologue in *S. aureus*. Both enzymes had originally been annotated as D,D-CP (*dacA*) but were recently shown to degrade tetra peptides from isolated PGN into tri peptides in vitro and were therefore renamed [50]. SCA_2445 could be the enzyme that creates tetra peptides, and tri peptides are then produced by SCA_1643. We tried to construct deletion mutants of SCA_1643 and SCA_2445 but were unsuccessful.

3.4. Influence of Sugars on the Muropeptide Composition

As we had observed an altered PGN pattern when we repressed plasmid gene expression with 25 mM glucose, we tested the influence of various carbon sources on the PGN pattern of *S. carnosus* TM300. We found an increase of tetra muropeptides when the cells of *S. carnosus* TM300 were grown with either 25 mM glucose (Figure 5, chromatogram 2) or fructose (Figure S5A). Again, tri muropeptides were still present in comparable amounts to these tetra muropeptides. No increase in tetra muropeptides was observed when supplemented with 25 mM xylose (Figure S5A), the standard gene induction conditions for plasmid pPTX [51,52] that served as a control.

In Gram-positive bacteria, the catabolite control protein A (CcpA), a global regulator of carbon source metabolism, regulates cellular processes that are influenced by the presence of glucose [53]. Therefore, we deleted the *ccpA* gene and analyzed the PGN composition again under low and high glucose concentrations. As expected, no elevated tetra peaks were observed in the *ccpA* deletion mutant under high glucose conditions. Instead, the muropeptide pattern was identical to the one obtained from cells grown in 5 mM glucose (Figure 5, chromatograms 3 and 4). Complementation with a plasmid constitutively expressing *ccpA* restored the original phenotype, showing that the appearance of tetra muropeptides can be traced back to the influence of glucose and fructose intermediate products on CcpA. Moreover, deletion of *ccpA* also affected cell growth. The deletion strain show a reduced growth rate in exponential phase and a severe decrease in colony size compared to the wild type strain, indicating a major role for CcpA in the metabolism of *S. carnosus* TM300.

Glucose and fructose are both metabolized to fructose-1,6-bisphosphate (FBP), an intermediate product of glycolysis. As alterations on the PGN pattern of *S. carnosus* TM300 did not only occur under high glucose concentrations, this effect could be rather explained by a general overflow metabolism instead of a glucose effect. However, glucose not only serves as a nutrient but also the expression of metabolic genes [54,55] and virulence factors [56] are influenced by glucose.

But how can glucose concentration influence the PGN composition? The increase in tetra muropeptides speaks again for a partial inhibition of a so far unknown LD-CP, although an increase in penta peptide structures was also detected. Taken together, this points to an influence of *ccpA* and *hlyD-ftsEX* on the stem peptide degrading enzyme(s) which is albeit not a complete inhibitory effect as tri stem peptides are also still present.

So far we do not understand why *S. carnosus* TM300 trims its stem peptides in a way that is also seen for other bacteria, but *S. aureus* does not. It was just shown that in *E. coli* the eight DD-CPs are active under different conditions. For example, PBP5 (*dacA*) is mainly active at neutral pH, while PBP6b is only expressed and active at acidic pH. Loss of either enzyme results in morphological defects when the cells are incubated at the respective pH. We, however, did not observe any obvious changes in the morphology of our strains during overexpression of the *hlyD-ftsE-ftsX* operon or under high glucose conditions. But the notion that even under these conditions tripeptides are present in similar amounts as the newly appearing penta or tetrapeptides can be interpreted as a hint for an important role of the tri peptides in the PGN of *S. carnosus* TM300.

4. Materials and Methods

For *strains*, *plasmids* and *oligonucleotides* used please refer to Supplementary Materials Table S1: Bacterial strains, Table S2: Plasmids and Table S3: Oligonucleotides.

4.1. Media

Basic medium (B medium) for *Staphylococci* consisted of Soy Peptone (10 g; Plato, Koblenz, Germany), Yeast Extract (5 g; Deutsche Hefewerke, Nuernberg, Germany), NaCl (5 g; Carl-Roth, Karlsruhe, Germany), Glucose (1 g; Carl Roth) and K_2HPO_4 (1 g; Applichem, Darmstadt, Germany). Deionized water was added to a final volume of 1 liter and pH was adjusted to 7.2.

LB medium for *E. coli* consisted of Peptone (10 g; Plato), Yeast Extract (5 g; Deutsche Hefewerke) and NaCl (5 g; Carl Roth). Deionized water was added to a final volume of 1 liter and pH was adjusted to 7.2. MacConkey agar was prepared according to the manufactures' instructions (Carl Roth). Minimal media M9 for staphylococci consisted of Na_2HPO_4 (6 g; Carl Roth), KH_2PO_4 (3 g; Fisher Chemicals), NH_4Cl (1 g; Merck Darmstadt, Germany) and NaCl (0.5 g; Carl Roth). Deionized water was added to a final volume of 1 L, the media was autoclaved and supplemented with thiamine (2 µg/mL; Sigma Aldrich, Munich, Germany), $MgSO_4$ (1 mM; Carl Roth) and casamino acids (0.2%; BD Bioscience, Heidelberg, Germany). Cells were routinely grown at 37 °C either in liquid culture in baffled Erlenmeyer flasks (1:5 ratio) with shaking or on 1.5% agar plates.

4.2. Reagents

Unless otherwise stated, all reagents were bought from Sigma-Aldrich.

4.3. Plasmid Construction for Deletion Mutants and Overexpression

Chromosomal DNA from *S. carnosus* and *S. aureus* was isolated [57] using lysostaphin (0.5 mg/mL) for cell lysis. SCA_1995-1997(*ftsX-ftsE-hlyD*): For deletion of the operon SCA_1995-1997 ,the pBT2 [58] knockout vector was used. For overexpression of HlyD, FtsE and FtsX, the genes SCA_1997, SCA_1995-1996 and SCA_1995-1997 were cloned into the xylose inducible plasmid pPTX [52] and cut with the same enzymes. SCA_0214 (putative LD-CP): For deletion, the knockout vector pGS1 was used [59]. The overexpression plasmid was constructed in the xylose inducible plasmid pPTX [52] and cut with the same enzymes. SCA_1342 (*ccpA*): For deletion, knockout vector pGS1was used [59]. For constitutive complementation, SCA_1342 was ligated into pRAB11-EF-TU, cut with the same enzymes. SAOUHSC01850 (*ccpA*) was deleted from *S. aureus* SA113 Δ*spa* using the pMAD knockout vector [60] and Gibson assembly [61] for cloning. For overexpression, pRAB11-EF-TU-SAOUHSC01850 was electroporated first into RN4220 and then into *S. aureus* SA113 Δ*spa* [62]. The correctness of all plasmids was confirmed by sequencing before transformation. *S. carnosus* TM300 and *S. aaureus* SA113 Δ*spa* were transformed by electroporation [62]; for *E. coli*, transformation chemocompetent cells were used [63].

4.4. Gene Deletion

All knockout procedures were performed according to the respective protocols of the vectors. While the pMAD system does not imply the usage of a resistance cassette, the other two knockout vectors were constructed with an *ermB* (erythromycin B) resistance cassette. Flanking of *ermB* with *loxP* sites enabled us to flox out the resistance cassette by the Cre recombinase constitutively produced by the vector pRAB1 [64]. This generated a marker-free mutant minimizing downstream effects caused by the resistance cassette.

4.5. Genomic Library

Chromosomal DNA from *S. carnosus* was isolated [57] using lysostaphin (0.5 mg/mL) for cell lysis. Genomic DNA was sheared using the nebulizer from the TOPO Shotgun Subcloning Kit (Invitrogen,

Carlsbad, CA, USA) and separated on a preparative agarose gel. Five pools of DNA from 1.7 to 3 kbp were isolated, cleaned and treated with Klenow fragment to generate blunt ends. DNA from each pool was used for ligation into pKT25 [65], which had been cut with *SmaI* and dephosphorylated by rAPid Alkaline Phosphatase (Roche, Mannheim, Germany). The resulting plasmids were transformed into NEB 5-alpha electrocompetent *E. coli* cells (New England Biolabs, Ipswich, MA, USA) according to the manufacturer's protocol. Ligation procedure was performed twice, resulting in ten transformations. Each transformation was plated on three LB/Kanamycin (50 µg/mL) plates (15 cm in diameter) and incubated overnight at 37 °C. All colonies from the same pool were combined and stored in 50% glycerol at −80 °C. From each pool, an aliquot was used to inoculate LB media for plasmid isolation ("prey" vectors). Over 80% of the plasmids contained genomic DNA inserts, and cell wall related genes like *pbpA*, *pbpF*, *pbp4*, *rodA* and *murJ* could each be amplified in at least one subpool. SCA_1084 (*pbp2*) was cloned into pUT18C [65] as "bait" vector.

4.6. Bacterial-Two-Hybrid Assays

The method of Karimova et al. was used [65]. The plasmids were co-transformed in *E. coli* BTH101, plated on LB agar plates containing 100 µg/mL ampicillin, 50 µg/mL kanamycin and 100 µg/mL streptomycin and incubated for 16 h at 37 °C. Ten colonies per each interaction tandem were transferred onto MacConkey agar plates (100 µg/mL ampicillin, 30 µg/mL kanamycin and 100 µg/mL streptomycin) and incubated for 24–48 h at 30 °C. To generate triplicates, the first three colonies per each interaction tandem were inoculated overnight in LB media containing 100 µg/mL ampicillin, 30 µg/mL kanamycin, 100 µg/mL streptomycin and 0.5 mM IPTG. Overnight cultures were diluted in H_2O_{bidest} (1:4) and cell density was measured at OD_{600}. Of each cell suspension, 100 µL was mixed with 20 µL 0.1% SDS, 40 µL chloroform and 1 mL Z buffer (70 mM $Na_2HPO_4 \times 12\ H_2O$, 30 mM $NaH_2PO_4\ H_2O$, 1 mM $MgSO_4$, 0.2 mM $MnSO_4$, pH 7, 100 mM β-mercaptoethanol). The cells were solubilized by pipetting 10–15 times. Of each supernatant, 100 µL was incubated with 20 µL ONPG solution (ortho-Nitrophenyl-β-galactoside; 4 mg/mL ONPG in Z-buffer without β-mercaptoethanol) for 10 min. ONPG served as substrate for the detection of β-galactosidase activity. The colorless substrate is cleaved to galactose and the yellow colored product ortho-nitrophenol. The reaction was stopped by adding 50 µL of 1 M Na_2CO_3 and the optical density was determined at 420 nm. The enzymatic activity of the β-galactosidase is given in units/mg dry weight bacteria and was calculated as follows:

Calculation of enzyme activity:

$$A = 200 \times (OD_{420} - OD_{420}\ \text{in control tube})/\text{minutes of incubation} \times \text{dilution factor}$$

Calculation of bacteria dry weight:

$$1\ \text{mL of culture at } OD_{600} = 1 \text{ corresponds to } 300\ \text{µg dry weight bacteria}$$

A negative control was performed by co-transforming the empty plasmids pKT25 and pUT18C into the host strain *E. coli* BTH101. The cut-off value for positive interactions was four times the negative control.

4.7. Peptidoglycan Analysis

The cells were grown in 20 mL BM for 8 h and peptidoglycan was isolated and analyzed by UPLC and UPLC/MS as previously described [37]. Precursors were isolated as published [66] and analyzed by UPLC-MS using the PGN method.

4.8. Overproduction of SCA_0214

Main cultures (20 mL B0 media supplemented with either 5 mM glucose for repression or 25 mM xylose for induction) were inoculated with overnight cultures to $OD_{578} = 0.05$. After 8 h culture, supernatant was used to isolate extracellular proteins using StrataClean beads (Agilent Technologies,

St. Clara, CA, USA). Intracellular proteins were extracted from pelleted cells. Cells were disrupted using a FastPrep®-24 (MP Biomedicals, Santa Ana, CA, USA) and 500 µL acid washed glass beads (0.22 mm in diameter, Sigma-Aldrich). Cells were treated 4 times at 6500 rpm for 30 s. After two cycles, the samples were placed on ice for 5 min to reduce potential heat that develops during FastPrep®-24 treatment and that could lead to protein denaturation. Afterwards, the tubes were centrifuged at 12,000 rpm for 5 min at RT. The supernatant contained the intracellular proteins. Proteins were analyzed by SDS-PAGE stained with Coomassie.

5. Conclusions

We could show that the PGN of the apathogenic bacterium *S. carnosus* TM300 differs from the well-studied PGN of the pathogen *S. aureus*. In TM300 free stem peptides are shortened to contain tri peptides only in contrast to the unmodified penta peptides of *S. aureus*. This suggests the activities of an LD- and a DD-CP. We could show, that the proposed DD-CP might be regulated by three enzymes that interact with the PGN synthase PBP2: HlyD, FtsE and FtsX. The overexpression of the respective operon results in the reappearance of penta stem peptides. The LD-CP seems to be regulated by the catabolite control protein A (*ccpA*) as high sugar concentrations result in the appearance of tetra stem peptides. Taken together, our results show that the PGN of *S. carnosus* can adapt to various conditions.

Supplementary Materials: The following are available online at www.mdpi.com/2079-6382/5/4/33/s1. Figure S1: Muropeptide structures of *S. aureus* and *S. carnosus* TM300; Figure S2: Growth behavior of *S. carnosus* TM300 Δ*hlyD-ftsEX*; Figure S3: Deletion of *hlyD-ftsEX* and overexpression of single genes does not influence the peptidoglycan pattern; Figure S4: Analysis of the *S. carnosus* TM300 Δ*0214::ermB* mutant and localization of the encoded protein; Figure S5: Influence of different sugars on the peptidoglycan of *S. carnosus* TM3; Figure S6: Influence of glucose on the peptidoglycan of *S. aureus* SA113 Δ*spa*; Table S1: Bacterial strains; Table S2: Plasmids; Table S3: Oligonucleotides.

Acknowledgments: This work was supported by the DFG via the SFB 766 and the University of Tuebingen: Promotion of Junior Researchers Program to Ute Bertsche. We thank Darya Belikova for excellent technical assistance, Friedrich Götz for helpful discussions and Christopher Schuster for critical reading of the manuscript.

Author Contributions: Julia Deibert and Ute Bertsche conceived and designed the experiments; Julia Deibert and Elif Koeksoy performed the experiments; Julia Deibert, Daniel Kühner, Mark Stahl and Ute Bertsche analyzed the data; Ute Bertsche wrote the paper.

Abbreviations

The following abbreviations are used in this manuscript:

BTH	Bacterial-Two-Hybrid
PGN	peptidoglycan
UPLC/MS	Ultra Performance Liquid Chromatography coupled to mass spectrometry
MurNAc	*N*-acetylmuramic acid
GlcNAc	*N*-acetylglucosamine
CP	carboxypeptidase

References

1. Schleifer, K.H.; Fischer, U. Description of a new species of the genus *Staphylococcus*: *Staphylococcus carnosus*. *Int. J. Syst. Bacteriol.* **1982**, *32*, 153–156. [CrossRef]

2. Niinivaara, F.P.; Pohja, M.S. Über die Reifung der Rohwurst. I. Mitt: Die Veränderung der Bakterienflora während der Reifung. *Z. Lebensm. Unters. Forsch.* **1956**, *104*, 413–422. (In German) [CrossRef]

3. Rosenstein, R.; Götz, F. Genomic differences between the food-grade *Staphylococcus carnosus* and pathogenic staphylococcal species. *Int. J. Med. Microbiol.* **2010**, *300*, 104–108. [CrossRef] [PubMed]

4. Rosenstein, R.; Nerz, C.; Biswas, L.; Resch, A.; Raddatz, G.; Schuster, S.C.; Götz, F. Genome analysis of the meat starter culture bacterium *Staphylococcus carnosus* TM300. *Appl. Environ. Microbiol.* **2009**, *75*, 811–822. [CrossRef] [PubMed]

5. Schleifer, K.H.; Kandler, O. Peptidoglycan types of bacterial cell walls and their taxonomic implications. *Bacteriol. Rev.* **1972**, *36*, 407–477. [PubMed]

6. Bera, A.; Biswas, R.; Herbert, S.; Götz, F. The presence of peptidoglycan O-acetyltransferase in various staphylococcal species correlates with lysozyme resistance and pathogenicity. *Infect. Immun.* **2006**, *74*, 4598–4604. [CrossRef] [PubMed]

7. Bera, A.; Herbert, S.; Jakob, A.; Vollmer, W.; Götz, F. Why are pathogenic staphylococci so lysozyme resistant? The peptidoglycan O-acetyltransferase OatA is the major determinant for lysozyme resistance of *Staphylococcus aureus*. *Mol. Microbiol.* **2005**, *55*, 778–787. [CrossRef] [PubMed]

8. Ruiz, N. Lipid flippases for bacterial peptidoglycan biosynthesis. *Lipid Insights* **2015**, *8*, 21–31. [CrossRef] [PubMed]

9. Mohammadi, T.; van Dam, V.; Sijbrandi, R.; Vernet, T.; Zapun, A.; Bouhss, A.; Diepeveen-de Bruin, M.; Nguyen-Disteche, M.; de Kruijff, B.; Breukink, E. Identification of FtsW as a transporter of lipid-linked cell wall precursors across the membrane. *EMBO J.* **2011**, *30*, 1425–1432. [CrossRef] [PubMed]

10. Mohammadi, T.; Sijbrandi, R.; Lutters, M.; Verheul, J.; Martin, N.; den Blaauwen, T.; de Kruijff, B.; Breukink, E. Specificity of the transport of Lipid II by FtsW in *Escherichia coli*. *J. Biol. Chem.* **2014**. [CrossRef] [PubMed]

11. Sham, L.-T.; Butler, E.K.; Lebar, M.D.; Kahne, D.; Bernhardt, T.G.; Ruiz, N. MurJ is the flippase of lipid-linked precursors for peptidoglycan biogenesis. *Science* **2014**, *345*, 220–222. [CrossRef] [PubMed]

12. Butler, E.K.; Tan, W.B.; Joseph, H.; Ruiz, N. Charge requirements of Lipid II flippase activity in *Escherichia coli*. *J. Bacteriol.* **2014**, *196*, 4111–4119. [CrossRef] [PubMed]

13. Figueiredo, T.A.; Sobral, R.G.; Ludovice, A.M.; Almeida, J.M.; Bui, N.K.; Vollmer, W.; de Lencastre, H.; Tomasz, A. Identification of genetic determinants and enzymes involved with the amidation of glutamic acid residues in the peptidoglycan of *Staphylococcus aureus*. *PLoS Pathog.* **2012**, *8*, e1002508. [CrossRef] [PubMed]

14. Münch, D.; Roemer, T.; Lee, S.H.; Engeser, M.; Sahl, H.G.; Schneider, T. Identification and in vitro analysis of the GatD/MurT enzyme-complex catalyzing lipid II amidation in *Staphylococcus aureus*. *PLoS Pathog.* **2012**, *8*, e1002509. [CrossRef] [PubMed]

15. Nakel, M.; Ghuysen, J.M.; Kandler, O. Wall peptidoglycan in *Aerococcus viridans* strains 201 Evans and ATCC 11563 and in *Gaffkya homari* strain ATCC 10400. *Biochemistry* **1971**, *10*, 2170–2175. [PubMed]

16. Goffin, C.; Ghuysen, J.M. Multimodular penicillin-binding proteins: An enigmatic family of orthologs and paralogs. *Microbiol. Mol. Biol. Rev.* **1998**, *62*, 1079–1093. [PubMed]

17. Pinho, M.G.; Errington, J. Recruitment of penicillin-binding protein PBP2 to the division site of *Staphylococcus aureus* is dependent on its transpeptidation substrates. *Mol. Microbiol.* **2005**, *55*, 799–807. [CrossRef] [PubMed]

18. Pinho, M.G.; Filipe, S.R.; de Lencastre, H.; Tomasz, A. Complementation of the essential peptidoglycan transpeptidase function of penicillin-binding protein 2 (PBP2) by the drug resistance protein PBP2A in *Staphylococcus aureus*. *J. Bacteriol.* **2001**, *183*, 6525–6531. [CrossRef] [PubMed]

19. Pinho, M.G.; de Lencastre, H.; Tomasz, A. An acquired and a native penicillin-binding protein cooperate in building the cell wall of drug-resistant staphylococci. *Proc. Natl. Acad. Sci. USA* **2001**, *98*, 10886–10891. [CrossRef] [PubMed]

20. Pereira, S.F.F.; Henriques, A.O.; Pinho, M.G.; de Lencastre, H.; Tomasz, A. Role of PBP1 in cell division of *Staphylococcus aureus*. *J. Bacteriol.* **2007**, *189*, 3525–3531. [CrossRef] [PubMed]

21. Pinho, M.G.; de Lencastre, H.; Tomasz, A. Cloning, characterization, and inactivation of the gene pbpC, encoding penicillin-binding protein 3 of *Staphylococcus aureus*. *J. Bacteriol.* **2000**, *182*, 1074–1079. [CrossRef] [PubMed]

22. Leski, T.A.; Tomasz, A. Role of penicillin-binding protein 2 (PBP2) in the antibiotic susceptibility and cell wall cross-linking of *Staphylococcus aureus*: Evidence for the cooperative functioning of PBP2, PBP4, and PBP2A. *J. Bacteriol.* **2005**, *187*, 1815–1824. [CrossRef] [PubMed]

23. Memmi, G.; Filipe, S.R.; Pinho, M.G.; Fu, Z.; Cheung, A. *Staphylococcus aureus* PBP4 is essential for β-lactam resistance in community-acquired methicillin-resistant strains. *Antimicrob. Agents Chemother.* **2008**, *52*, 3955–3966. [CrossRef] [PubMed]

24. KEGG: Kyoto Encyclopedia of Genes and Genomes. Available online: http://www.genome.jp/kegg/ (accessed on 6 August 2016).

25. Omasits, U.; Ahrens, C.H.; Müller, S.; Wollscheid, B. Protter: Interactive protein feature visualization and integration with experimental proteomic data. *Bioinformatics* **2014**, *30*, 884–886. [CrossRef] [PubMed]

26. Tzagoloff, H.; Novick, R. Geometry of cell division in *Staphylococcus aureus*. *J. Bacteriol.* **1977**, *129*, 343–350. [PubMed]

27. Monteiro, J.M.; Fernandes, P.B.; Vaz, F.; Pereira, A.R.; Tavares, A.C.; Ferreira, M.T.; Pereira, P.M.; Veiga, H.; Kuru, E.; VanNieuwenhze, M.S.; et al. Cell shape dynamics during the staphylococcal cell cycle. *Nat. Commun.* **2015**. [CrossRef] [PubMed]

28. Aarsman, M.E.; Piette, A.; Fraipont, C.; Vinkenvleugel, T.M.; Nguyen-Disteche, M.; den Blaauwen, T. Maturation of the *Escherichia coli* divisome occurs in two steps. *Mol. Microbiol.* **2005**, *55*, 1631–1645. [CrossRef] [PubMed]

29. Söderström, B.; Daley, D.O. The bacterial divisome: More than a ring? *Curr. Genet.* **2016**. [CrossRef] [PubMed]

30. Schmidt, K.L.; Peterson, N.D.; Kustusch, R.J.; Wissel, M.C.; Graham, B.; Phillips, G.J.; Weiss, D.S. A predicted ABC transporter, FtsEX, is needed for cell division in *Escherichia coli*. *J. Bacteriol.* **2004**, *186*, 785–793. [CrossRef] [PubMed]

31. Bajaj, R.; Bruce, K.E.; Davidson, A.L.; Rued, B.E.; Stauffacher, C.V.; Winkler, M.E. Biochemical characterization of essential cell division proteins FtsX and FtsE that mediate peptidoglycan hydrolysis by PcsB in *Streptococcus pneumoniae*. *Microbiol. Open* **2016**. [CrossRef] [PubMed]

32. Sham, L.-T.; Jensen, K.R.; Bruce, K.E.; Winkler, M.E. Involvement of FtsE ATPase and FtsX extracellular loops 1 and 2 in FtsEX-PcsB complex function in cell division of *Streptococcus pneumoniae* D39. *mBio* **2013**. [CrossRef] [PubMed]

33. Sham, L.T.; Barendt, S.M.; Kopecky, K.E.; Winkler, M.E. Essential PcsB putative peptidoglycan hydrolase interacts with the essential FtsXSpn cell division protein in *Streptococcus pneumoniae* D39. *Proc. Natl. Acad. Sci. USA* **2011**, *108*, E1061–E1069. [CrossRef] [PubMed]

34. Yang, D.C.; Peters, N.T.; Parzych, K.R.; Uehara, T.; Markovski, M.; Bernhardt, T.G. An ATP-binding cassette transporter-like complex governs cell-wall hydrolysis at the bacterial cytokinetic ring. *Proc. Natl. Acad. Sci. USA* **2011**, *108*, E1052–E1060. [CrossRef] [PubMed]

35. Meisner, J.; Montero Llopis, P.; Sham, L.T.; Garner, E.; Bernhardt, T.G.; Rudner, D.Z. FtsEX is required for CwlO peptidoglycan hydrolase activity during cell wall elongation in *Bacillus subtilis*. *Mol. Microbiol.* **2013**, *89*, 1069–1083. [CrossRef] [PubMed]

36. Glauner, B.; Höltje, J.-V.; Schwarz, U. The composition of the murein of *Escherichia coli*. *J. Biol. Chem.* **1988**, *263*, 10088–10095. [PubMed]

37. Kühner, D.; Stahl, M.; Demircioglu, D.D.; Bertsche, U. From cells to muropeptide structures in 24 h: Peptidoglycan mapping by UPLC-MS. *Sci. Rep.* **2014**. [CrossRef] [PubMed]

38. De Jonge, B.L.; Chang, Y.S.; Gage, D.; Tomasz, A. Peptidoglycan composition of a highly methicillin-resistant *Staphylococcus aureus* strain. The role of penicillin binding protein 2A. *J. Biol. Chem.* **1992**, *267*, 11248–11254. [PubMed]

39. Murakami, K.; Fujimura, T.; Doi, M. Nucleotide sequence of the structural gene for the penicillin-binding protein 2 of *Staphylococcus aureus* and the presence of a homologous gene in other staphylococci. *FEMS Microbiol. Lett.* **1994**, *117*, 131–136. [CrossRef] [PubMed]

40. Lovering, A.L.; de Castro, L.H.; Lim, D.; Strynadka, N.C. Structural insight into the transglycosylation step of bacterial cell-wall biosynthesis. *Science* **2007**, *315*, 1402–1405. [CrossRef] [PubMed]

41. De Leeuw, E.; Graham, B.; Phillips, G.J.; ten Hagen-Jongman, C.M.; Oudega, B.; Luirink, J. Molecular characterization of *Escherichia coli* FtsE and FtsX. *Mol. Microbiol.* **1999**, *31*, 983–993. [CrossRef] [PubMed]

42. Shivers, R.P.; Dineen, S.S.; Sonenshein, A.L. Positive regulation of *Bacillus subtilis* ackA by CodY and CcpA: Establishing a potential hierarchy in carbon flow. *Mol. Microbiol.* **2006**, *62*, 811–822. [CrossRef] [PubMed]

43. Sonenshein, A.L. Control of key metabolic intersections in *Bacillus subtilis*. *Nat. Rev. Microbiol.* **2007**, *5*, 917–927. [CrossRef] [PubMed]

44. Lopez, J.M.; Thoms, B. Role of sugar uptake and metabolic intermediates on catabolite repression in *Bacillus subtilis*. *J. Bacteriol.* **1977**, *129*, 217–224. [PubMed]

45. De Jonge, B.L.; Chang, Y.S.; Gage, D.; Tomasz, A. Peptidoglycan composition in heterogeneous Tn551 mutants of a methicillin-resistant *Staphylococcus aureus* strain. *J. Biol. Chem.* **1992**, *267*, 11255–11259. [PubMed]

46. Takacs, C.N.; Hocking, J.; Cabeen, M.T.; Bui, N.K.; Poggio, S.; Vollmer, W.; Jacobs-Wagner, C. Growth medium-dependent glycine incorporation into the peptidoglycan of *Caulobacter crescentus*. *PLoS ONE* **2013**, *8*, e57579. [CrossRef] [PubMed]

47. Zhou, X.; Cegelski, L. Nutrient-dependent structural changes in *S. aureus* peptidoglycan revealed by solid-state NMR spectroscopy. *Biochemistry* **2012**, *51*, 8143–8153. [CrossRef] [PubMed]

48. Schülein, R.; Gentschev, I.; Möllenkopf, H.J.; Goebel, W. A topological model for the haemolysin translocator protein HlyD. *Mol. Gen. Genet.* **1992**, *234*, 155–163. [PubMed]

49. Steele, A.L.; Young, S. A descriptive study of Myers-Briggs personality types of professional music educators and music therapists with comparisons to undergraduate majors. *J. Music Ther.* **2011**, *48*, 55–73. [CrossRef] [PubMed]

50. Hoyland, C.N.; Aldridge, C.; Cleverley, R.M.; Duchene, M.C.; Minasov, G.; Onopriyenko, O.; Sidiq, K.; Stogios, P.J.; Anderson, W.F.; Daniel, R.A.; et al. Structure of the LdcB LD-carboxypeptidase reveals the molecular basis of peptidoglycan recognition. *Structure* **2014**, *22*, 949–960. [CrossRef] [PubMed]

51. Peschel, A.; Ottenwalder, B.; Götz, F. Inducible production and cellular location of the epidermin biosynthetic enzyme EpiB using an improved staphylococcal expression system. *FEMS Microbiol. Lett.* **1996**, *137*, 279–284. [CrossRef] [PubMed]

52. Popella, P.; Krauss, S.; Ebner, P.; Nega, M.; Deibert, J.; Götz, F. VraH is a third component of the *Staphylococcus aureus* VraDEH system involved in gallidermin and daptomycin resistance and pathogenicity. *Antimicrob. Agents Chemother.* **2016**. [CrossRef] [PubMed]

53. Henkin, T.M.; Grundy, F.J.; Nicholson, W.L.; Chambliss, G.H. Catabolite repression of alpha-amylase gene expression in *Bacillus subtilis* involves a trans-acting gene product homologous to the *Escherichia coli lacI* and *galR* repressors. *Mol. Microbiol.* **1991**, *5*, 575–584. [CrossRef] [PubMed]

54. Collins, F.M.; Lascelles, J. The effect of growth conditions on oxidative and dehydrogenase activity in *Staphylococcus aureus*. *J. Gen. Microbiol.* **1962**, *29*, 531–535. [CrossRef] [PubMed]

55. Strasters, K.C.; Winkler, K.C. Carbohydrate Metabolism of *Staphylococcus aureus*. *J. Gen. Microbiol.* **1963**, *33*, 213–229. [CrossRef] [PubMed]

56. Seidl, K.; Stucki, M.; Ruegg, M.; Goerke, C.; Wolz, C.; Harris, L.; Berger-Bächi, B.; Bischoff, M. Staphylococcus aureus CcpA affects virulence determinant production and antibiotic resistance. *Antimicrob. Agents Chemother.* **2006**, *50*, 1183–1194. [CrossRef] [PubMed]

57. Marmur, J. A procedure for the isolation of deoxyribonucleic acid from micro-organisms. *J. Mol. Biol.* **1961**, *3*, 208–218. [CrossRef]

58. Brückner, R. Gene replacement in *Staphylococcus carnosus* and *Staphylococcus xylosus*. *FEMS Microbiol. Lett.* **1997**, *151*, 1–8. [CrossRef]

59. Krismer, B.; Nega, M.; Thumm, G.; Götz, F.; Peschel, A. Highly efficient *Staphylococcus carnosus* mutant selection system based on suicidal bacteriocin activation. *Appl. Environ. Microbiol.* **2012**, *78*, 1148–1156. [CrossRef] [PubMed]

60. Arnaud, M.; Chastanet, A.; Debarbouille, M. New vector for efficient allelic replacement in naturally nontransformable, low-GC-content, gram-positive bacteria. *Appl. Environ. Microbiol.* **2004**, *70*, 6887–6891. [CrossRef] [PubMed]

61. Gibson, D.G.; Young, L.; Chuang, R.Y.; Venter, J.C.; Hutchison, C.A., 3rd; Smith, H.O. Enzymatic assembly of DNA molecules up to several hundred kilobases. *Nat. Methods* **2009**, *6*, 343–345. [CrossRef] [PubMed]

62. Lofblom, J.; Kronqvist, N.; Uhlen, M.; Stahl, S.; Wernerus, H. Optimization of electroporation-mediated transformation: *Staphylococcus carnosus* as model organism. *J. Appl. Microbiol.* **2007**, *102*, 736–747. [CrossRef] [PubMed]

63. Dagert, M.; Ehrlich, S.D. Prolonged incubation in calcium chloride improves the competence of *Escherichia coli* cells. *Gene* **1979**, *6*, 23–28. [CrossRef]

64. Leibig, M.; Krismer, B.; Kolb, M.; Friede, A.; Götz, F.; Bertram, R. Marker removal in Staphylococci via Cre recombinase and different *lox* sites. *Appl. Environ. Microbiol.* **2008**, *74*, 1316–1323. [CrossRef] [PubMed]

65. Karimova, G.; Pidoux, J.; Ullmann, A.; Ladant, D. A bacterial two-hybrid system based on a reconstituted signal transduction pathway. *Proc. Natl. Acad. Sci. USA* **1998**, *95*, 5752–5756. [CrossRef] [PubMed]

66. Kohlrausch, U.; Höltje, J.-V. One-step purification procedure for UDP-N-acetylmuramyl-peptide murein precursors from *Bacillus cereus*. *FEMS Microbiol. Lett.* **1991**, *62*, 253–257. [CrossRef] [PubMed]

7

Exploring the Effect of Phage Therapy in Preventing *Vibrio anguillarum* Infections in Cod and Turbot Larvae

Nanna Rørbo [1], Anita Rønneseth [2], Panos G. Kalatzis [1,3] (iD), Bastian Barker Rasmussen [4] (iD), Kirsten Engell-Sørensen [5], Hans Petter Kleppen [6], Heidrun Inger Wergeland [2], Lone Gram [4] (iD) and Mathias Middelboe [1,*] (iD)

[1] Marine Biological Section, University of Copenhagen, 3000 Helsingør, Denmark; nanna_ir@hotmail.com (N.R.); panos.kalatzis@bio.ku.dk (P.G.K.)

[2] Department of Biology, University of Bergen, 5020 Bergen, Norway; anita.ronneseth@uib.no (A.R.); heidrun.wergeland@uib.no (H.I.W.)

[3] Institute of Marine Biology, Biotechnology and Aquaculture, Hellenic Centre for Marine Research, 71003 Heraklion, Greece

[4] Department of Biotechnology and Biomedicine, Technical University of Denmark, 2800 Kongens Lyngby, Denmark; bbara@bio.dtu.dk (B.B.R.); gram@bio.dtu.dk (L.G.)

[5] Fishlab, 8270 Højbjerg, Denmark; kes@fishlab.dk

[6] ACD Pharmaceuticals AS, 8376 Leknes, Norway; hans.kleppen@acdpharma.com

* Correspondence: mmiddelboe@bio.ku.dk

Abstract: The aquaculture industry is suffering from losses associated with bacterial infections by opportunistic pathogens. *Vibrio anguillarum* is one of the most important pathogens, causing vibriosis in fish and shellfish cultures leading to high mortalities and economic losses. Bacterial resistance to antibiotics and inefficient vaccination at the larval stage of fish emphasizes the need for novel approaches, and phage therapy for controlling *Vibrio* pathogens has gained interest in the past few years. In this study, we examined the potential of the broad-host-range phage KVP40 to control four different *V. anguillarum* strains in Atlantic cod (*Gadus morhua* L.) and turbot (*Scophthalmus maximus* L.) larvae. We examined larval mortality and abundance of bacteria and phages. Phage KVP40 was able to reduce and/or delay the mortality of the cod and turbot larvae challenged with *V. anguillarum*. However, growth of other pathogenic bacteria naturally occurring on the fish eggs prior to our experiment caused mortality of the larvae in the unchallenged control groups. Interestingly, the broad-spectrum phage KVP40 was able to reduce mortality in these groups, compared to the nonchallenge control groups not treated with phage KVP40, demonstrating that the phage could also reduce mortality imposed by the background population of pathogens. Overall, phage-mediated reduction in mortality of cod and turbot larvae in experimental challenge assays with *V. anguillarum* pathogens suggested that application of broad-host-range phages can reduce *Vibrio*-induced mortality in turbot and cod larvae, emphasizing that phage therapy is a promising alternative to traditional treatment of vibriosis in marine aquaculture.

Keywords: *Vibrio anguillarum*; phage therapy; aquaculture; fish larvae; challenge trials

1. Introduction

Vibrionaceae is a genetic and metabolic diverse family of heterotrophic bacteria which are widespread in aquatic environments around the world [1]. Several vibrios are able to infect a wide range of aquatic animals and constitute therefore a large problem in aquaculture [2]. One of the most important is *Vibrio anguillarum*, which causes the disease vibriosis and is responsible for large-scale losses in the aquaculture industry [3,4]. Chemotherapy against vibriosis is associated with a major concern due to the risk of antibiotic-resistance developing in the pathogenic bacteria [5]. Vaccines against vibrio have been successful in preventing disease [6,7], however, they are often not useful at the larval stage, as the immune system is not fully developed. Therefore, alternative methods for the control and treatment of *V. anguillarum* infections in fish larvae and fry are needed. The use of bacteriophages (phages) has been explored in several studies as a treatment of pathogens in aquaculture [4,8–13]. Pereira et al. [4] and Mateus et al. [11] did in vitro assays with phages infecting different bacteria responsible for the diseases vibriosis and furunculosis and showed that both single-phage suspensions and phage cocktails could inactivate the bacteria [4,11]. However, often regrowth of phage tolerant bacteria was observed within 24 h after phage treatment [11,13]. Phage addition to shrimp larvae infected with *V. harveyi* caused a reduction in the pathogen load and significantly increased shrimp survival compared to untreated controls groups as well as parallel treatments with antibiotics [8,9]. Another study on zebrafish larvae infected with *V. anguillarum* [12] also found significantly enhanced larvae survival after phage addition. Successful phage treatment in Atlantic salmon (*Salmo salar* L.) infected with *V. anguillarum* strain PF4 was found for phage CHOED, resulting in complete elimination of pathogen-induced mortality when phages were added at a high multiplicity of infection [10]. Together, the previous experimental approaches demonstrate that phage therapy can be a feasible alternative method to control specific *Vibrio* pathogens in aquaculture. However, the use of phages is complicated by the fact that multiple strains of the *Vibrio* pathogens with different phage susceptibility patterns may coexist in aquaculture environments [14]. The implications of strain diversity for the efficiency of phage control may be overcome either by combining several phages which target a broad range of pathogenic hosts, or to use a broad-host-range phage which can infect multiple strains within a given species or even multiple species [15]. The phage KVP40 represents a broad-host-range phage which infects at least eight species of *Vibrio* sp. (*V. parahaemolyticus*, *V. alginolyticus*, *V. natriegens*, *V. cholerae*, *V. mimicus*, *V. anguillarum*, *V. splendidus*, and *V. fluvialis*) and one *Photobacterium* sp. (*P. leignathi*) [16]. All of these species contain a 26-kDa outer membrane protein named OmpK, which is a receptor for phage KVP40 [17].

The application of phages for controlling pathogens may be hampered by the development of phage resistance in the bacteria [18], and several mechanisms have been described in *V. anguillarum* which can eliminate or reduce bacterial sensitivity to phages and thus limit the efficiency and duration of phage control [19].

The aim of this study was to examine the effect of phage KVP40 on the survival of turbot and cod larvae challenged with four different *V. anguillarum* strains. Larval mortality and abundance of bacteria and phages were quantified to determine the potential of using phage KVP40 to control *V. anguillarum* infections during the early larval stage. In general, phage KVP40 was able to reduce or delay the mortality of both turbot and cod larvae in all the challenge trials and reduce larval mortality imposed by the background population of pathogens.

The results demonstrated that phage KVP40 reduced the mortality imposed by the added pathogens as well as other *Vibrio* pathogens already present in the environment during the initial 1–4 days of the experiment, emphasizing the potential of using phages to reduce turbot and cod mortality at the larval stage.

2. Results

2.1. Phage Effect on Turbot Mortality in Vibrio Challenge Trials

2.1.1. Turbot Challenge Trial 1

In general, larval mortality was high in all treatments, including the nonchallenged controls where a maximum mortality of 86% (i.e., 103 dead larvae out of 120) was found (Figure 1), indicating that the eggs were associated with unknown bacterial pathogens prior to the challenge trial. Challenging the turbot eggs with *V. anguillarum* resulted in higher mortalities for all four strains (Figure 1), emphasizing that the added *V. anguillarum* pathogens increased larval mortality. Strain PF430-3 was the most virulent of the four strains, with 100% larval mortality after 3 days, whereas strains PF7, 90-11-286, and 4299 caused 97%–100% mortality after 4 and 5 days of challenge. Subsequent quantification of the abundance of colony forming bacteria in the water used for transportation of the fish eggs confirmed the presence of a microbial community associated with the eggs (see Section 2.5).

Despite the presence of other pathogen communities associated with the eggs/larvae, addition of phage KVP40 had a significant positive effect on larval survival in all the challenge treatments during all or part of the trials. When challenged with strain PF430-3, the maximum relative reduction in mortality was 29% ($p < 0.05$) one day after phage addition (Figure 1a; Table 1). The delay in mortality only lasted for 3 days, and the mortality reached almost 100% mortality at day 5 (Figure 1a). When challenged with strain PF7 or strain 90-11-286 (Figure 1b,c), the maximum phage-induced reduction in mortality was 47% obtained 1 and 2 days (Table 1), respectively, after addition of KVP40 and a significant effect of the phage on mortality was observed for 3–4 days ($p < 0.05$). The effect of phage addition was largest in the treatment group with strain 4299, where the larval mortality remained below 66% throughout the 8-day trial, corresponding to an average of 36% reduction in larval mortality compared to larvae challenged with *V. anguillarum* ($p < 0.05$) (Figure 1d).

Interestingly, larval mortality in the KVP40 controls (addition of phage but not *V. anguillarum*) showed the lowest larval mortality, reaching 65% at day 4 and remaining at that level (Figure 1). This significant reduction in mortality compared to the nonchallenged control (i.e., 86% mortality in larvae not exposed to *V. anguillarum* or phage) suggested that phage KVP40 was able to control part of the unknown pathogen community, thereby increasing the larval survival. This was later confirmed by analysis of phage susceptibility of bacteria initially associated with the eggs (see Section 2.5 below).

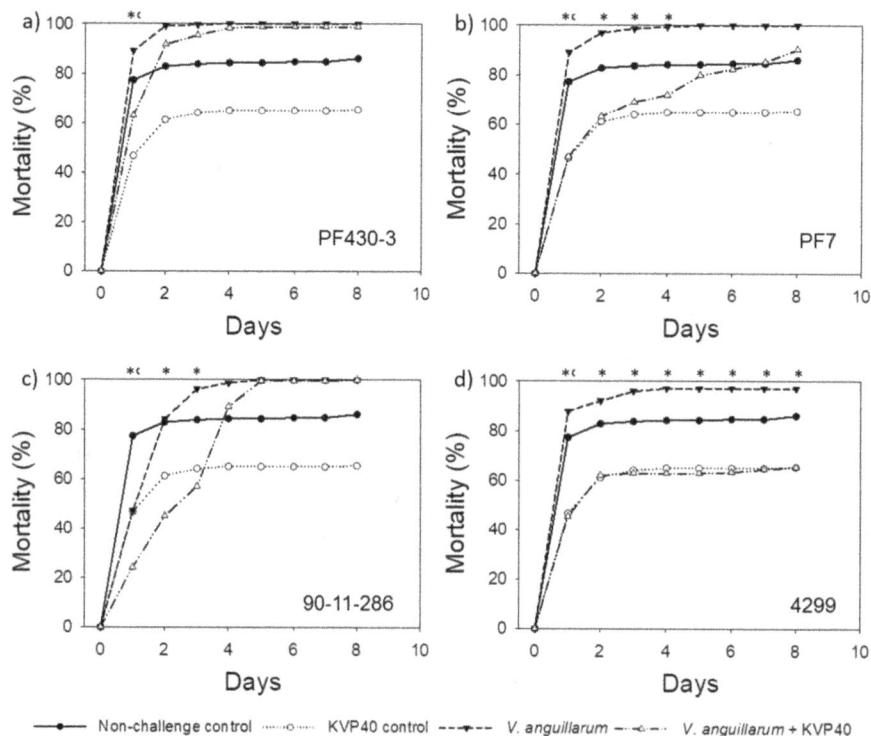

Figure 1. Cumulative percent mortality over time in turbot challenge trial 1: (**a**) strain PF430-3; (**b**) strain PF7; (**c**) strain 90-11-286; (**d**) strain 4299. Significant difference in mortality between cultures "*V. anguillarum*" and "*V. anguillarum* + KVP40" for individual time points is indicated by *. Significant difference in mortality between cultures "Nonchallenge control" and "KVP40 control" is indicated by [c].

Table 1. Overview of the percent reduction in mortality caused by phage KVP40 addition in the four experiments. The maximum relative reduction and reduction at the end of the experiment (final) is shown.

V. *anguillarum* Strains	Relative Reduction * in Larval Mortality in the Presence of Phages (%)							
	Turbot Challenge Trial				Cod Challenge Trial			
	1		2		1		2	
	Max.	Final	Max.	Final	Max.	Final	Max.	Final
PF430-3	29	N/S [1]	60	N/S [1]	79	N/S [1]	86	N/ [1]
PF7	47	N/S [1]	53	N/S [1]	75	43	59	32
90-11-286	47	N/S [1]	92	N/S [1]	−119	N/S [1]	49	N/S [1]
4299	48	33	45	N/S [1]	N/D [2]	N/D [2]	82	72

* The relative reduction in mortality is calculated as difference in mortality between *V. anguillarum* and *V. anguillarum* + phage treatment, divided by the mortality in the *V. anguillarum* treatment. [1] N/S: not significant, [2] N/D: not determined.

2.1.2. Turbot Challenge Trial 2

The relatively high fraction of low-quality eggs and high mortality in the control group led us to repeat the challenge experiments in an attempt to optimize the egg quality and in order to verify the indications of positive effects of phages for larval mortality in replicate experiments.

Also in the second challenge trial with turbot larvae, a high mortality (71%) was observed in the nonchallenged control groups after 5 days (Figure 2), indicating pathogenic effects of the bacterial background community in the turbot eggs. In contrast to turbot challenge trial 1, the mortality caused by the background bacteria was not observed immediately, and mortality in the control groups gradually increased during the first 4 days, indicating growth of the pathogenic bacteria. Addition of *V. anguillarum* strains increased larval mortality in all four treatments, resulting in mortalities between 72% and 98% after 4–5 days of incubation. As in turbot challenge trial 1, addition of phage KVP40 had significant positive effects on the larval survival. However, in this case, the phage addition delayed the mortality by 2–4 days relative to the treatment with *V. anguillarum* alone.

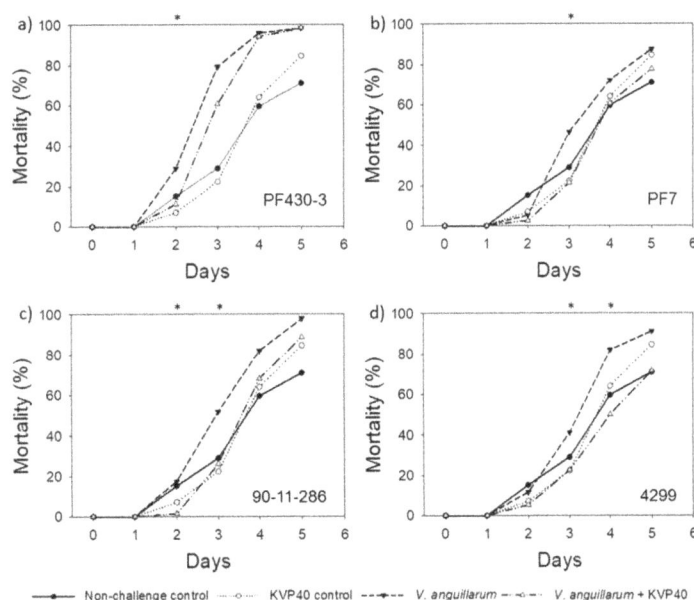

Figure 2. Cumulative percent mortality over time in turbot challenge trial 2: (**a**) strain PF430-3; (**b**) strain PF7; (**c**) strain 90-11-286; (**d**) strain 4299. Significant difference in mortality between cultures "*V. anguillarum*" and "*V. anguillarum* + KVP40" for individual time points is indicated by *.

When challenged with strain PF430-3, the addition of phages reduced mortality from 29% to 11% 2 days after phage addition (Figure 2a), corresponding to a maximum phage-mediated reduction in mortality of 60% ($p < 0.05$, Table 1). The delay in mortality lasted until day 4, where mortality approached 100% mortality as in the treatment without phage (Figure 2a). Phage addition to the larvae challenged with strain PF7 and strain 90-11-286 resulted in a significant 3-day delay in mortality with a maximum reduction in mortality of 53% and 92%, respectively, after 2–3 days relative to the larvae challenged with *V. anguillarum* alone ($p < 0.05$ (Figure 2b,c; Table 1). As in the turbot challenge trial 1, the larvae challenged with strain 4299 were best protected by phage addition, with a maximum relative reduction in mortality of 45% ($p < 0.05$) obtained 3 days after phage addition (Table 1), and a continued reduction in larval mortality of 22% relative to the larvae challenged with bacteria alone throughout the experiment (Figure 2d).

2.2. Abundance of Bacteria and Phages in Turbot Challenge Trial 2

In all the treatments in turbot challenge trial 2, the total count of colony forming bacteria (CFU) increased exponentially over time for the first 2–4 days (Figure 3).

The number of infective KVP40 phages increased about 100-fold reaching 1–5×10^{10} PFU mL^{-1} in all the treatment groups where KVP40 was added, with no significant differences between cultures with and without the addition of *Vibrio* pathogens. This indicated that the background bacteria supported phage proliferation and that addition of *V. anguillarum* only had a minor effect on phage production.

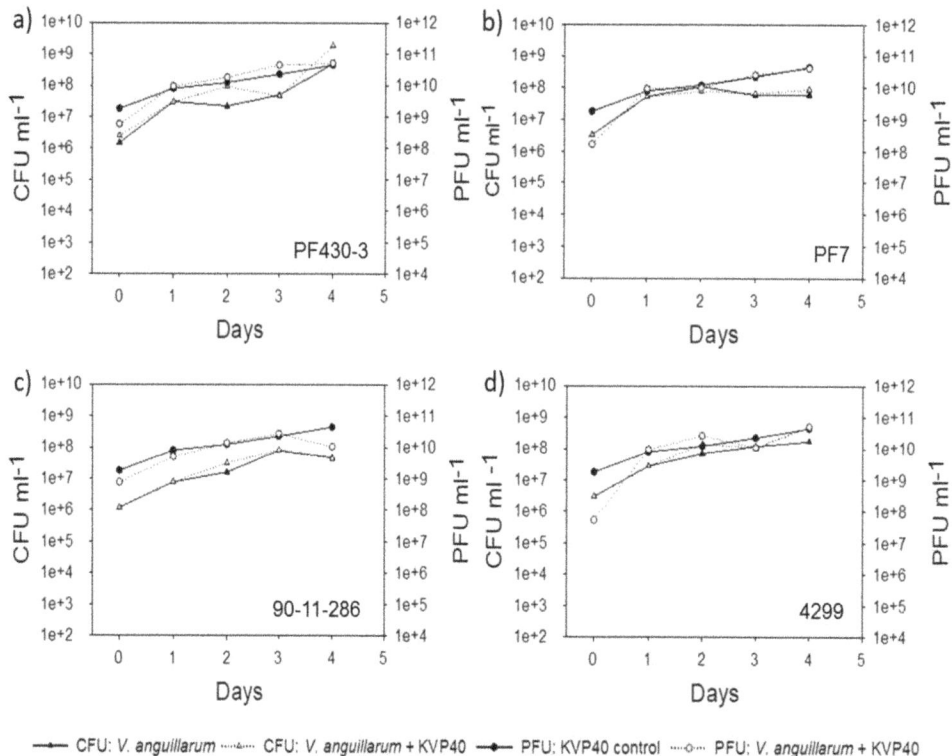

Figure 3. Bacterial abundance (CFU mL^{-1}) and phage abundance (PFU mL^{-1}) in turbot challenge trial 2: (a) strain PF430-3; (b) strain PF7; (c) strain 90-11-286; (d) strain 4299.

2.3. Phage Effect on Cod Mortality in Vibrio Challenge Trials

2.3.1. Cod Challenge Trial 1

The cod larvae mortality in the nonchallenged controls remained low throughout the trial (<10%) (Figure 4), and the addition of *Vibrio anguillarum* strains increased mortality significantly (Figure 4).

Strain PF430-3 and strain 90-11-286 increased mortality to 82% and 78%, respectively, after 11 days (Figure 4a,c), whereas the mortality was 41% in the treatment with strain PF7 (Figure 4b).

The addition of phage KVP40 had significant positive effects on larval survival in the larvae exposed to strain PF430-3 and strain PF7. For strain PF430-3, the mortality was reduced from 24% to 5% in the phage added cultures after 5 days, corresponding to maximal relative reduction in mortality by phage KVP40 of 79% compared to the larvae only challenged with *V. anguillarum* ($p < 0.05$; Table 1). The significant phage-induced reduction in mortality lasted to day 8 (Figure 4a). Phage KVP40 addition to strain PF7 reduced relative larval mortality by 75% compared to the larvae only challenged with *V. anguillarum* ($p < 0.05$) after 8 days (Table 1), and the significant phage-mediated reduction in mortality remained throughout the 11-day trial (Figure 4b). Surprisingly, the addition of phage KVP40 increased larval mortality significantly in the cultures challenged with strain 90-11-286 with a maximum increase in mortality of 119 ($p < 0.05$) reached at day 6 (Figure 4c; Table 1). The negative effect of phage addition was significant from day 5 to day 10, with the mortality reaching 100% in the phage treated cultures at day 11.

Despite the low mortality in the nonchallenged control treatment, the reduced larval mortality in the phage KVP40 controls (addition of phage but not *V. anguillarum*) (<7%) compared with the nonchallenged control group without phages again indicated a positive effect of the phages in reducing the original pathogenic bacterial load in the trials.

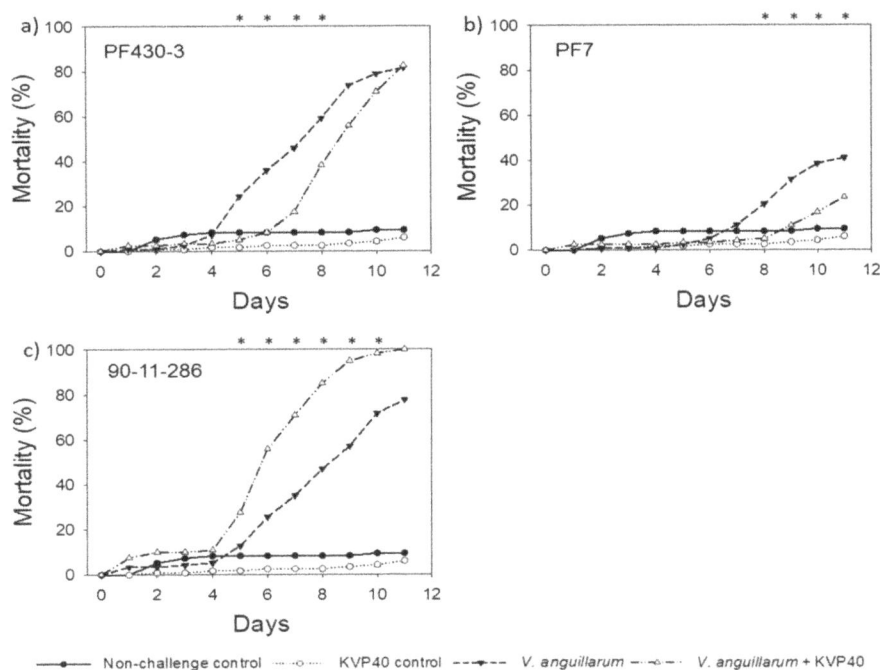

Figure 4. Cumulative percent mortality over time in cod challenge trial 1: (**a**) strain PF430-3; (**b**) strain PF7; (**c**) strain 90-11-286. Significant difference in mortality between cultures "*V. anguillarum*" and "*V. anguillarum* + KVP40" for individual time points is indicated by *.

2.3.2. Cod Challenge Trial 2

As for the turbot experiments, the challenge trials with cod were repeated to examine the reproducibility of the first results using a new batch of eggs. The second challenge trial with cod larvae confirmed the high virulence of strains PF430-3 and 90-11-286 obtained in cod challenge trial 1, whereas strain PF7 caused less mortality in cod challenge trial 2. Strain 4299 was not very virulent to the cod larvae (Figure 5). A gradual increase in mortality was observed in larvae challenged with strains PF430-3, PF7, and 90-11-286, which reached mortalities of 74% to 91% after 11 days post challenge (Figure 5a–c). Challenge with strain 4299 did not increase mortality compared to the nonchallenged control level, suggesting that this strain had very low virulence to cod (Figure 5d). The nonchallenged control showed an increase in mortality from 5% to 15% between days 2 and 3, followed by a more gradual increase to 35% mortality at day 11 (Figure 5).

Addition of phage KVP40 had a significant positive effect on cod larvae survival in all the treatments (Table 1). In the larvae challenged with strain PF430-3, phage addition kept larval mortality below 27% for 6 days, with a maximum reduction in mortality of 86% ($p < 0.05$) obtained 4 days after phage addition (Table 1). The reduced mortality lasted from day 2 to day 9, and after day 10 the mortality reached almost the same level as in the cultures without phages (Figure 5a). When challenged with strain PF7, the maximal effect of phage addition was a reduction in mortality of 59% ($p < 0.05$) obtained 6 days after phage addition (Table 1). The delay in mortality lasted throughout the trial, with the difference being significant from day 5 and onwards (Figure 5b). In the treatments challenged with strain 90-11-286, the maximal reduction in mortality was 49% ($p < 0.05$) obtained 6 days after phage addition (Table 1). The mortality then increased but remained below the nonphage treated group throughout the experiment (Figure 5c). Phage KVP40 very efficiently reduced mortality of larvae challenged with strain 4299, with a maximum reduction of 82% ($p < 0.05$) after 5 days (Table 1), and a significant reduction in mortality (mortality always < 12%) throughout the trial (Figure 5d).

The relatively high initial mortality in the nonchallenged control from day 1 to day 3 compared with corresponding nonchallenge control group in cod challenge trial 1, and compared with the lower and more gradual increase in mortality in the group challenged with strain 4299, suggested the presence of a high fraction of low-quality eggs in this specific control group. As in the previous trials, the phage-added controls showed a lower mortality than in the nonchallenged controls, again suggesting a positive effect of phage KVP40 in controlling other pathogens growing up during the trials (Figure 5).

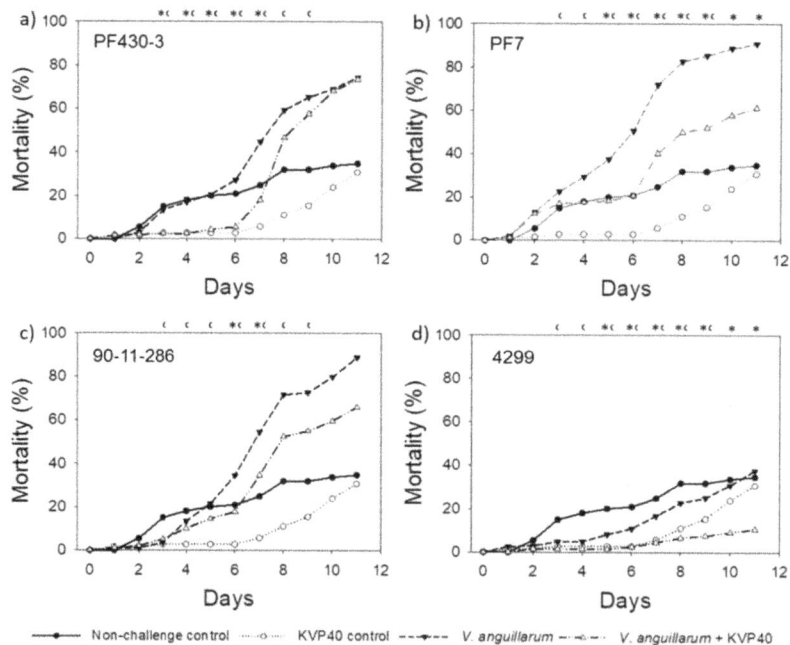

Figure 5. Cumulative percent mortality over time in cod challenge trial 2: (a) strain PF430-3; (b) strain PF7; (c) strain 90-11-286; (d) strain 4299. Significant difference in mortality between cultures "*V. anguillarum*" and "*V. anguillarum* + KVP40" for individual time points is indicated by *. Significant difference in mortality between cultures "Nonchallenge control" and "KVP40 control" is indicated by ᶜ.

2.4. Abundance of Bacteria and Phages in Cod Challenge Trials

2.4.1. Cod Challenge Trial 1

The total abundance of colony forming microorganisms increased approximately 10-fold in all *Vibrio* challenged larval groups from approx. 10^5 to 10^6 CFU mL^{-1} (Figure 6). Addition of phages only reduced the bacterial load in the strain PF7 challenged larval group and only during the first 2 days (Figure 6b). In contrast to this, total CFU counts increased after addition of phage KVP40 in larval groups challenged with strain PF430-3 and strain 90-11-286. Especially in the challenge with strain 90-11-286, a > 10-fold increase in colony forming bacteria was observed (Figure 6c) in accordance with the increased larval mortality in this treatment (Figure 4c). The phage abundance was approximately 10^7 PFU mL^{-1} in all phage-added treatments and remained stable during the 4 days when PFU was measured.

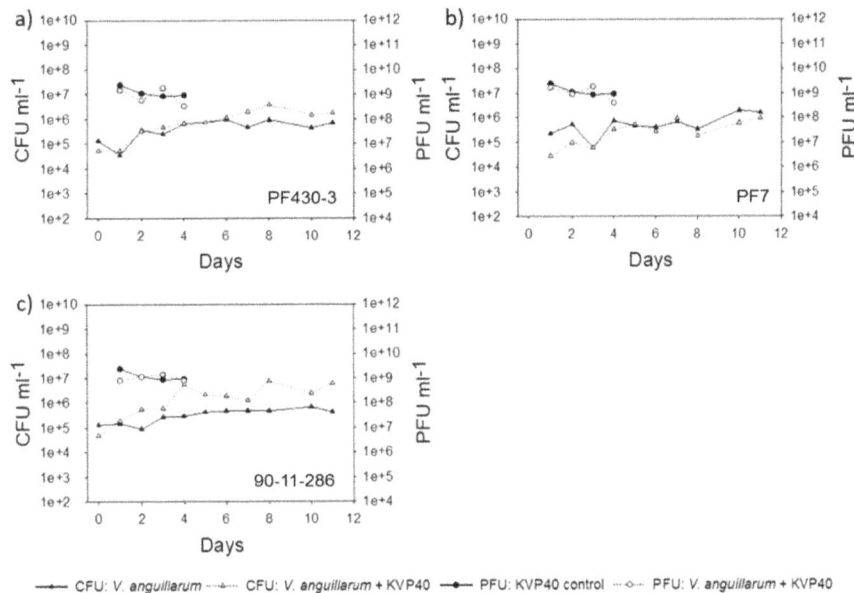

Figure 6. Bacterial abundance (CFU mL^{-1}) and phage abundance (PFU mL^{-1}) in cod challenge trial 1: (**a**) strain PF430-3; (**b**) strain PF7; (**c**) strain 90-11-286.

2.4.2. Cod Challenge Trial 2

The *V. anguillarum* load was approximately 10-fold higher in the second than in the first cod challenge trial and the CFU counts were approximately 10^6 CFU mL^{-1} in the *Vibrio* challenged groups (Figure 7).

In all the groups, addition of phage KVP40 reduced the bacterial counts significantly from day 0. In the groups challenged with strain PF430-3 and strain PF7, a significant phage-mediated reduction (approximately 1 log reduction) in the *V. anguillarum* pathogens was maintained for the first 8–9 days, followed by an increase in total CFU which then reached values close to the bacteria-alone group at day 11 (Figure 7a,b). For the group challenged with strain 90-11-286, phage reduction of the *Vibrio* pathogen was rather short. After 3 days, the bacterial abundance had reached the same level as in the bacteria-only group (Figure 7c). In the group challenged with strain 4299, the addition of phage KVP40 caused a 100-fold reduction in total CFU counts, indicating a strong phage control of the pathogen. However, after day 8, total bacterial cell counts increased 100-fold and reached numbers similar to the group without phage (Figure 7d). Phages were added at an initial concentration of 1.75×10^9 PFU mL^{-1} and the abundance of phage remained stable throughout the trial, both in the absence and presence of the *Vibrio* hosts (Figure 7).

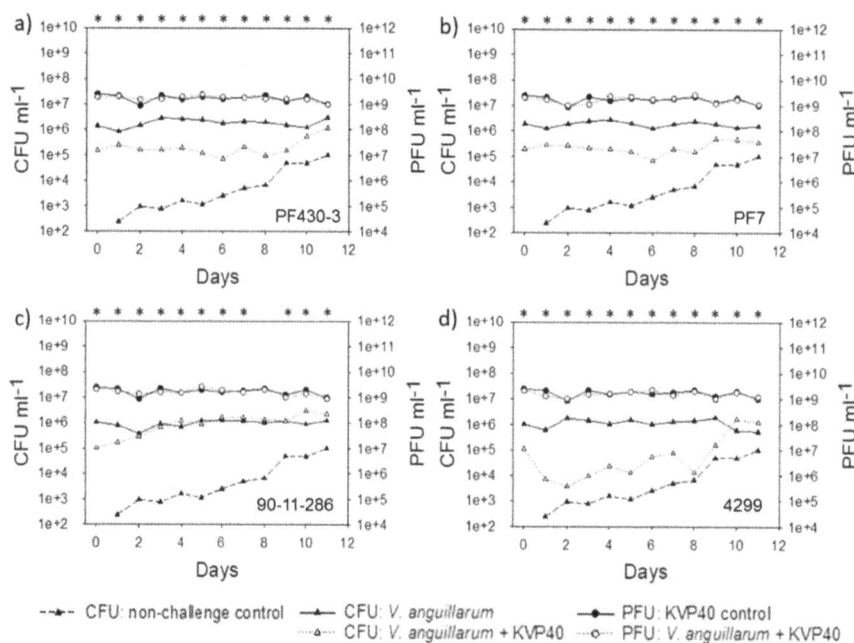

Figure 7. Bacterial abundance (CFU mL^{-1}) and phage abundance (PFU mL^{-1}) in cod challenge trial 2: (**a**) strain PF430-3; (**b**) strain PF7; (**c**) strain 90-11-286; (**d**) strain 4299. Significant difference in CFU between cultures "CFU: *V. anguillarum*" and "CFU: *V. anguillarum* + KVP40" for individual time points is indicated by *.

2.5. Abundance and Phage KVP40 Susceptibility of Bacterial Background Communities Associated with the Turbot Eggs

During the second turbot trial, the abundance of colony-forming bacteria in water used for transportation of the fish eggs was determined to shed light on the observed positive effect of phage KVP40 on unchallenged control groups. Different general and *Vibrio*-promoting growth media were used. In all the experiments, there was a high load of bacteria associated with the eggs, and a general increase in their abundance over time was found (Table 2). The high abundance of colonies growing on TCBS plates (up to >10^8 CFU mL^{-1}) indicated that a large fraction of these background communities were presumptive *Vibrio* or *Vibrio*-related species.

Table 2. Abundance of the bacterial background community (CFU mL^{-1}) associated with the fish eggs, in turbot challenge trial 2, and cultured on different media. Day 0: water the eggs were transported in for 24 h; Day 11: water in the wells of the live nonchallenged larvae.

Growth Substrate	Day 0 (CFU mL^{-1})	Day 11 (CFU mL^{-1})
LB media	2×10^7	9.39×10^6
TCBS media	2×10^6	1.5×10^8
Marine agar	N/D [1]	2.89×10^8

[1] N/D: not determined.

The susceptibility to phage KVP40 was tested in 40 isolates obtained from the water containing the turbot eggs during transportation used for challenge trial 1 by quantification of the growth reduction relative to a control culture without phage KVP40 (Figure 8). The results showed that 35 out of 40 isolated showed a growth reduction, indicating that the majority of the colony-forming cells originating from the water used for transporting the eggs were susceptible to phage KVP40.

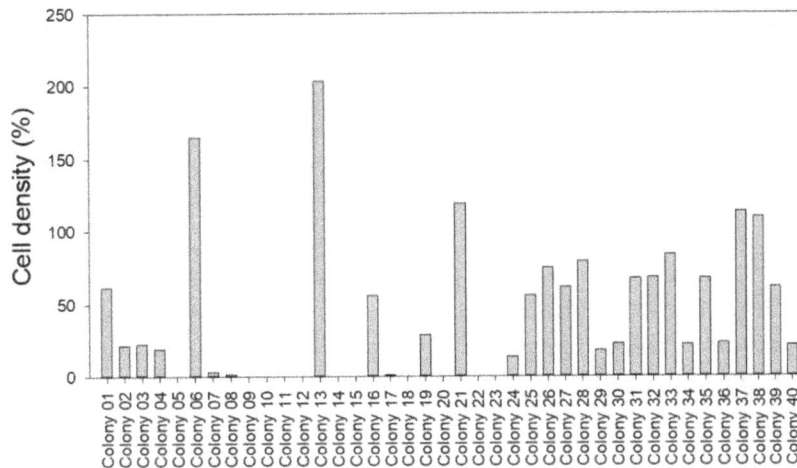

Figure 8. Quantification of phage KVP40-induced inhibition/promotion of cell growth in cultures of bacteria isolated from water used for transport of eggs used in turbot challenge trial 1. Phage-induced growth inhibition/promotion was determined as the percent cell density in cultures added phage KVP40 relative to control cultures without phage KVP40 (100%) after 3 h incubation.

3. Discussion

In general, the addition of phage KVP40 reduced or delayed the mortality of turbot and cod larvae challenged with *V. anguillarum*, with the largest effect observed for strain 4299, where the relative turbot and cod mortality was reduced by 22–33% and 72%, respectively, by the end of the experiment. In most of the challenges, the positive effect of phage KVP40 addition on larval survival was maintained throughout the incubation period. However, incubation with strain PF430-3 showed a temporary effect of phage addition on mortality and larval mortality reached the same level as in the bacterial challenges (without phage) after 4–10 days. Since the phage was maintained in high concentrations throughout the experiment, it is likely that strain PF430-3 was protected against infection, which supports previous observations that strain PF430-3 can reduce its susceptibility to phage KVP40 by forming aggregates or biofilm, creating spatial refuges [20].

In addition to the specific *V. anguillarum* pathogens, other pathogens already associated with the fish eggs prior to the experiments were present in the experiments. This allowed an assessment of the effects of phages on both the mortality caused by the *V. anguillarum* strains and the mortality imposed by the natural background pathogen communities. The decrease in mortality recorded for all the phage controls (without *V. anguillarum*) compared to the nonchallenge controls (without phage and *V. anguillarum*) demonstrated a strong effect of phage KVP40 on the initial bacterial pathogen communities associated with the eggs. This was supported by the observation that >85% of the isolated colonies originating from the background bacterial community were susceptible to phage KVP40.

Despite the large fraction of phage susceptible strains, the bacterial abundance increased in all the incubations over time, and only in cod challenge trial 2 did addition of phage KVP40 reduce the bacterial abundance for multiple days. This suggested that during the experiment, pathogens that were not infected by KVP40 (i.e., non-*Vibrio* pathogens and possibly phage-resistant *V. anguillarum* strains) replaced the phage susceptible strains, and thus were the main cause of mortality in the experiments. This was supported by the increased effects of phages on mortality in cod challenge trial 2, where the eggs were pretreated with 25% glutaraldehyde. These results emphasized that the growth of other pathogens than *V. anguillarum* was the main cause of mortality in the experiments that were not pretreated with glutaraldehyde, and that phage KVP40 was able to significantly reduce mortality imposed by the added *V. anguillarum* strains.

Consequently, even though the presence of a bacterial background pathogen community masked the effect of phage KVP40 on the added *V. anguillarum* strains, it at the same time provided a more realistic demonstration of how the addition of phage KVP40 will affect an infected aquaculture system. These results emphasized the potential of phage KVP40 to control not only the added host strains but also a broader range of pathogens present in the rearing facilities. Similar results were obtained for the two broad-host-range KVP40-like phages φSt2 and φGrn1 infecting the fish pathogens *V. alginolyticus* [21]. These phages were able to reduce the natural *Vibrio* load present in *Artemia* live feed cultures used in fish hatcheries. The current study is, however, the first demonstration of a positive effect of phage application on larval survival by reducing the natural microbiota, rather than exclusively focusing on the effects of one added pathogen. While the composition of the background microbiota was not analyzed in the current study, previous studies have found that bacterial communities associated with cod and turbot eggs in rearing units were dominated by *Pseudomonas*, *Alteromonas*, *Aeromonas*, and *Flavobacterium* [22], but also *Vibrio* has been shown to be prevalent in these environments [23]. In our study, the high fraction of bacteria growing on *Vibrio*-selective TCBS medium combined with the high susceptibility to phage KVP40 suggested that the background bacterial community was dominated by *Vibrio* or *Vibrio*-related species, as the phage KVP40 has been shown to infect at least eight *Vibrio* species and one *Photobacterium* [16]. This was also supported by preliminary analysis of the microbiome associated with the turbot eggs used in challenge trial 2, which showed dominance of *Vibrio* species (Dittmann, unpublished results). The differences in mortality in the control treatments (nonchallenged control and KVP40 control) between different experiments may therefore reflect differences in the composition of background bacterial community, representing differences in virulence and KVP40 susceptibility. Further, higher incubation temperature of the turbot than cod eggs may also have increased bacteria-induced mortality in the turbot experiments. In one of the treatments (cod challenge trial 1 with strain 90-11-286), addition of phage KVP40 increased larval mortality (Figure 4c). Specific secondary metabolites or toxins released during cell lysis may potentially inhibit larval growth [24]. However, since this was not observed in any of the other treatments, it is not likely that the viral lysates affected the cod larvae. Alternatively, the viral lysates may have stimulated growth of other specific pathogens already present in the experiment, as also indicated by the enhanced bacterial growth in the phage added culture (Figure 6c). Previous studies have shown that lysogenization of *V. harveyi* with phage VHS1 increased the virulence of the bacterium against black tiger shrimp (*Penaus monodon*) by the phage encoded toxin associated with hemocyte agglutination ([25]). There has not been any indication of lysogenization of *Vibrio* pathogens with phage KVP40, and the production of a KVP40-encoded toxin is therefore not a likely explanation for the observed increase in larval mortality in this experiment.

Our results support previous attempts to control pathogens in aquaculture by use of phages. A challenge trial in Atlantic salmon using *V. anguillarum* strain PF4, a close relative to strain PF430-3 used in the current study [13], showed 100% survival using the phage CHOED, independent of the original multiplicity of infection (MOI) [10]. The efficiency of this phage on fish survival compared to the current study most likely relates to the fact that larger fish are more robust against infections by co-occurring pathogens than larvae. A delay in mortality after phage addition was also observed by Imbeault et al. [26] and Verner-Jeffreys et al. [27] in brook trout and Atlantic salmon, respectively, infected with *A. salmonicida* using different phages. While Imbeault et al. [26] were able to delay the onset of disease and reduce the mortality to 10%, Verner-Jeffreys et al. [27] also demonstrated a delay in the mortality, but only observed a temporary effect of the phages in survival.

Previous in vivo challenge studies with a positive outcome of phage therapy were conducted on >5 day old larvae [12] or fish averaging 15–25 grams [10], while our study was conducted on eggs which hatched during the course of the challenge trials. Eggs and newly hatched larvae are more sensitive to the infection by pathogenic *V. anguillarum* and other pathogens than late stages due to the inefficient protection provided by the intestinal microflora associated with their gut mucosa, which constitutes a primary barrier [28]. Despite the general frailty of newly hatched larvae, we demonstrated a significant phage-mediated reduction in mortality of cod and turbot larvae in experimental challenge trials with *V. anguillarum* pathogens in combination with the natural pathogenic bacteria associated with the incubated fish eggs. These results emphasize that phage therapy is a promising approach to reduce pathogen load and mortality in marine larviculture.

4. Materials and Methods

4.1. Bacterial Strains and Growth Conditions

The four *V. anguillarum* strains—PF4303-3, PF7, 90-11-286, and 4299—used in this study were isolated in Chile, Denmark, and Norway [10,13,29,30]. The bacteria were stored at −80 °C in Luria-Bertani (LB) medium with 15% glycerol. Before each assay, the strains were inoculated on LB plates and grown overnight at 24 °C. Then, one colony was transferred to 4 mL LB medium and grown overnight at 24 °C with agitation (200 rpm).

4.2. Phage Infectivity and Production

The broad-host-range phage KVP40 [16], which previously has been shown to infect the *V. anguillarum* strains PF430-3, 90-11-286, and 4299 [13], was tested on *V. anguillarum* strain PF7 using the double-layer agar assay [14] with minor modifications. The double-layer agar assay in brief: 100 µL phage lysate was mixed with 300 µL bacterial cells and incubated for 30 min at 24 °C. The mixture was added to 4 mL of 45 °C top agar (LB with 0.4% agar) and poured onto a LB 1.5% agar plate, which was placed for incubation at 24 °C overnight. The next day, the presence of phages in the form of clear plaques in the top agar was detected. KVP40 was produced and purified by ACD Pharmaceuticals AS (Leknes, Norway).

4.3. Eggs and Larvae

Eggs from turbot and cod were used in the challenge trials. The eggs for turbot challenge trial 1 were obtained from Stolt Sea Farm (Galicia, Spain), with 48 h of transport before conducting the challenge trial at the University of Bergen (Bergen, Norway). The eggs for turbot challenge trial 2 were obtained from France Turbot, hatchery L'Epine (Noirmoutier Island, France), with 24 h of transport before conducting the challenge trial at the Technical University of Denmark (Lyngby, Denmark). The eggs for cod challenge trial 1 and cod challenge trial 2 were obtained from the Institute of Marine Research, Austevoll Research Station (Storebø, Norway), with 1 hour of transport before conducting the challenge trial at the University of Bergen (Bergen, Norway). The eggs in cod challenge trial 2 were disinfected with 25% glutaraldehyde at the Institute of Marine Research, Austevoll Research Station before being transported to the University of Bergen for the challenge trial.

4.4. Phage Therapy Assays

Challenge trials with turbot and cod larvae were established as outlined in Table 3. For each of the *V. anguillarum* strains tested, eggs were distributed in 10 24-well dishes with 2 mL sterile filtered (0.2 µm) and autoclaved, oxygenated 80% sea water and 1 egg well^{-1}. In group 1 (*V. anguillarum* only), five 24-well plates were inoculated with 100 µL *V. anguillarum* culture in each well. Prior to addition, the bacterial culture had been grown overnight, washed twice in sterile sea water (ssw), and resuspended in ssw to a final concentration of 0.5–1 × 10^6 CFU mL^{-1}. In group 2 (*V. anguillarum* + phage KVP40), five 24-well plates were inoculated with *V. anguillarum* as above and 50 µL of phage KVP40 was added to each well to a final concentration of 0.5–8 × 10^8 PFU mL^{-1}, resulting in a multiplicity of infection (MOI) of ~5–100. The five 24-well plates in group 3 (nonchallenged control) were only inoculated with 100 µL autoclaved, oxygenated 80% ssw, whereas in group 4 (phage KVP40 control), each well also contained 50 µL of phage KVP40. Plates were then incubated in an air-conditioned room of 15.5 °C and 5.5 °C for turbot and cod, respectively, which are optimal conditions for larval development in the two species. The eggs in groups 1, 2, and 4 had bacteria and/or phages added to them immediately after their distribution in the wells (=day 0 of the experiment). Due to large variation in the viability of the eggs used for the experiment, the challenge trials were done twice for both fish species in an attempt to confirm the results at different egg qualities. The challenge trials lasted for 8 days for turbot challenge trial 1, 5 days for turbot challenge trial 2, and for

11 days for cod. The mortality was monitored daily. The quality of the eggs varied considerably depending on transportation time and handling, resulting in differences in egg mortality prior to hatching. The initial egg mortality was calculated for each 24-well plate and then averaged for all 50 24-well plates used in the individual experiments. Of the 1200 eggs used in each experiment, the average fraction of eggs that died prior to hatching amounted to 0% and 30.3% in turbot challenge trials 1 and 2, respectively, and 4.9% and 23.2% in cod challenge trials 1 and 2, respectively. These eggs were excluded from the analysis. The effect of phage addition on larval mortality was calculated as a relative reduction [31], corresponding to the reduction in mortality in treatments to which both phage KVP40 and *V. anguillarum* were added relative to the mortality in treatments with *V. anguillarum* alone (i.e., the difference in mortality between the two treatments in percentage of the mortality in the incubations without phage.

Table 3. Experimental design and addition *V. anguillarum* and phage KVP40.

Group	Treatment	*V. anguillarum* (CFU mL^{-1})	Phage KVP40 (PFU mL^{-1})	Replicate Wells
1	*V. anguillarum* only	$0.5–1 \times 10^6$	-	5×24 wells $\times 4$ strains
2	*V. anguillarum* + phage KVP40	$0.5–1 \times 10^6$	$0.5–12 \times 10^8$	5×24 wells $\times 4$ strains
3	Nonchallenge control	-	-	5×24 wells
4	Phage KVP40 control	-	$0.5–12 \times 10^8$	5×24 wells

The concentration of bacteria and phages was monitored daily except in turbot challenge trial 1, where neither was monitored. In turbot challenge trial 2, the concentrations were only monitored for half of the experiment, while the phage concentration was only monitored for 3 days in cod challenge trial 1. To determine the bacterial concentration, dilutions were inoculated on LB agar plates (in cod challenge trial 2, the dilutions were inoculated on marine agar plates and on selective thiosulfate-citrate-bile salts-sucrose (TCBS) plates), which incubated overnight at 24 °C. To determine the phage concentration, the double-layer agar assay was used as described earlier. The culture medium was LB, the host strain was *V. anguillarum* strain PF430-3 $\Delta vanT$ [19], and the plates were incubated overnight at 24 °C.

4.5. Bacterial Background Community and Susceptibility Assays

In order to characterize the bacterial background, different media were used in the challenge trials. The water used for the transport of the eggs in turbot challenge trial 1 was spread on TCBS plates at day 4. A total of 40 colonies were picked and transferred to LB medium and grown overnight at 24 °C with agitation (200 rpm). The bacteria had their optical density at 600 nm (OD$_{600}$), measured using Novaspec Plus Visible Spectrophotometer after 1 hour in the presence and in the absence of KVP40. The sterile 80% sea water with the live nonchallenged control larvae in turbot challenge trial 2 were inoculated on LB, TCBS, and marine agar plates at day 11. The plates incubated overnight at 24 °C before determining the bacterial concentration. Throughout cod challenge trial 2, the bacterial concentration was determined on both marine agar and TCBS plates.

4.6. Statistical Analysis

Differences between challenged larvae with and without phage therapy and between the controls (nonchallenge control and KVP40 control) for each time point were analyzed by chi-squared tests using the software R (R foundation for statistical computing). A value of $p < 0.05$ were considered statistically significant.

5. Conclusions

The significant positive effect of phage KVP40 on larval survival during hatching and initial growth observed in the current experiment demonstrates the potential in using phages to reduce pathogen load in cod and turbot hatcheries and may also be a strategy to improve egg quality and survival during transport from egg producers to hatcheries. It is obvious, however, that the effect of the phage addition on mortality is temporary, and we suggest that a more efficient and long-term control of the pathogens may be obtained using a cocktail of different phages that target a broader range of pathogens.

Author Contributions: N.R., A.R. and M.M. designed the experiments; N.R. and A.R. performed turbot challenge trial 1 and cod challenge trial 1, P.G.K. and B.B.R. performed turbot challenge trial 2, N.R., A.R., P.G.K. and B.B.R. performed cod challenge trial 2; N.R. and M.M. analyzed the data; K.E.-S., H.P.K., H.I.W., L.G. and M.M. contributed reagents/materials/analysis tools; N.R. and M.M. wrote the paper with contributions from all authors.

Acknowledgments: The study was supported by the Danish Council for Strategic Research (ProAqua project 12-132390) and the Danish Research Council for Independent Research (Project # DFF-7014-00080).

References

1. Thompson, F.L.; Iida, T.; Swings, J. Biodiversity of Vibrios. *Microbiol. Mol. Biol. Rev.* **2004**, *68*, 403–431. [CrossRef] [PubMed]

2. Actis, L.A.; Tolmasky, M.E.; Crosa, J.H. Vibriosis. In *Fish Diseases and Disorders*; Woo, P.T.K., Bruno, D.W., Eds.; CAB International: Oxfordshire, UK, 2011; pp. 570–605.

3. Frans, I.; Michiels, C.W.; Bossier, P.; Willems, K.A.; Lievens, B.; Rediers, H. Vibrio anguillarum as a fish pathogen: Virulence factors, diagnosis and prevention. *J. Fish Dis.* **2011**, *34*, 643–661. [CrossRef] [PubMed]

4. Pereira, C.; Silva, Y.J.; Santos, A.L.; Cunha, A.; Gomes, N.C.M.; Almeida, A. Bacteriophages with potential for inactivation of fish pathogenic bacteria: Survival, host specificity and effect on bacterial community structure. *Mar. Drugs* **2011**, *9*, 2236–2255. [CrossRef] [PubMed]

5. Karunasagar, I.; Pai, R.; Malathi, G.R.; Karunasagar, I. Mass mortality of Penaeus monodon larvae due to antibiotic-resistant Vibrio harveyi infection. *Aquaculture* **1994**, *128*, 203–209. [CrossRef]

6. Bricknell, I.R.; Bowden, T.J.; Verner-Jeffreys, D.W.; Bruno, D.W.; Shields, R.J.; Ellis, A.A.E. Susceptibility of juvenile and sub-adult Atlantic halibut (*Hippoglossus hippoglossus* L.) to infection by Vibrio anguillarum and efficacy of protection induced by vaccination. *Fish Shellfish Immunol.* **2000**, *10*, 319–327. [CrossRef] [PubMed]

7. Mikkelsen, H.; Lund, V.; Larsen, R.; Seppola, M. Vibriosis vaccines based on various sero-subgroups of Vibrio anguillarum O2 induce specific protection in Atlantic cod (*Gadus morhua* L.) juveniles. *Fish Shellfish Immunol.* **2011**. [CrossRef] [PubMed]

8. Vinod, M.G.; Shivu, M.M.; Umesha, K.R.; Rajeeva, B.C.; Krohne, G.; Karunasagar, I.; Karunasagar, I. Isolation of Vibrio harveyi bacteriophage with a potential for biocontrol of luminous vibriosis in hatchery environments. *Aquaculture* **2006**. [CrossRef]

9. Karunasagar, I.; Shivu, M.M.; Girisha, S.K.; Krohne, G.; Karunasagar, I. Biocontrol of pathogens in shrimp hatcheries using bacteriophages. *Aquaculture* **2007**, *268*, 288–292. [CrossRef]

10. Higuera, G.; Bastías, R.; Tsertsvadze, G.; Romero, J.; Espejo, R.T. Recently discovered Vibrio anguillarum phages can protect against experimentally induced vibriosis in Atlantic salmon, Salmo salar. *Aquaculture* **2013**, *392*, 128–133. [CrossRef]

11. Mateus, L.; Costa, L.; Silva, Y.J.; Pereira, C.; Cunha, A.; Almeida, A. Efficiency of phage cocktails in the inactivation of Vibrio in aquaculture. *Aquaculture* **2014**, *424*, 167–173. [CrossRef]

12. Silva, Y.J.; Costa, L.; Pereira, C.; Mateus, C.; Cunha, Â.; Calado, R.; Gomes, N.C.M.; Pardo, M.A.; Hernandez, I.; Almeida, A. Phage therapy as an approach to prevent Vibrio anguillarum infections in fish larvae production. *PLoS ONE* **2014**. [CrossRef] [PubMed]

13. Tan, D.; Gram, L.; Middelboe, M. Vibriophages and their interactions with the fish pathogen vibrio anguillarum. *Appl. Environ. Microbiol.* **2014**, *80*, 3128–3140. [CrossRef] [PubMed]

14. Stenholm, A.R.; Dalsgaard, I.; Middelboe, M. Isolation and characterization of bacteriophages infecting the fish pathogen *Flavobacterium psychrophilum. Appl. Environ. Microbiol.* **2008**, *74*, 4070–4078. [CrossRef] [PubMed]

15. Letchumanan, V.; Chan, K.G.; Pusparajah, P.; Saokaew, S.; Duangjai, A.; Goh, B.H.; Ab Mutalib, N.S.; Lee, L.H. Insights into bacteriophage application in controlling vibrio species. *Front. Microbiol.* **2016**, *7*. [CrossRef] [PubMed]

16. Matsuzaki, S.; Tanaka, S.; Koga, T.; Kawata, T. A broad-host-range vibriophage, KVP40, isolated from sea water. *Microbiol. Immunol.* **1992**. [CrossRef]

17. Inoue, T.; Matsuzaki, S.; Tanaka, S. A 26-kDa outer membrane protein, OmpK, common to Vibrio species is the receptor for a broad-host-range vibriophage, KVP40. *FEMS Microbiol. Lett.* **1995**, *125*, 101–105. [CrossRef] [PubMed]

18. Labrie, S.J.; Samson, J.E.; Moineau, S. Bacteriophage resistance mechanisms. *Nat. Rev. Microbiol.* **2010**, *8*, 317–327. [CrossRef] [PubMed]

19. Tan, D.; Svenningsen, S.L.; Middelboe, M. Quorum sensing determines the choice of antiphage defense strategy in *Vibrio anguillarum*. *MBio* **2015**, *6*, e00627. [CrossRef] [PubMed]

20. Tan, D.; Dahl, A.; Middelboe, M. Vibriophages differentially influence biofilm formation by *Vibrio anguillarum* strains. *Appl. Environ. Microbiol.* **2015**, *81*, 4489–4497. [CrossRef] [PubMed]

21. Kalatzis, P.G.; Bastías, R.; Kokkari, C.; Katharios, P. Isolation and characterization of two lytic bacteriophages, φst2 and φgrn1; Phage therapy application for biological control of vibrio alginolyticus in aquaculture live feeds. *PLoS ONE* **2016**, *11*. [CrossRef] [PubMed]

22. Hansen, G.H.; Olafsen, J.A. Bacterial colonization of cod (*Gadus morhua* L.) and halibut (*Hippoglossus hippoglossus*) eggs in marine aquaculture. *Appl. Environ. Microbiol.* **1989**, *55*, 1435–1446. [PubMed]

23. Austin, B. Taxonomy of bacteria isolated from a coastal marine fish-rearing unit. *J. Appl. Bacteriol.* **1982**, *53*, 253–268. [CrossRef]

24. Goodridge, L.D. Designing phage therapeutics. *Curr. Pharm. Biotechnol.* **2010**, *11*, 15–27. [CrossRef] [PubMed]

25. Khemayan, K.; Prachumwat, A.; Sonthayanon, B.; Intaraprasong, A.; Sriurairatana, S.; Flegel, T.W. Complete genome sequence of virulence-enhancing siphophage VHS1 from Vibrio harveyi. *Appl. Environ. Microbiol.* **2012**, *78*, 2790–2796. [CrossRef] [PubMed]

26. Imbeault, S.; Parent, S.; Lagacé, M.; Carl, F.; Blais, J. Using bacteriophages to prevent furunculosis caused by Aeromonas salmonicida in farmed brook trout. *J. Aquat. Anim. Health* **2006**, *18*, 203–214. [CrossRef]

27. Verner–Jeffreys, D.W.; Algoet, M.; Pond, M.J.; Virdee, H.K.; Bagwell, N.J.; Roberts, E.G. Furunculosis in Atlantic salmon (*Salmo salar* L.) is not readily controllable by bacteriophage therapy. *Aquaculture* **2007**, *270*, 475–484. [CrossRef]

28. Hansen, G.H.; Olafsen, J.A. Bacterial interactions in early life stages of marine cold water fish. *Microb. Ecol.* **1999**, *38*, 1–26. [CrossRef] [PubMed]

29. Skov, M.N.; Pedersen, K.; Larsen, J.L. Comparison of pulsed-field gel electrophoresis, ribotyping, and plasmid profiling for typing of *Vibrio anguillarum* serovar O1. *Appl. Environ. Microbiol.* **1995**, *61*, 1540–1545. [PubMed]

30. Mikkelsen, H.; Schrøder, M.B.; Lund, V. Vibriosis and atypical furunculosis vaccines; efficacy, specificity and side effects in *Atlantic cod, Gadus morhua* L. *Aquaculture* **2004**. [CrossRef]

31. Ranganathan, P.; Pramesh, C.; Aggarwal, R. Common pitfalls in statistical analysis: Absolute risk reduction, relative risk reduction, and number needed to treat. *Perspect. Clin. Res.* **2016**, *7*. [CrossRef] [PubMed]

8

Geographic Variation in Antibiotic Consumption—Is It Due to Doctors' Prescribing or Patients' Consulting?

Marte Meyer Walle-Hansen [1],[*] [ID] **and Sigurd Høye** [2]

[1]   Bærum Hospital, Vestre Viken Hospital Trust, 3019 Drammen, Norway
[2]   Antibiotic Centre for Primary Care, Department of General Practice, Institute of Health and Society, University of Oslo, 0315 Oslo, Norway; sigurd.hoye@medisin.uio.no
[*]   Correspondence: marte@hansencorp.eu

Abstract: Antibiotic consumption varies greatly between Norwegian municipalities. We examine whether this variation is associated with inhabitants' consultation rates or general practitioners' (GP) prescription rates. Our study comprises consultations and antibiotic prescriptions for respiratory tract infections (RTIs) in general practice in all Norwegian municipalities with over 5000 inhabitants in 2014. Data was collected from The Norwegian Prescription Database, The Directorate of Health's system for control and payment of health reimbursements registry and Norway Statistics. Consultation rates and prescription rates were categorised in age- and gender specific quintiles and the effect on antibiotic consumption was analysed using a Poisson regression model. We found that inhabitants with RTIs received 42% more prescriptions if they belonged to a municipality with high consultation rates compared to low consultation rates [incidence rate ratio (IRR) 1.42 (95% CI 1.41–1.44)] and 48% more prescriptions if they belonged to a municipality with high prescription rates versus low prescription rates [IRR 1.48 (95% KI 1.47–1.50)]. Our results demonstrate that inhabitants' consultation rates and GPs' prescription rates have about equal impact on the number of RTI antibiotics prescribed at municipality level. These findings highlight the importance of interventions targeting patients as well as doctors in efforts to reduce unnecessary antibiotic consumption.

Keywords: antibiotic resistance; general practice; respiratory tract infections; drug consumption; pharmacoepidemiology

1. Introduction

Antibiotics are an integral part of modern health care. The use of antibiotics, especially wide spectrum antibiotics, increases the risk of antimicrobial resistance both at national and local levels [1,2]. Scandinavian countries still have relatively low levels of antimicrobial resistance but this situation is threatened by an increasing relative use of broad spectrum antibiotics and import of resistant bacteria from abroad [3].

All inhabitants in Norway are entitled to a general practitioner (GP). GP offices, alongside accident and emergency units (A&Es), nursing homes, child health clinics and school health services make up most of Norwegian primary care. Most A&Es offer access 24 h a day year-round. Some GP offices offer appointments in the evenings on selected week days. Our study therefore includes consultations conducted after hours and on weekends.

Around 85% of all antibiotics in Norway measured in defined daily dose (DDD) are prescribed in primary care [3,4]. Around half of this amount is prescribed to treat respiratory tract infections (RTIs) [3], although the clinical benefit of antibiotic treatment is modest for most RTIs [5]. Several studies have explored ways to lower RTI antibiotic consumption in general practice. Interventions have especially targeted the antibiotic prescriber, aiming to reduce their prescription rate [6].

European countries show significant differences in antibiotic usage [7]. Variations in health care organisation and epidemiology cannot fully account for these differences [8]. Norwegian municipalities also show great variation in terms of antibiotics use per inhabitants and the number of prescriptions per municipality shows little variation over time [3,9]. Latitude and municipality population size has been shown to covariate with consumption but this effect may well be a surrogate for undisclosed variables such as different patient expectations, geographical distance between patient and health care provider and differing GP prescribing habits [10].

Retrospective analyses have demonstrated that time periods with lower rates of antibiotic consumption coincide with time periods where people frequent their doctor less often [11,12]. Many of the conditions for which patients visit their doctor are safely managed in the home with symptomatic treatment. This is especially relevant to RTIs. Antibiotic consumption is dependent both on the patients' tendency to visit a doctor and the doctors' tendency to prescribe antibiotics. The relative significance of these variables is not known.

To ensure a more sustainable use of antibiotics it is important to understand the mechanisms contributing to geographic differences in consumption. The aim of this study is to investigate to what degree geographic variations in antibiotic consumption for RTIs is associated with differences in inhabitants' health seeking behaviour and GPs' prescription behaviour.

2. Results

The data set comprises 3,364,585 inhabitants with a total of 1,037,278 primary care consultations for RTIs by the course of 2014. Study population details are provided in Table 1. There was a total of 738,646 RTI antibiotic prescriptions dispensed in the same year. RTI consultations, GPs' prescription rates and RTI antibiotic prescriptions are summarised in Table 2. There was a weighted mean of 311 RTI consultations per 1000 inhabitants, making up 10.3% of all primary care consultations in 2014. GPs' prescribed a weighted mean of 779 RTI prescriptions per 1000 RTI consultations and the rate increased with increasing age for both genders. There was a weighted mean of 220 RTI prescriptions dispensed per 1000 inhabitants the same year.

Table 1. Number of included females and males by age group.

Age	Number of Included Females	Number of Included Males	Total
0–9 years	201,493	212,574	414,067
10–19 years	212,673	224,929	437,602
20–29 years	201,200	214,863	416,063
30–79 years	968,954	983,760	1,952,713
80 years or older	90,299	53,843	144,142
Total	1,674,618	1,689,968	3,364,585

Table 2. Respiratory tract infections (RTI) consultations per 1000 inhabitants, RTI antibiotic prescription per 1000 RTI consultations and RTI antibiotic prescriptions per 1000 inhabitants in 198 Norwegian municipalities in Norway in 2014.

Age	Gender	RTI Consultations per 1000 Inhabitants (SD)	RTI Antibiotic Prescriptions per 1000 RTI Consultations (SD)	RTI Antibiotic Prescriptions per 1000 Inhabitants (SD)
0–9 years	Female	604 (129)	356 (67)	217 (66)
	Male	672 (139)	345 (67)	234 (73)
10–19 years	Female	295 (56)	570 (107)	166 (40)
	Male	206 (46)	552 (134)	110 (27)
20–29 years	Female	352 (58)	797 (123)	278 (52)
	Male	209 (43)	809 (177)	165 (35)

Table 2. *Cont.*

Age	Gender	RTI Consultations per 1000 Inhabitants (SD)	RTI Antibiotic Prescriptions per 1000 RTI Consultations (SD)	RTI Antibiotic Prescriptions per 1000 Inhabitants (SD)
30–79 years	Female	307 (44)	853 (136)	260 (48)
	Male	211 (29)	940 (146)	197 (36)
80 years or older	Female	282 (66)	896 (238)	243 (66)
	Male	353 (100)	972 (293)	325 (94)
	Total [1]	311 (145)	779 (236)	220 (62)

[1] Weighted mean.

Effect on the Total Use of Antibiotics

The findings from the Poisson regression analysis are summarised in Table 3. The outcome of interest was RTI antibiotic prescriptions per 1000 inhabitants. We found a lower risk of getting a prescription in males [incidence rate ratio (IRR) 0.78]. The risk of getting a prescription for treatment of an RTI was highest among preschool age and late retirement age.

Table 3. The effect on total use of antibiotics for RTIs, mixed linear Poisson regression model.

Variable	Antibiotic Prescriptions for Treatment of RTI		
	Incidence [1]	IRR	95% CI
GPs' prescription rates			
1st quintile	187	1	
2nd quintile	201	1.11	1.10–1.12
3rd quintile	216	1.20	1.19–1.22
4th quintile	233	1.32	1.30–1.33
5th quintile	258	1.48	1.47–1.50
Inhabitants' consultation rates			
1st quintile	184	1	
2nd quintile	208	1.11	1.10–1.12
3rd quintile	225	1.18	1.17–1.20
4th quintile	227	1.29	1.27–1.30
5th quintile	246	1.42	1.41–1.44
Age			
0–9 years	229	1	
10–19 years	137	0.62	0.61–0.63
20–29 years	218	0.99	0.98–1.00
30–79 years	232	1.01	1.01–1.02
≥80 years	277	1.18	1.16–1.19
Gender			
Female	247	1	
Male [2]	192	0.78	0.78

[1] Weighted incidence: antibiotic prescriptions per 1000 inhabitants per year. [2] Additional decimal values: Male IRR = 0.7808, 95% CI = 0.776–0.784. GPs' prescription rates: municipality-level antibiotic prescriptions per 1000 consultations per year. Inhabitants' consultation rates: municipality-level consultations per 1000 inhabitants per year. IRR is adjusted for age and gender. All p-values < 0.05.

Inhabitants with RTIs received 42% more prescriptions if they belonged to a municipality with high consultation rates versus low consultation rates (5th versus 1st quintile of consultation rates, (IRR) 1.42 (95% CI 1.41–1.44)). Furthermore, inhabitants with RTIs received 48% more prescriptions if they belonged to a municipality with high prescription rates versus low prescription rates (5th versus 1st quintile of prescription rates, IRR 1.48 (95% CI 1.47–1.50). Total numbers per municipality on RTI prescriptions, RTI consultations and RTI prescriptions per consultation are demonstrated in Figures 1–3.

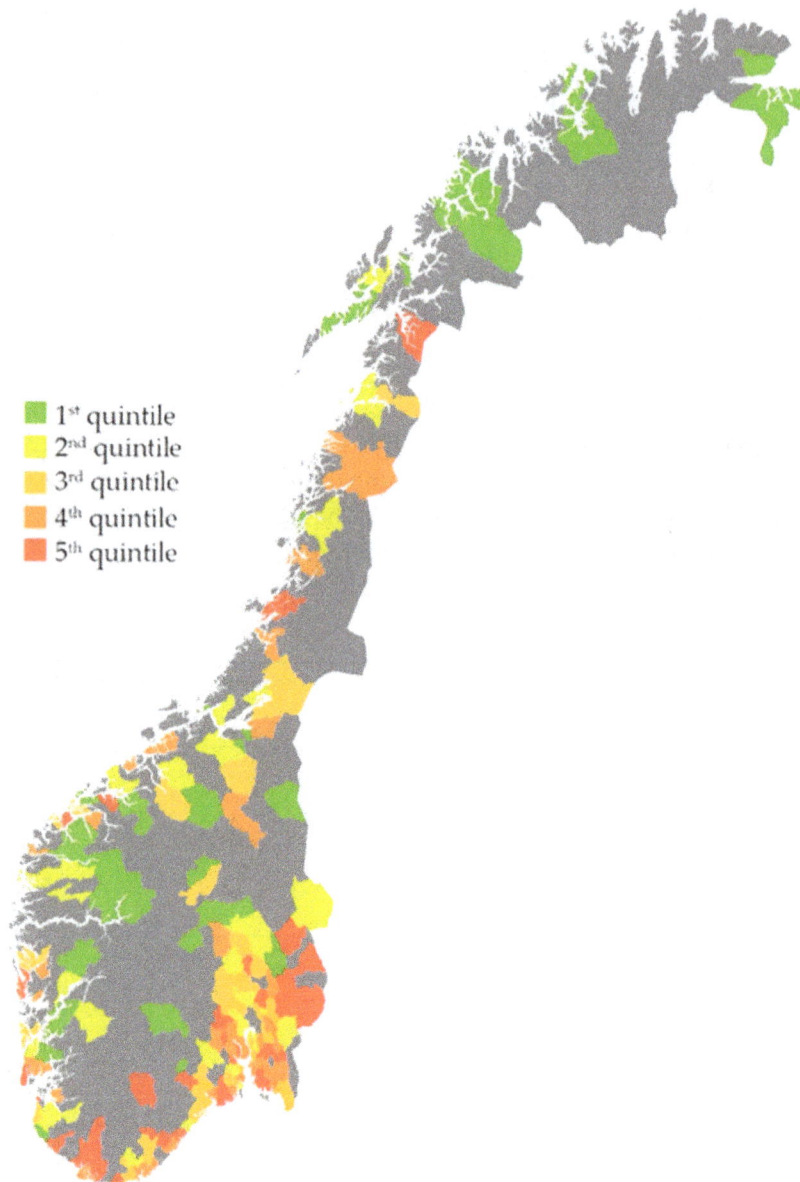

Figure 1. RTI antibiotic prescriptions per 1000 inhabitants in 198 Norwegian municipalities. Quintile 1: 76–186 prescriptions. Quintile 2: 186–209 prescriptions. Quintile 3: 209–224 prescriptions. Quintile 4: 224–246 prescriptions. Quintile 5: 246–331 prescriptions [13].

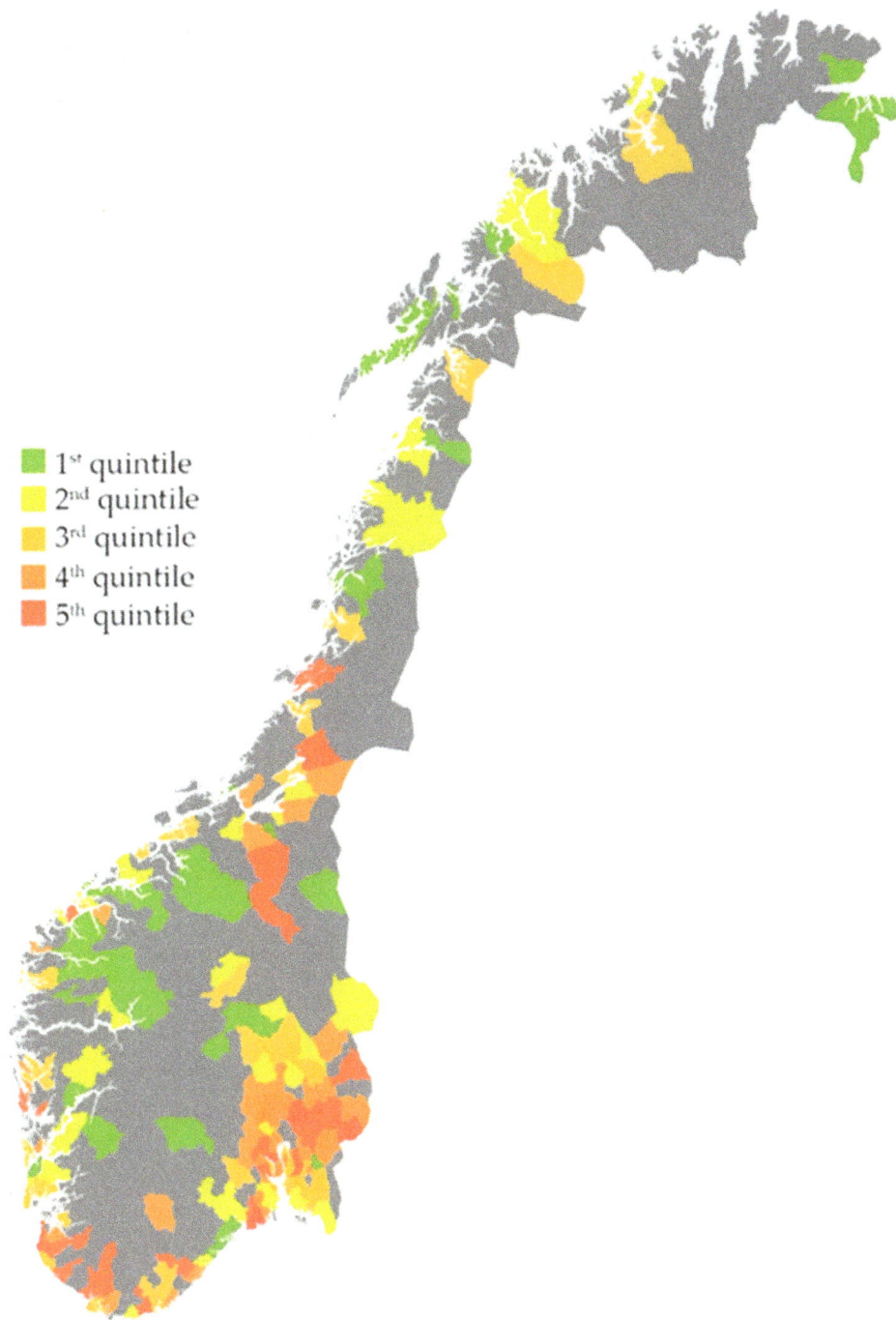

Figure 2. RTI consultations per 1000 inhabitants in 198 Norwegian municipalities. Quintile 1: 158–263 consultations. Quintile 2: 266–293 consultations. Quintile 3: 294–314 consultations. Quintile 4: 315–344 consultations. Quintile 5: 344–412 consultations [13].

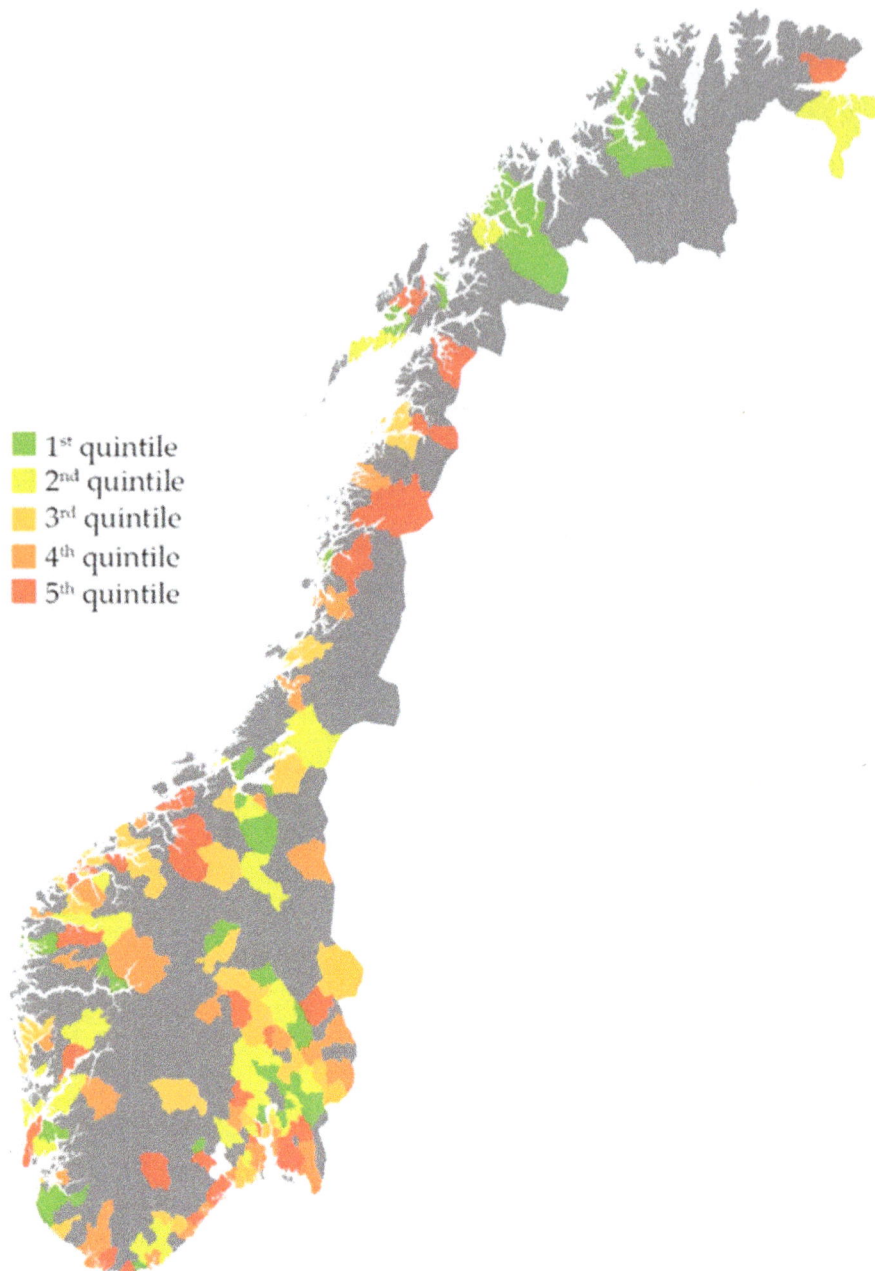

Figure 3. RTI antibiotic prescriptions per 1000 RTI consultations in 198 Norwegian municipalities. Quintile 1: 271–634 prescriptions per 1000 RTI consultations. Quintile 2: 636–688 prescriptions per 1000 RTI consultations. Quintile 3: 688–736 prescriptions per 1000 RTI consultations. Quintile 4: 738–792 prescriptions per 1000 RTI consultations. Quintile 5: 793–1146 prescriptions per 1000 RTI consultations [13].

3. Discussion

3.1. Main Findings

Our study demonstrates that at a municipality level, inhabitants' consultation rates and GPs' prescription rates were almost equally associated with the number of RTI antibiotics prescribed.

3.2. Strengths

A municipality with less than 5000 inhabitants may be served by only a few GPs in Norway. By excluding such municipalities our aim was to reduce bias from doctors with markedly different prescription behaviour. Data were collected from national registries and covered more than 66% of the Norwegian population. In NorPD, the number of registered prescriptions is linked to the dispensing of a prescription from a pharmacy, thereby avoiding bias from delayed prescriptions that are not dispensed. In KUHR, the number and types of consultations that are registered are linked to reimbursements to health care providers. The financial incentives by reporting is high and we therefore assume that the numbers form KUHR are realistic.

3.3. Limitations

This study has some limitations. Data on consultations are collected from primary care (GP offices, A&Es), while data on prescriptions include all prescriptions dispensed outside institutions, including prescriptions from outpatient clinics or from specialist practices. A Danish study has shown that GPs prescribe about 75% of all antibiotic prescriptions dispensed at pharmacies [14]. Although GPs prescribe most antibiotics, our study does not adjust for geographic variation in density of specialists, which is therefore an unmeasured confounder in the study. The indication or diagnosis leading to a prescription is not registered in NorPD. We have linked RTI antibiotics with RTI consultations based on predefined ICPC-2 codes and ATC codes. This limiting of antibiotics included by use of predefined codes may have introduced bias. The method is vulnerable because antibiotics commonly indicated for RTIs have other indications, for example skin infections and sexually transmittable infections. We have not included telephone consultations or reiterations of prescriptions. Due to these factors, the calculated antibiotic prescription rate in our study is considerably higher than what is found when exploring electronic patient records from Norwegian general practice [15]. Our data are grouped on a municipality level. The results of the study therefore provide limited insight to the behaviour of individual GPs or patients. Furthermore, we did not include patient comorbidity as a confounding variable.

Moreover, this study does not address factors that affect health seeking behaviour or GP prescription behaviour in a municipality. Such factors are demonstrated to include the travel distance to the health care provider, socio-economic status, cultural differences in disease coping strategies and attitudes towards using antibiotics among inhabitants, as well as characteristics of the GP practice [16–18]. Studies have also demonstrated the association between overuse of antibiotics and increased patient re-attendance, leading to more prescriptions of antibiotics [19]. In our model, the variables are adjusted, so that the IRR is the mutual importance of prescription rates and consultation rates. Our model does not, however, identify which patients are frequently consulting primary care and which doctors are high prescribers. We have merely studied the effect of consultation rates and GPs' prescription rates in themselves, regardless of factors that explain them. Despite these limitations we believe the results are useful and realistic when comparing to what degree consultation rates and prescription rates contribute to differences in antibiotic consumption in different municipalities.

3.4. Comparison with Existing Literature

Previous Norwegian studies report that RTI consultations comprise 11.7–15.0% of all consultations in primary care [15,20]. Our study finds lower consultation rates for RTIs with a share of 10.3% of all consultations. Furthermore, the share of RTI prescriptions has been reported as 51.3–57.7% of all dispensed antibiotic prescriptions in Norway [21,22]. This is in line with our findings of RTI prescriptions comprising 49.9% of all dispensed antibiotic prescriptions.

From 1994 to 2000 the number of antibiotic prescriptions for RTIs in British primary care was almost cut by half. In the same period, doctors had become more restrictive prescribers but a more important explanation to the reduction was that the population less often sought medical attention for

RTIs [11,12]. Our results are in line with this; not only chronological variations but also geographical variations, can to a large extent be explained by variations in health seeking behaviour.

A recently published study has investigated the characteristics of patients consulting their GPs for suspected RTIs. These same characteristics did not seem to affect the doctor's subsequent decision to prescribe antibiotics [23]. Patients report that the most important reasons to attend their GP include symptom relief and assurance, not necessarily an antibiotic prescription [24]. These findings stress that patients attending their GP with a suspected RTI are not necessarily the patients with most benefit of antibiotics.

It has been said that the most important risk factor for receiving an unnecessary antibiotic prescription is consulting a doctor [25]. In our opinion, patients' health seeking behaviours have been underappreciated, both as an explanation and a factor affecting the large number of unnecessary antibiotic prescriptions made in primary care.

4. Materials and Methods

4.1. Data Collection

The number of antibiotic prescriptions were collected from The Norwegian Prescription Database (NorPD) [26]. NorPD at the Norwegian Institute of Public Health monitors all drugs dispensed by prescription outside institutions (hospitals, nursing homes) in Norway. The number of primary care consultations were collected from the Directorate of Health's system for control and payment of health reimbursements (KUHR) registry [27]. The KUHR registry is a national database collecting data on the number and types of consultations as a part of the reimbursement system for health care providers. Population statistics including age and gender were collected from Statistics Norway (SSB) [28]. All data were on a municipality level and from 2014.

4.2. Inclusion and Exclusion Criteria

A total of 428 municipalities existed in Norway in 2014 [29], with a median number of inhabitants of 4600. In small municipalities, there may be long travel distances to pharmacies and GP offices and A&Es may provide patients with antibiotics directly. Such consumptions are not registered in NorPD. To ensure data validity and avoid missing numbers, only municipalities with 5000 inhabitants or more in 2014 were included ($n = 202$). The four largest municipalities (Oslo, Bergen, Trondheim, Stavanger) were excluded from the study because we expected a higher share of private health care providers from which data on consultations are not registered in KUHR. A total of 198 municipalities were included in the study.

4.3. Variable Definition

Age was categorised as early childhood (0–9 years), late childhood and adolescence (10–19 years), young adults (20–29 years), adult and early retirement age (30–79 years) and late retirement age (>80 years). A primary care consultation was defined as either an appointment at a GP office, a home visit or a consultation at an A&E unit. A consultation for an RTI was defined as a consultation registered with one of the following International Classification of Primary Care 2 (ICPC-2) codes: R01–05, R07–29, R71, R72, R74, R75, R76, R77, R78, R80, R81, R82, R83, H01, H71, H72, H74 (Table 4) [30]. This is the same definition as has been used in earlier research on RTIs in Norwegian ambulatory care [31]. Antibiotics with RTIs as the presumed most frequent indication were defined as an RTI antibiotic (Table 5). Inhabitants' consultation rates for RTIs were defined as the number of RTI consultations per 1000 inhabitants per year. GPs' prescription rates for RTIs were defined as the number of antibiotic prescriptions for treatment of RTI per 1000 RTI consultations per year.

Table 4. International Classification of Primary Care 2 (ICPC-2) codes and corresponding descriptions.

ICPC-2 Code	Description
R01	Pain respiratory system
R02	Shortness of breath/dyspnoea
R03	Wheezing
R04	Breathing problem, other
R05	Cough
R07	Sneezing/nasal congestion
R08	Nose symptom/complaint other
R09	Sinus symptom/complaint
R21	Throat symptom/complaint
R23	Voice symptom/complaint
R24	Haemoptysis
R25	Sputum/phlegm abnormal
R26	Fear of cancer respiratory system
R27	Fear of respiratory disease, other
R28	Limited function/disability (r)
R29	Respiratory symptom/complaint, other
R71	Whooping cough
R72	Strep throat
R74	Upper respiratory infection acute
R75	Sinusitis acute/chronic
R76	Tonsillitis acute
R77	Laryngitis/tracheitis acute
R78	Acute bronchitis/bronchiolitis
R80	Influenza
R81	Pneumonia
R82	Pleurisy/pleural effusion
R83	Respiratory infection other
H01	Ear pain/earache
H71	Acute otitis media/myringitis
H72	Serous otitis media
H74	Chronic otitis media

Table 5. Classification of antibiotic prescriptions by Anatomical Therapeutic Chemical (ATC)-codes.

ICPC-2 Code	Description
J01AA02	Doxycycline
J01CA04	Amoxicillin
J01CE02	Phenoxymethylpenicillin
J01FA	Macrolides

4.4. Missing Data

SSB contained no missing data. In NorPD, to ensure anonymity of inhabitants in a municipality, data was reported as missing if the number of prescriptions were less than 5 for a given age and gender group. This resulted in 0.15% of data reported as missing for RTI prescriptions. 6.11% of data were missing for RTI consultations.

4.5. Modelling

We have used a mixed Poisson regression model to evaluate the effect of age, gender, GPs' prescription rates and inhabitants' consultation rates on the outcome of interest, which was RTI antibiotic prescriptions per 1000 inhabitants. Different age groups show varying consumption rates of antibiotics (Table 1). To account for this, inhabitants' consultation rates and GPs' prescription rates were categorised by age and gender adjusted quintiles before being included in the model. Quintiles were chosen as fewer groups would provide less accuracy and additional groups would make the calculations extensive. A mixed model was used to account for the clustering of data on a municipality level. The two software packages used for analysis were Microsoft Excel for Windows version 14, IBM SPSS Statistics for Windows version 22.0 and STATA/SE version 14.1 for Windows.

4.6. Ethics

Data was collected from national registries. The raw data set contained the total number of persons, prescriptions and consultations for each gender and age group per municipality. The data was not linked to personal identification numbers. Furthermore, if the number of consultations or prescriptions for a given age and gender group was less than 5, the registry described this number as anonymous. As all data were anonymous and aggregated, no study approval was applied for.

5. Conclusions

Inhabitants' consultation rates and GPs' prescription rates have an almost equally strong association with differences in antibiotic consumption between Norwegian municipalities. Our study highlights the importance of targeting both patients and doctors in efforts to reduce unnecessary antibiotic prescriptions in primary care.

Acknowledgments: The authors would like to thank Ibrahimu Mdala at the Antibiotic Centre for Primary Care, University of Oslo for statistical analysis and Hege Salvesen Blix, at the Norwegian Institute of Public Health for comments and aid in draft revisions. We also wish to acknowledge the services of the NorPD, KUHR registry and Norway Statistics.

Author Contributions: For research articles with several authors, a short paragraph specifying their individual contributions must be provided. The following statements should be used "S.H. conceived and designed the experiments; S.H. and M.M.W.-H. performed the experiments; S.H. and M.M.W.-H. analyzed the data; S.H. and M.M.W.-H. contributed reagents/materials/analysis tools; S.H. and M.M.W.-H. wrote the paper".

References

1. Goossens, H.; Ferech, M.; Stichele, R.V.; Elseviers, M.; Grp, E.P. Outpatient antibiotic use in Europe and association with resistance: A cross-national database study. *Lancet* **2005**, *365*, 579–587. [CrossRef]
2. Thapa, B. Antimicrobial resistance: A global threat. Available online: https://www.nepjol.info/index.php/IJIM/article/view/7405/5998 (accessed on 15 January 2017).
3. Usage of Antimicrobial Agents and Occurrence of Antimicrobial Resistance in Norway. Available online: https://unn.no/Documents/Kompetansetjenester,%20-sentre%20og%20fagr%C3%A5d/NORM%20-%20Norsk%20overv%C3%A5kingssystem%20for%20antibiotikaresistens%20hos%20mikrober/Rapporter/NORM_NORM-VET_2016.pdf (accessed on 6 January 2017).
4. WHO Collaborating Centre for Drug Statistics Methodology NIoPH. Definition and General Considerations. Available online: https://www.whocc.no/ddd/definition_and_general_considera/ (accessed on 15 January 2017).
5. Sundsfjord, A.; Simonsen, G.S. Antibiotikaresistens. Available online: http://www.antibiotikaiallmennpraksis.no/index.php?action=showtopic&topic=bytMNets&j=1 (accessed on 5 May 2017).
6. Van der Velden, A.W.; Pijpers, E.J.; Kuyvenhoven, M.M.; Tonkin-Crine, S.K.; Little, P.; Verheij, T.J. Effectiveness of physician-targeted interventions to improve antibiotic use for respiratory tract infections. *Br. J. Gen. Pract.* **2012**, *62*, e801–e807. [CrossRef] [PubMed]
7. Adriaenssens, N.; Coenen, S.; Versporten, A.; Muller, A.; Minalu, G.; Faes, C.; Vankerckhoven, V.; Aerts, M.; Hens, N.; Molenberghs, G.; et al. European Surveillance of Antimicrobial Consumption (ESAC): Outpatient antibiotic use in Europe (1997–2009). *J. Antimicrob. Chemother.* **2011**, *66*. [CrossRef] [PubMed]
8. Deschepper, R.; Grigoryan, L.; Lundborg, C.S.; Hofstede, G.; Cohen, J.; Kelen, G.V.; Deliens, L.; Haaijer-Ruskamp, F.M. Are cultural dimensions relevant for explaining cross-national differences in antibiotic use in Europe? *BMC Health Serv. Res.* **2008**, *8*. [CrossRef] [PubMed]
9. Helsenorge.no. Forekomst av Antibiotikabehandling. Available online: https://helsenorge.no/Kvalitetsindikatorer/legemidler/forekomst-av-antibiotikabehandling (accessed on 6 January 2017).
10. Haugen, P.; Skov Simonsen, G.; Primicerio, R.; Furberg, A.S.; Smabrekke, L. Antibiotics to outpatients in Norway-Assessing effect of latitude and municipality population size using quantile regression in a cross-sectional study. *Pharm. Stat.* **2017**, *17*, 4–11. [CrossRef] [PubMed]

11. Ashworth, M.; Latinovic, R.; Charlton, J.; Cox, K.; Rowlands, G.; Gulliford, M. Why has antibiotic prescribing for respiratory illness declined in primary care? A longitudinal study using the General Practice Research Database. *J. Public Health* **2004**, *26*, 268–274. [CrossRef] [PubMed]

12. Fleming, D.M.; Ross, A.M.; Cross, K.W.; Kendall, H. The reducing incidence of respiratory tract infection and its relation to antibiotic prescribing. *Br. J. Gen. Pract.* **2003**, *53*, 778–783. [PubMed]

13. Norway_Municipalities_2010_blank.svg: Kåre-Olav Derivative Work: Røed. Available online: https://creativecommons.org/licenses/by-sa/2.0 (accessed on 27 February 2018).

14. Aabenhus, R.; Siersma, V.; Hansen, M.P.; Bjerrum, L. Antibiotic prescribing in Danish general practice 2004–2013. *J. Antimicrob. Chemother.* **2016**, *71*, 2286–2294. [CrossRef] [PubMed]

15. Gjelstad, S.; Straand, J.; Dalen, I.; Fetveit, A.; Strom, H.; Lindbaek, M. Do general practitioners' consultation rates influence their prescribing patterns of antibiotics for acute respiratory tract infections? *J. Antimicrob. Chemother.* **2011**, *66*, 2425–2433. [CrossRef] [PubMed]

16. Wang, K.Y.; Seed, P.; Schofield, P.; Ibrahim, S.; Ashworth, M. Which practices are high antibiotic prescribers? *A cross-sectional analysis. Br. J. Gen. Pract.* **2009**, *59*, e315–e320. [CrossRef] [PubMed]

17. Raknes, G.; Morken, T.; Hunskar, S. Travel distance and the utilisation of out-of-hours services. *J. Nor. Med. Assoc.* **2014**, *134*, 2151–2155.

18. Deschepper, R.; Vander Stichele, R.H.; Haaijer-Ruskamp, F.M. Cross-cultural differences in lay attitudes and utilisation of antibiotics in a Belgian and a Dutch city. *Patient Educ. Couns.* **2002**, *48*, 161–169. [CrossRef]

19. Little, P.; Gould, C.; Williamson, I.; Warner, G.; Gantley, M.; Kinmonth, A.L. Reattendance and complications in a randomised trial of prescribing strategies for sore throat: The medicalising effect of prescribing antibiotics. *BMJ* **1997**, *315*, 350–352. [CrossRef] [PubMed]

20. Grimsmo, A.; Hagman, E.; Faikø, E.; Matthiessen, L.; Njálsson, T. Patients, diagnoses and processes in general practice in the Nordic countries. An attempt to make data from computerised medical records available for comparable statistics. *Scand. J. Prim. Health Care* **2001**, *19*, 76–82. [PubMed]

21. Straand, J.; Rokstad, K.S.; Sandvik, H. Prescribing systemic antibiotics in general practice: A report from the M re & Romsdal Prescription Study. *Scand. J. Prim. Health Care* **1998**, *16*, 121–127. [PubMed]

22. Gjelstad, S.; Dalen, I.; Lindbæk, M. GPs' antibiotic prescription patterns for respiratory tract infections—Still room for improvement. *Scand. J. Prim. Health Care* **2009**, *27*, 208–215. [CrossRef] [PubMed]

23. Mehta, N.; Schilder, A.; Fragaszy, E.; E R Evans, H.; Dukes, O.; Manikam, L.; Little, P.; Smith, S.C.; Hayward, A. Antibiotic prescribing in patients with self-reported sore throat. *J. Antimicrob. Chemother.* **2016**, *72*, 914–922. [CrossRef] [PubMed]

24. McNulty, C.A.; Nichols, T.; French, D.P.; Joshi, P.; Butler, C.C. Expectations for consultations and antibiotics for respiratory tract infection in primary care: The RTI clinical iceberg. *Br. J. Gen. Pract.* **2013**, *63*, e429–e436. [CrossRef] [PubMed]

25. Høye, S. Don't ask your doctor. *J. Nor. Med. Assoc.* **2014**, *134*, 1341.

26. The Norwegian Prescription Database. About the Norwegian Prescription Database. Available online: http://www.norpd.no/Viktig.aspx (accessed on 6 January 2017).

27. The Norwegian Ministry of Health and Care Services. *Proposition 106 L—Changes in the Personal Health Data Filing System Act and other regulations (Municipal Patient and User Registry) [TNMoHaC. Prop. 106 L—Endringer i Helseregisterloven m.m. (Kommunalt Pasient- og Brukerregister m.m.)]*; The Norwegian Ministry of Health and Care Services: Oslo, Norway, 2015.

28. Statistics Norway. About Us. Available online: http://ssb.no/en/omssb/om-oss (accessed on 6 January 2017).

29. Store Norske Leksikon. Kommuner i Norge. Available online: https://snl.no/Kommuner_i_Norge (accessed on 6 January 2017).

30. WHO (World Health Organization). *International Classification of Primary Care*, 2nd ed.; Oxford University Press: Oxford, UK, 1998.

31. Gjelstad, S.; Hoye, S.; Straand, J.; Brekke, M.; Dalen, I.; Lindbaek, M. Improving antibiotic prescribing in acute respiratory tract infections: Cluster randomised trial from Norwegian general practice (prescription peer academic detailing (Rx-PAD) study). *BMJ* **2013**, *347*, f4403. [CrossRef] [PubMed]

9

Reevaluation of the Acute Cystitis Symptom Score, a Self-Reporting Questionnaire: Patient-Reported Outcome Assessment

Jakhongir F. Alidjanov [1,2] ⓘD, Kurt G. Naber [3,*,†], Ulugbek A. Abdufattaev [1], Adrian Pilatz [2] and Florian M. Wagenlehner [2]

[1]   State Institution "Republican Specialized Scientific-Practical Medical Center of Urology", Tashkent 100109, Uzbekistan; jakhonghir@hotmail.com (J.F.A.); abdufattaev@gmail.com (U.A.A.)

[2]   Clinic of Urology, Pediatric Urology, and Andrology, Justus Liebig University, 35392 Giessen, Germany; pilatz@t-online.de (A.P.); Florian.Wagenlehner@chiru.med.uni-giessen.de (F.M.W.)

[3]   Department of Urology, School of Medicine, Technical University of Munich, 80333 Munich, Germany

*   Correspondence: kurt@nabers.de

†   Current address: Karl-Bickleder-Str. 44c, 94315 Straubing, Germany.

Abstract: This study aimed to reevaluate the Acute Cystitis Symptom Score (ACSS). The ACSS is a self-reporting questionnaire for the clinical diagnosis of acute uncomplicated cystitis (AC) and the assessment of symptomatic changes after therapy in female patients with AC. The part II of the present study was to reevaluate the utility of the different domains of the ACSS after therapy. The applicability of these domains in assessing changes in symptoms, as a function of time, in this population was investigated. The ACSS was evaluated in 48 female patients (mean age 31.1 ± 10.6) in the Uzbek and Russian languages, who returned after therapy and filled in part B of the ACSS, which corresponds to part A with the additional "Dynamics" domain. Descriptive statistics were used, where suitable. The reduction of typical symptoms and quality of life assessment between first and follow-up visit correlated significantly with answers in the "Dynamics" domain. *Success/Cure* and *Non-success/Failure* could be clearly differentiated by the scores obtained in "Typical" and "Quality of Life" domains. The ACSS has proven to be a useful instrument to clinically diagnose AC in women. It is also a suitable instrument for patient-reported outcome measures, with applicability both in daily practice and clinical studies. Slight modifications in the "Dynamics" domain will even increase the applicability.

Keywords: cystitis; female; quality of life; urinary tract infection; Acute Cystitis Symptom Score; questionnaire; patient-reported outcome

1. Introduction

The Acute Cystitis Symptom Score (ACSS) was developed and validated as a simple and self-reporting questionnaire for diagnosing acute uncomplicated cystitis (AC) in female patients by assessing typical and differential symptoms, quality of life, and additional health conditions, which may play an important role in such a clinical setting. The evaluation in 286 women in Uzbek and Russian languages, which also included the results of the 58 women in whom the preliminary slightly different questionnaire: Urinary Symptoms and the Quality of Life Assessment Tool (USQOLAT), was applied, has been published earlier [1,2]. Part I of the report on the evaluation of the 228 women in whom only the current ACSS in Uzbek and Russian language was applied, deals mainly with the diagnostics of AC [3]. The studies were performed in Uzbekistan. Although Uzbek is the official language, Russian as the second language remains in widespread use, with the majority of the population speaking both languages. Both evaluations revealed significant differences in the scores in the domain with typical symptoms and with the quality of life between female patients with AC and controls. As an optimal threshold to predict AC, a total score of six points in the domain of typical symptoms can be established. In part of the patients, a follow-up visit was performed. The overall symptom score decreased significantly when comparing before and after therapy [1,2].

The present study refers to the subgroup of 48 female patients with AC, in whom part A (first visit) and part B (follow-up visit) of the current ACSS in Uzbek and Russian languages were applied, because they also participated in a follow up visit, to study in more detail the suitability of the ACSS as a practical instrument for patient-reported outcome assessment.

2. Patients and Methods

2.1. Clinical Procedures

The development of the ACSS and the total study population were described earlier in details [3]. A subgroup of 48 patients (mean age 31.10, standard deviation 10.64, range 19–63) who returned to a follow-up visit was also asked to fill in the part B (follow-up form) of the ACSS (Supplementary Figures S1 and S2). All participants signed written informed consent before filling in the questionnaire. Data from filled-in paper-form questionnaires were then recorded in an electronic form using PC software specially developed for the purpose of recording, storing, and processing inputted data (e-USQOLAT). Besides medical history and clinical evaluation in all patients, microscopic analysis of the urinary sediment and urine culture were performed at the first visit. Otherwise, the study was performed under conditions of clinical practice, where no specific treatment modalities and follow up visits were required to be included in the study.

At the follow-up visit, the patients were asked to fill in the follow-up part (part B) of the ACSS containing the same questions as the diagnostic part (part A) in the domains of typical and differential symptoms, quality of life, and additional health conditions. In addition, part B includes a domain "Dynamics" with five questions concerning overall evolution and changes of the symptomatology (Table 1). During the follow-up visit in 42/48 (87.5%) patients in addition to clinical evaluation also microscopic urinalysis was performed, whereas urine culture was performed only to the physician's discretion, e.g., in case of treatment failure.

Table 1. Answers from 48 female patients at follow-up visit in the "Dynamics" domain of part B of the Acute Cystitis Symptom Score (ACSS) Questionnaire.

Score	Answer	Follow-Up Visit n = 48 (100%)
0	Yes, I feel myself great better (All symptoms went off)	12 (25.0%)
1	Yes, I feel myself much better (Majority of symptoms were solved)	26 (54.2%)
2	Yes, I feel myself somewhat better (Some symptoms are remaining)	8 (16.7%)
3	No changes, I feel about the same (All symptoms are remaining)	2 (4.2%)
4	Yes, I feel worse (My condition is declining)	0 (0.0%)

2.2. Statistical Analysis

Ordinary descriptive statistics were used for demographic characteristics of the study respondents. Calculation of Cronbach's alpha [4] was used for assessment of internal consistency for the part B of the ACSS. Nonparametric Wilcoxon's signed rank test [5] was used for comparative analysis of variables for related samples and parametric paired t-test was used for a reassessment of statistical significance [6]. Means and 95% confidence intervals were calculated. A p-value equal or lower than 0.05 was considered statistically significant. Substantive significance (effect size) was estimated by the modified correlation coefficient (r) proposed by Rosenthal and Rosnow [7] using Z value retrieved from the Wilcoxon's signed-rank test. IBM SPSS for Windows, Version 22.0 (IBM Corp., Armonk, NY, USA) was used for statistical analysis and graphical presentations of the results.

3. Results

3.1. Study Population

Of a total of 107 patients with AC, 48 (44.9%) had a subsequent follow-up visit after 5.08 ± 2.71 (range 3–18; median 4.00; IQR (IQR—interquartile range) (3.25–6.00) days of therapy. The Uzbek Cyrillic version of the ACSS was filled in by 38/48 (79.2%) of the patients. The remaining 10/48 patients (20.8%) filled in the Russian version. The mean (SD) age of the patients was 31.1 (10.6) years; range 19 to 63 years; nine (18.8%) of them were pregnant. During the follow-up visit, 42 of the (87.5%) 48 subjects had a microscopic urinalysis performed. However, urine culture was done at the physician's discretion.

3.2. Dynamics

The responses of the 48 female patients treated for AC in the "Dynamics" domain at the follow-up visit (ACSS part B) are shown in Table 1. All symptoms went off in 12 (25.0%); the majority of symptoms went off in 26 (52.2%); some symptoms still remained in 8 (16.7%), and all symptoms remained in two (4.2%) patients. In none of the patients, the condition declined.

3.3. Reliability of the Follow-Up form of the ACSS

Internal consistency of the follow-up form of the ACSS, including the "Dynamics" domain, was 0.92 (95% CI: 0.89 to 0.95). Values of internal consistency for ACSS "if item deleted" and item-total correlations are presented in Table 2.

Table 2. Values of current internal consistency, alpha 'if item deleted' and item-total correlations for ACSS items.

Items of the ACSS		Correlation Between Item and Entire ACSS	
	Dynamics	Dynamics	Cronbach's Alpha If Item Deleted
Typical	Frequency	0.83	0.91
Typical Differential	Urgency	0.62	0.92
	Painful urination	0.63	0.91
	Incomplete bladder emptying	0.77	0.91
	Suprapubic pain	0.63	0.91
	Visible blood in urine	0.80	0.91
	Flank pain	0.40	0.92
Differential Quality of Life (QoL)	Vaginal discharge	0.52	0.93
	Urethral discharge	0.19	0.93
	Feeling of chill/fever	0.40	0.92
	General discomfort	0.40	0.92
QoL	Impairment of everyday activity	0.82	0.91
	Impairment of social activity	0.86	0.91

Current Cronbach's alpha = 0.92 (95% CI: 0.89 to 0.95).

3.4. ACSS Scores at First and Follow-Up Visits

In Table 3, the mean scores and 95% confidence intervals (CI), effect sizes correlation coefficient (r) of the ACSS items, and subscales in 48 female patients at first and follow-up visits are presented. The scores of all ACSS items and subscales were significantly ($p < 0.05$) reduced from the first visit to the follow-up visit, except for "urethral discharge" in the "Differential" domain. Figure 1a–i shows the distributions of scores in the Typical Symptoms and the Quality of Life domains in 48 female patients with AC at the first and the follow-up visit.

Table 3. Mean scores and 95% confidence intervals (CI), effect sizes correlation coefficient (r) of ACSS items, and subscales in 48 female patients at first and follow-up visit.

ACSS Items		Mean Scores (95% CI)			p-Value	Effect Size r
		First Visit	Follow-Up Visit	Difference Between Scores		
Typical	Frequency	2.06 (1.82 to 2.31)	0.52 (0.29 to 0.75)	−1.68 (−1.94 to −1.42)	0.000	−0.82
	Urgency	2.02 (1.75 to 2.29)	0.46 (0.23 to 0.69)	−1.56 (−1.87 to −1.26)	0.000	−0.79
	Painful urination	2.29 (2.08 to 2.51)	0.46 (0.28 to 0.64)	−1.83 (−2.10 to −1.57)	0.000	−0.85
	Incomplete bladder emptying	1.92 (1.70 to 2.13)	0.44 (0.21 to 0.66)	−1.48 (−1.74 to −1.22)	0.000	−0.82
	Suprapubic pain	1.81 (1.58 to 2.05)	0.44 (0.25 to 0.63)	−1.38 (−1.63 to −1.12)	0.000	−0.82
	Visible blood in urine	0.71 (0.45 to 0.96)	0.15 (−0.02 to 0.32)	−0.56 (−0.84 to −0.29)	0.001	−0.50
Differential	Flank pain	1.27 (0.99 to 1.55)	0.60 (0.41 to 0.80)	−0.67 (−0.92 to −0.42)	0.000	−0.61
	Vaginal discharge	0.38 (0.18 to 0.57)	0.19 (0.03 to 0.34)	−0.19 (−0.33 to −0.05)	0.013	−0.36
	Urethral discharge	0.25 (0.10 to 0.40)	0.08 (0.00 to 0.16)	−0.17 (−0.34 to 0.01)	0.059	−0.27
	Feeling of chill/fever [a]	0.26 (0.09 to 0.43)	0.07 (−0.01 to 0.14)	−0.20 (−0.34 to −0.05)	0.014	−0.36
QoL	General discomfort	2.04 (1.86 to 2.22)	0.52 (0.30 to 0.74)	−1.52 (−1.78 to −1.26)	0.000	−0.82
	Impairment of everyday activity	1.88 (1.70 to 2.05)	0.50 (0.28 to 0.72)	−1.38 (−1.63 to −1.12)	0.000	−0.81
	Impairment of social activity	1.77 (1.57 to 1.97)	0.50 (0.28 to 0.72)	−1.27 (−1.52 to −1.03)	0.000	−0.80

ACSS Subscales	Mean total Scores and (95% CI)			p-Value	Effect Size r
	First Visit	Follow-Up Visit	Difference Between Scores		
"Main Symptoms" [b]	6.37 (5.85 to 6.90)	1.44 (0.90 to 1.98)	−4.94 (−5.56 to −4.31)	0.00	−0.86
"Five Typical Symptoms" [c]	10.10 (9.27 to 10.93)	2.31 (1.44 to 3.18)	−8.75 (−8.75 to −6.84)	0.00	0.86
"Typical"	10.81 (9.89 to 11.73)	2.46 (1.52 to 3.39)	−8.35 (−9.42 to 7.29)	0.00	−0.86
"Differential" [a]	2.13 (1.66 to 2.61)	0.85 (0.51 to 1.19)	−1.28 (−1.63 to −0.94)	0.00	−0.77
"Quality of Life (QoL)"	5.69 (5.21 to 6.17)	1.52 (0.87 to 2.17)	−4.17 (−4.86 to −3.47)	0.00	−0.82
"Typical" and "QoL"	16.50 (15.24 to 17.76)	3.98 (2.45 to 5.51)	−12.52 (−14.15 to −10.89)	0.00	−0.86
Total ACSS [a]	18.37 (16.97 to 19.77)	4.65 (2.93 to 6.37)	−13.72 (−15.46 to −11.98)	0.00	−0.86

[a] Based on sum of scores of 46 cases with non-missing values; [b] "Main Symptoms" include "Typical" 1-3: frequency, urgency, painful urination; [c] "Five Typical Symptoms" includes "Typical" with the exclusion of one symptom (visible blood in the urine).

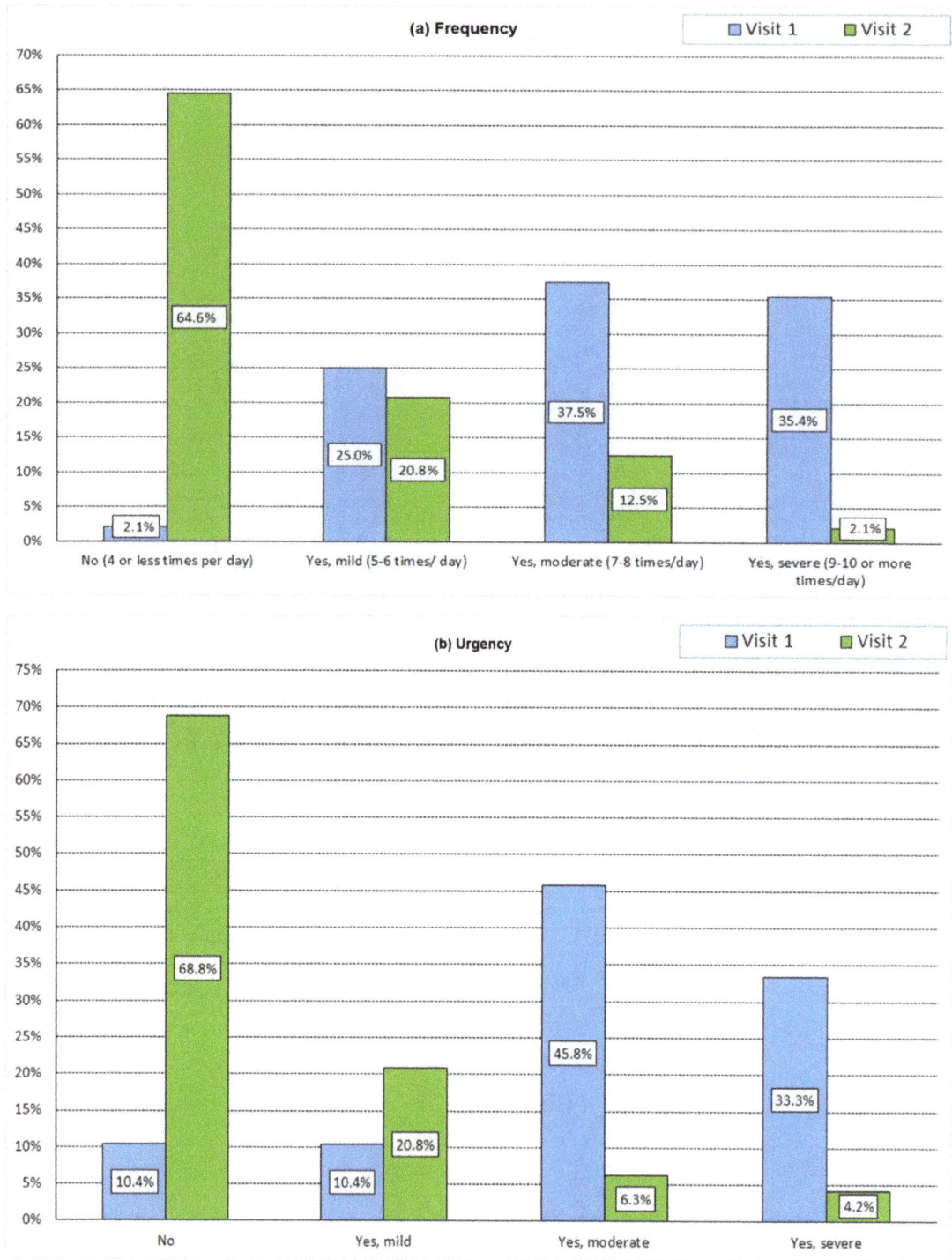

Figure 1. *Cont.*

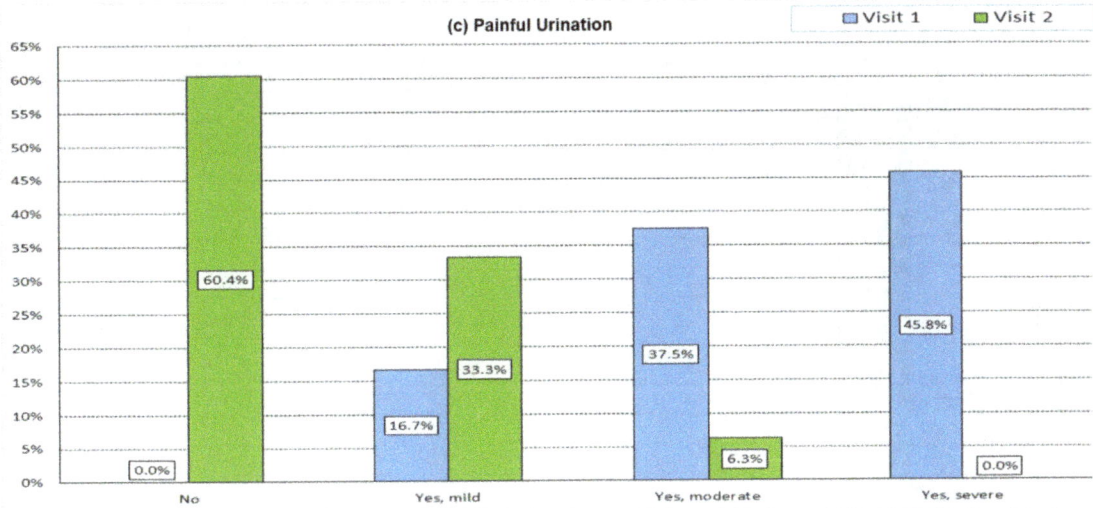

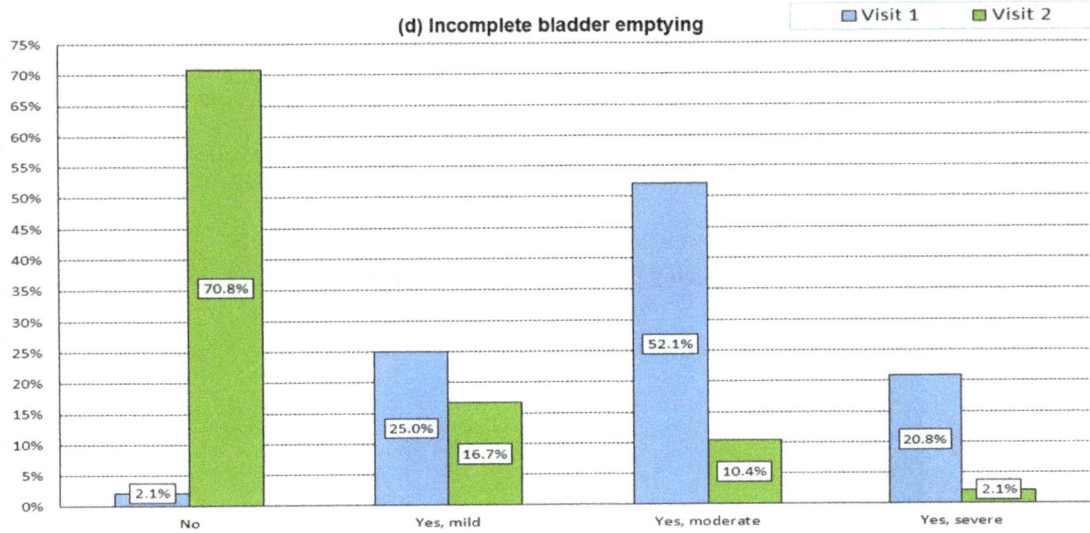

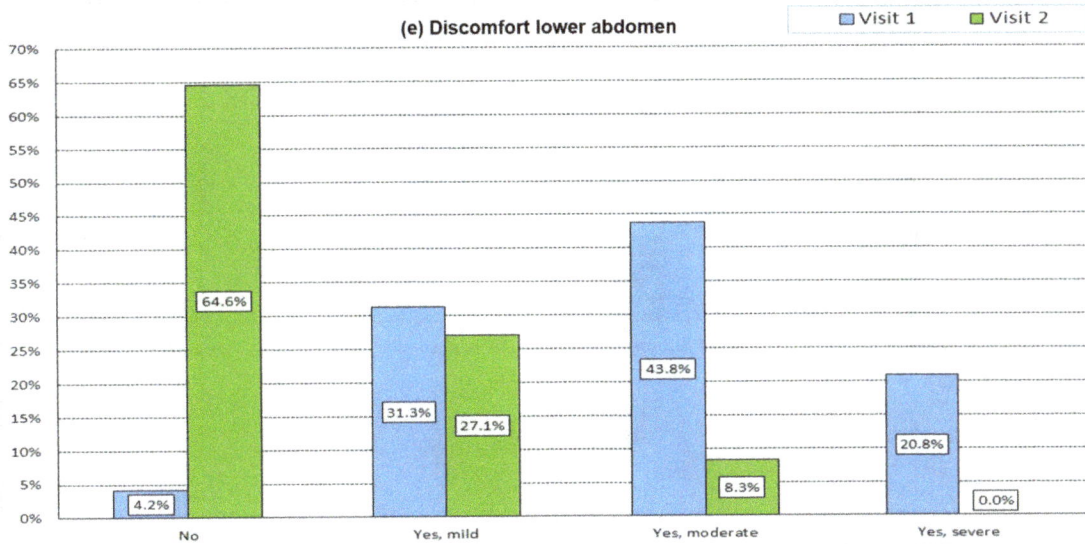

(c) Painful Urination

(d) Incomplete bladder emptying

(e) Discomfort lower abdomen

Figure 1. *Cont.*

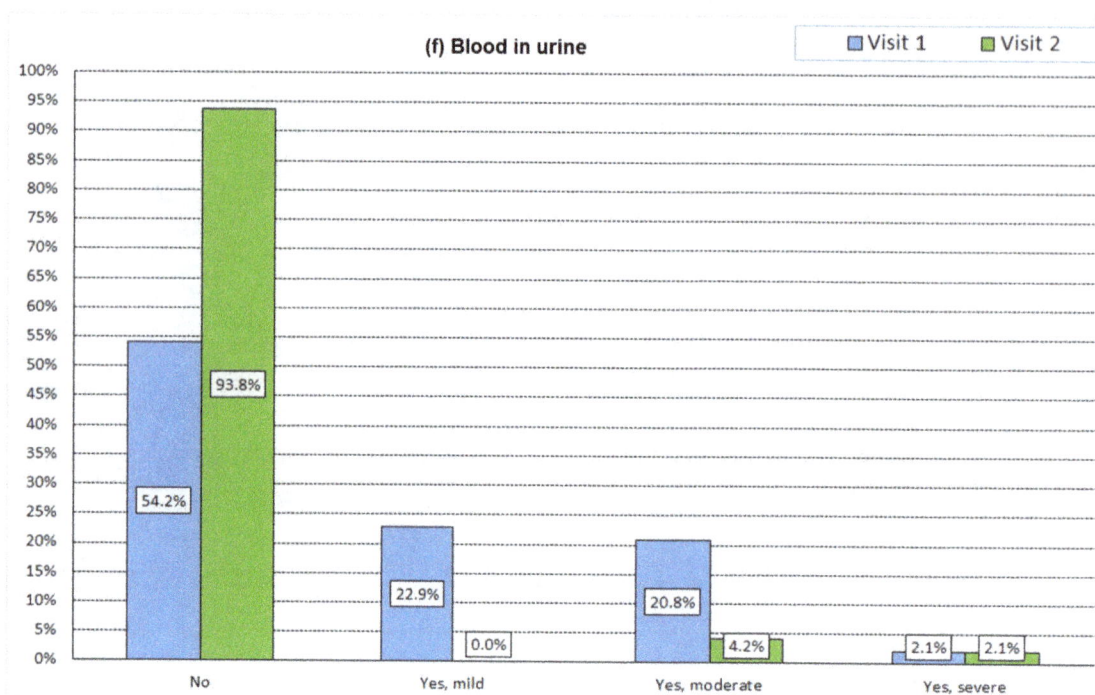

(f) Blood in urine

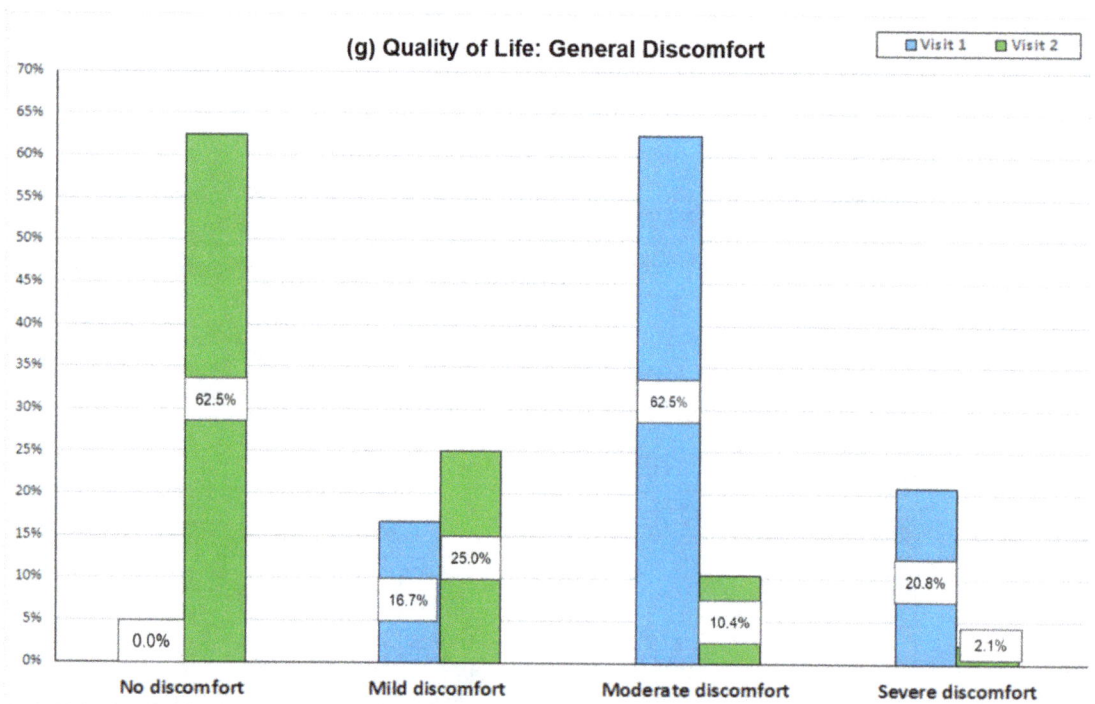

(g) Quality of Life: General Discomfort

Figure 1. *Cont.*

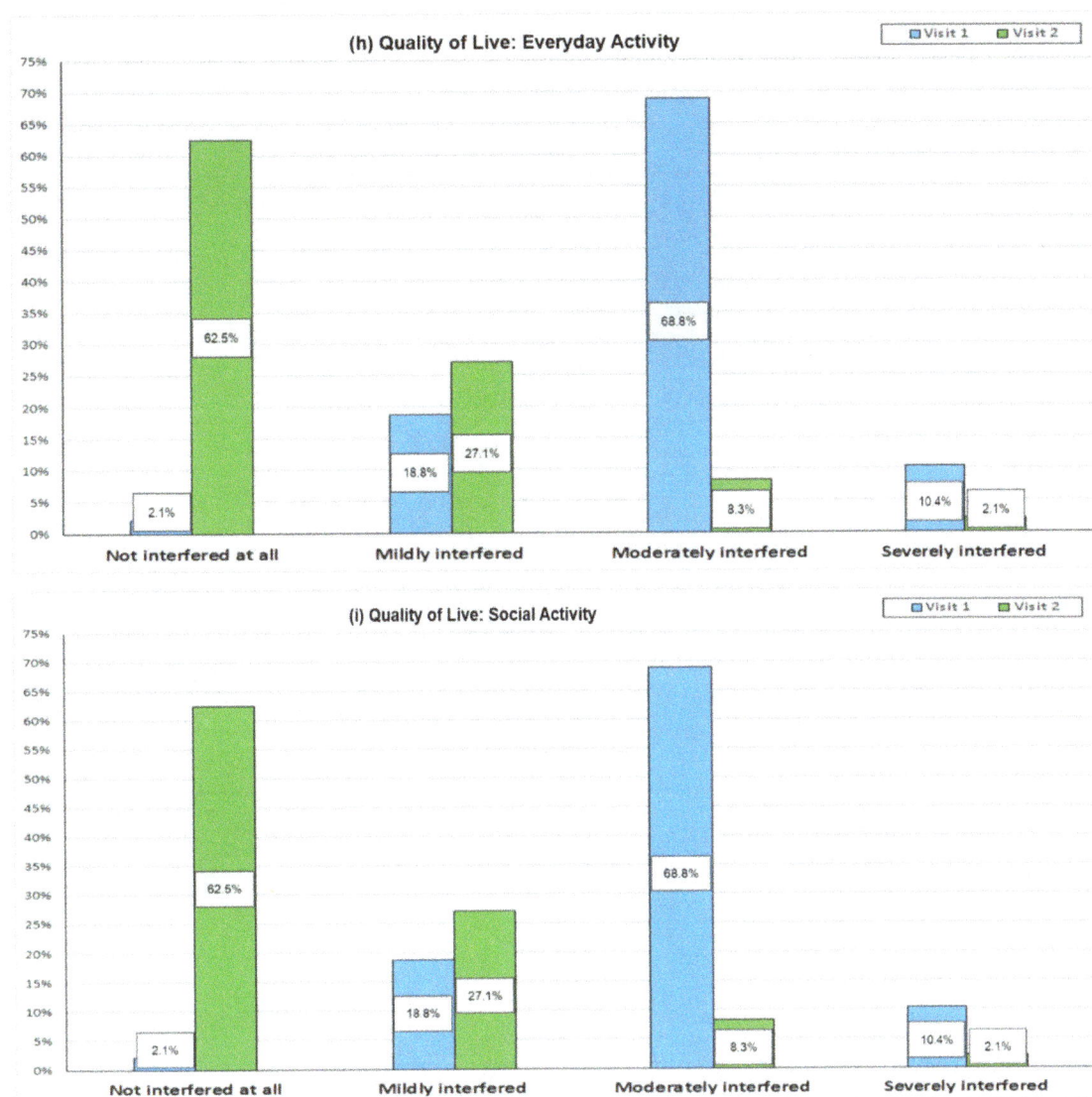

Figure 1. Distribution of scores at visit 1 and follow-up svisit in 48 female patients with AC. (**a**) Frequency; (**b**)Urgency; (**c**) Painful urination; (**d**) Incomplete bladder emptying; (**e**) Discomfort lower abdomen; (**f**) Blood in urine; (**g**) Quality of Life: General Discomfort; (**h**) Quality of Live: Everyday Activity; (**i**) Quality of Live: Social Activity.

3.5. Correlation between Symptom Scores and Outcome

The correlations between the differences of various symptom scores and scores in 'Dynamics' found in 48 female patients between first and follow-up visit are shown in Table 4. The correlations were statistically significant ($p < 0.05$, two-sided) for all typical symptoms (except frequency), quality of life and the corresponding subscales. There were, however, no significant correlations between the differences of scores in the 'Differential' domain, such as flank pain, vaginal discharge, urethral discharge, and feeling febrile, which can be expected because these symptoms are only used for differential diagnosis and not for the patient-reported outcome.

Table 4. Correlation between scores of "Dynamics" domain and differences in scores for ACSS items in 48 female patients between first and follow-up visit.

	ACSS Items	Spearman's Rho	p-Value [a]
Typical	Frequency	0.27	0.067
	Urgency	0.34	0.017
	Painful urination	0.4	0.005
	Incomplete bladder emptying	0.375	0.009
	Suprapubic pain	0.409	0.004
	Visible blood in urine	0.301	0.037
Differential [b]	Flank pain	0.079	0.594
	Vaginal discharge	0.061	0.682
	Urethral discharge	−0.059	0.689
	Feeling of chill/fever	0.088	0.563
QoL	General dyscomfort	0.581	0.000
	Impairment of everyday activity	0.613	0.000
	Impairment of social activity	0.499	0.000

Table 4. *Cont.*

ACSS Items	Spearman's Rho	p-Value [a]
Differences in scores for ACSS Subscales	Spearman's Rho	p
"Main Symptoms" [c]	0.435	0.002
"Five Typical Symptoms" [d]	0.514	0.000
"Typical"	0.508	0.000
"Differential"	0.152	0.312
"QoL"	0.606	0.000
"Typical" plus "QoL"	0.598	0.000
Total ACSS score	0.624	0.000

QoL-Quality of Life; [a] significant = $p \leq 0.05$; [b] Non-obligatory item "Hyperthermia" (Please indicate if measured) was not included into the analysis because majority of patients (60–95.2%) missed to check this item during their follow-up visit; [c] "Main Symptoms" include "Typical" 1–3; frequency, urgency, painful urination; [d] "Five Typical Symptoms" include "Typical" with the exclusion of one symptom (visible blood in the urine).

3.6. Clinical Outcome Categories

The scores of the specific ACSS items at the follow-up visit and the correlations of the "Typical" and its subgroups, "Main Symptoms'"and "Five Typical Symptoms," "Quality of Life," "Typical" plus "Quality of Life," and total ACSS domains with the scores of the "Dynamics" domain are shown in Table 5. The "Five Typical Symptoms" subscale of "Typical," although not used for diagnostics, was also tested here for the outcome, because the sixth symptom (visible blood in urine) of "Typical" is only typical in the minority of patients suffering from a specific hemorrhagic cystitis. The results showed statistically significant correlations between the scores of all specific items and the corresponding subscales (except visible blood in urine) as mentioned before with the scores of the "Dynamics" domain.

Table 5. Mean scores and 95% confidence intervals (CI) of ACSS items and subscales in 48 female patients according to scores of the "Dynamics" domain at the follow up visit.

ACSS Items		Mean Scores (95% CI)					p-Value
		Total	Dynamics = 0	Dynamics = 1	Dynamics = 2	Dynamics = 3	Dynamics
		n = 48	n = 12	n = 26	n = 8	n = 2	0 + 1 vs. 2 + 3
Typical	Frequency	0.52 (0.29 to 0.75)	0.00 (constant)	0.46 (0.20 to 0.72)	1.38 (0.49 to 2.26)	1.00 (−11.71 to 13.71)	0.008
	Urgency	0.46 (0.23 to 0.69)	0.00 (constant)	0.35 (0.15 to 0.54)	1.13 (−0.01 to 2.26)	2.00 (constant)	0.018
	Painful urination	0.46 (0.28 to 0.64)	0.00 (constant)	0.35 (0.15 to 0.54)	1.13 (0.83 to 1.42)	2.00 (constant)	0.000
	Incomplete bladder emptying	0.44 (0.21 to 0.66)	0.00 (constant)	0.35 (0.12 to 0.57)	1.00 (0.00 to 2.00)	2.00 (constant)	0.018
	Suprapubic pain	0.44 (0.25 to 0.63)	0.00 (constant)	0.35 (0.12 to 0.57)	1.13 (0.59 to 1.66)	1.50 (−4.85 to 7.85)	0.000
	Visible blood in urine	0.15 (−0.02 to 0.32)	0.00 (constant)	0.00 (constant)	0.63 (−0.37 to 1.62)	1.00 (−11.71 to 13.71)	0.154
QoL	General discomfort	0.52 (0.30 to 0.74)	0.00 (constant)	0.38 (0.15 to 0.62)	1.50 (0.73 to 2.27)	1.50 (−4.85 to 7.85)	0.000
	Impairment of everyday activity	0.50 (0.28 to 0.72)	0.00 (constant)	0.35 (0.12 to 0.57)	1.50 (0.87 to 2.13)	1.50 (−4.85 to 7.85)	0.000
	Impairment of social activity	0.50 (0.28 to 0.72)	0.00 (constant)	0.35 (0.12 to 0.57)	1.50 (0.87 to 2.13)	1.50 (−4.85 to 7.85)	0.000
ACSS subscales		Mean scores (95% CI)					
"Main Symptoms" [a]		1.44 (0.90 to 1.98)	0.00 (constant)	1.15 (0.72 to 1.59)	3.63 (1.63 to 5.62)	5.00 (−7.71 to 17.71)	0.000
"Five Typical Symptoms" [b]		2.31 (1.44 to 3.18)	0.00 (constant)	1.85 (1.10 to 2.59)	5.75 (2.73 to 8.77)	8.50 (−10.56 to 27.56)	0.000
"Typical"		2.46 (1.52 to 3.39)	0.00 (constant)	1.85 (1.10 to 2.59)	6.38 (3.25 to 9.50)	9.50 (3.15 to 15.85)	0.000
"Quality of Life (QoL)"		0.85 (0.51 to 1.19)	0.00 (constant)	1.08 (0.40 to 1.75)	4.50 (2.55 to 6.45)	4.50 (−14.56 to 23.56)	0.000
"Typical" and "QoL"		1.52 (0.87 to 2.17)	0.00 (constant)	2.92 (1.63 to 4.22)	10.88 (5.95 to 15.80)	14.00 (−11.41 to 39.41)	0.000
Total ACSS		3.98 (2.45 to 5.51)	0.42 (−0.01 to 0.84)	3.08 (1.97 to 4.20)	12.63 (7.51 to 17.74)	17 (constant)	0.000

[a] "Main Symptoms" include "Typical" 1–3; frequency, urgency, painful urination; [b] "Five Typical Symptoms" include "Typical" with the exclusion of one symptom (visible blood in the urine).

3.7. Patient-Reported Outcome Assessment

To differentiate the patient-reported clinical outcome into the two categories, *Success* and *Non-success*, several rational possibilities may be discussed. The differentiation according to the scores obtained by the "Dynamics" domain alone was not convincing enough (Figures 2–4). If *Success* would be defined only by a score of 0, the number would have been unrealistically too low. If, however, *Success* is defined as a score of 1 or less, then the number seems to be adequate (Table 6, Mode 1).

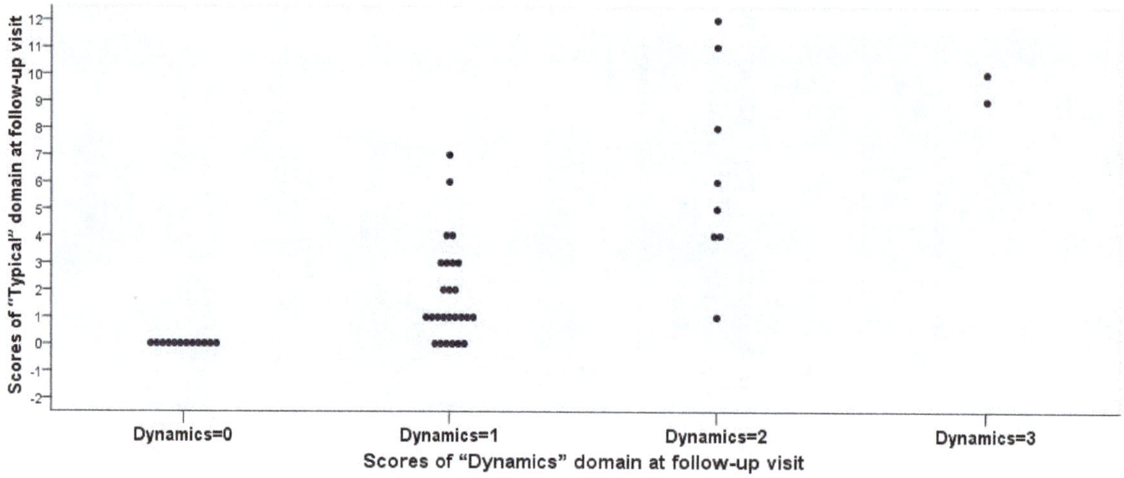

Figure 2. Individual scores for "Typical" versus "Dynamics" domain obtained from 48 female patients at the follow-up visit.

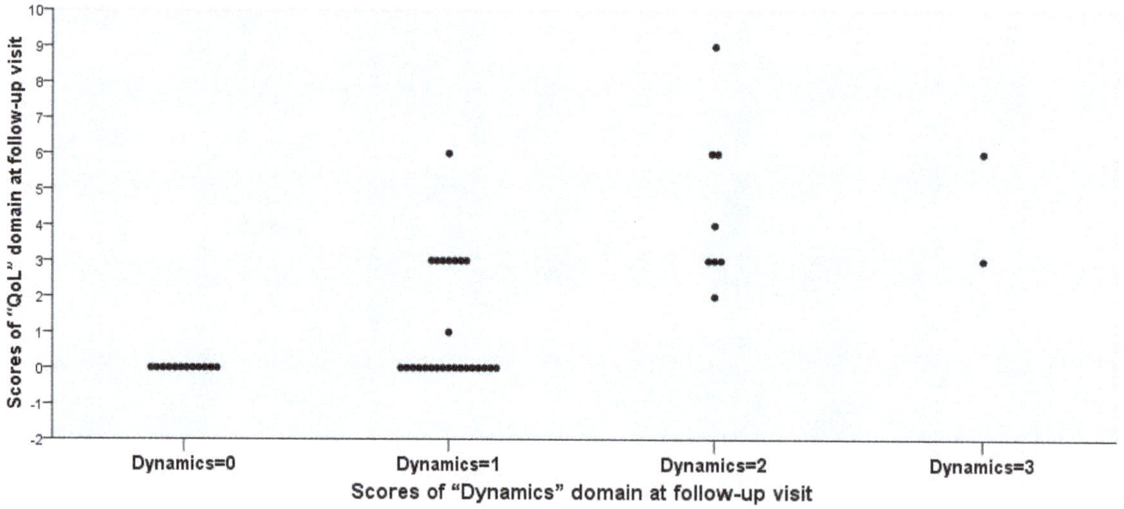

Figure 3. Individual scores for "Quality of Life (QoL)" versus "Dynamics" domain obtained from 48 female patients at the follow-up visit.

A differentiation between *Success* and *Non-success* can also be performed without using the "Dynamics" domain in various ways using the individual patients' scores of the "Typical" and its subgroups, "Main Symptoms" and "Five Typical Symptoms," "Quality of Life," and "Typical" plus "Quality of Life" subscales, because a good correlation was seen between "Typical" and "Quality of Life" (Figure 5). In addition, it is reasonable to assume that in patients showing *Success* the scores of each specific item in the "Typical" or "Quality of Life" domains should not exceed 1 (mild) (Table 6).

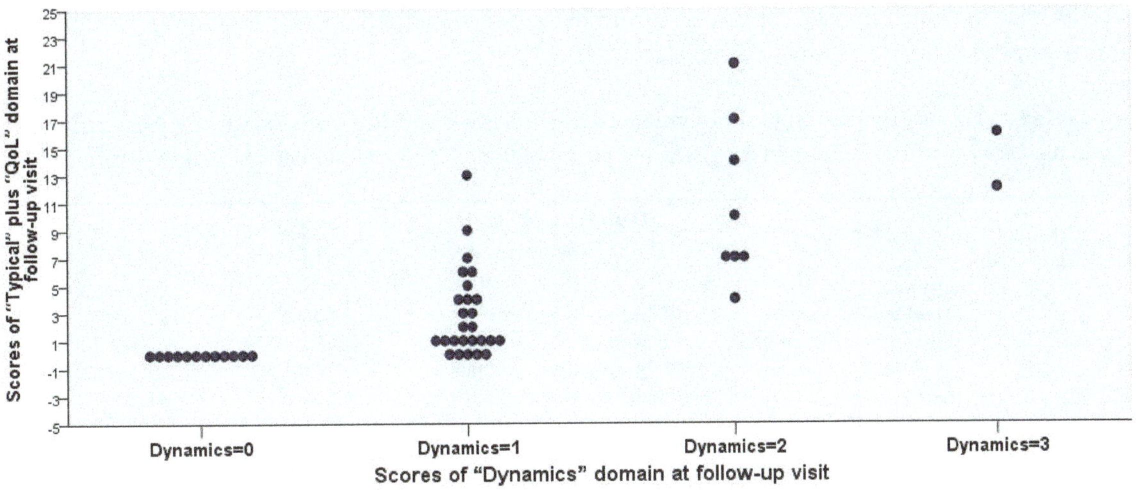

Figure 4. Individual scores for "Typical" plus "Quality of Life (QoL)" versus "Dynamics" domain obtained from 48 female patients at the follow-up visit.

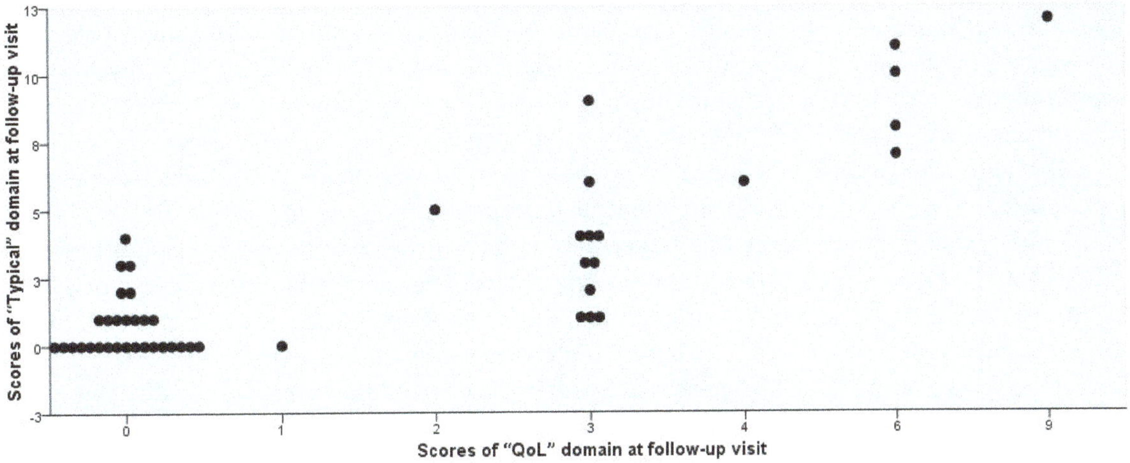

Figure 5. Individual scores for "Typical" versus "Quality of Life (QoL)" domain obtained from 48 female patients at the follow-up visit. .

In Table 6 the evaluation according to the four modes—Nr. 3, 4, 6, and 7—showed exactly the same numbers (37/11 *Success/Non-success*), which also represented the same patients. By the mode Nr. 2 (Main Symptoms) two additional patients were rated as a success, in total 39 patients. Both of these two patients were 30 years of age, had a total score in the "Typical" domain of 17, pyuria, bacteriuria of $\geq 10^5$ CFU/mL with *Escherichia coli* as uropathogen, and both also had visible blood in the urine with a score of 2 (moderate), thus having a hemorrhagic cystitis. At the follow-up visit at Day 3, one patient still had visible blood in her urine (severe) and suprapubic pain (moderate), although her total score of the Main Symptoms was reduced to 1 (mild painful urination). The other patient complaint at the follow-up visit at Day 5 about the moderate incomplete emptying of the bladder and suprapubic pain, although her total score of the Main Symptoms was reduced to 3 (mild frequency, urgency, and painful urination). Most likely in both cases, the follow-up visit was too early to demonstrate the final success of the treatment. Nevertheless, this evaluation demonstrates that with the Main Symptoms alone the success rate at a given visit may be overestimated at least in a few patients. We recommend to use the evaluation by the mode Nr. 4 ('Typical' domain score not more than 4 with no item more than 1)—or alternatively by the mode Nr. 3 (Five Typical Symptoms)—as standard to differentiate between *Success* and *Non-success,* which may be confirmed by either using the mode Nr. 6 or 7 including also the scores obtained in the "Quality of Life" domain.

Table 6. Various possibilities to differentiate between *Success* and *Non-success* in 48 female patients treated for acute uncomplicated cystitis using part B of the ACSS. QoL = Quality of Life; N—number.

Mode	Domain (s)	Definition of *Success* (Scores)	*Success* N (%)	*Non-Success* N (%)
1	Dynamics	≤ 1	38 (79.2%)	10 (20.8%)
2	Main Symptoms [a]	≤ 3, but no item >1 (mild)	39 (81.2%)	9 (18.8%)
3	Five Typical Symptoms [b]	≤ 4, but no item >1 (mild)	37 (77.1%)	11 (22.9%)
4	Typical	≤ 4, but no item >1 (mild)	37 (77.1%)	11 (22.9%)
5	QoL	≤ 3, but no item >1 (mild)	42 (87.5%)	6 (12.5%)
6	Typical plus QoL	≤ 7, but no item >1 (mild)	37 (77.1%)	11 (22.9%)
7 [c]	Typical/QoL	$\leq 4/\leq 3$, but no item >1 (mild)	37 (77.1%)	11 (22.9%)

[a] "Main Symptoms" include "Typical" 1–3: frequency, urgency, painful urination; [b] "Five Typical Symptoms" include "Typical" with the exclusion of one symptom (visible blood in the urine); [c] recommended as overall optimal balanced to differentiate between *Success* and *Non-Success.*

4. Discussion

In the past the primary aim of clinical studies on female patients with uncomplicated acute cystitis (AC) was the eradication of bacteriuria at the test-of-cure visit and the clinical outcome was used as confirmation. In such a classical study [8] for inclusion a positive culture was defined as isolation of a uropathogen in quantities $\geq 10^5$ colony-forming units (CFU)/mL urine with pyuria, defined as ≥ 10 leukocytes/mm^3, and bacteriologic response was assessed as *eradication* ($<10^4$ CFU/mL of original uropathogen), *persistence* ($\geq 10^4$ CFU/mL of original uropathogen), *superinfection* ($\geq 10^5$ CFU/mL of a uropathogen other than the original pathogen at any time during active therapy), and *new infection* ($\geq 10^5$ CFU/mL of a uropathogen other than the original pathogen at any time after the end of therapy).

In contrast, Stamm et al. [9] had already shown that the traditional diagnostic criterion, $\geq 10^5$ CFU/mL of midstream urine, has a very high degree of diagnostic specificity (99%) but a very low level of sensitivity (51%), which means that only 51% of symptomatic women with lower urinary tract infections (UTI) could be identified, whose bladder urine—obtained by suprapubic aspiration or by catheter—contained coliforms. The authors found the best diagnostic criterion to be $\geq 10^2$ CFU/mL (sensitivity, 95%; specificity, 85%) and suggested that clinicians and microbiologists should alter their approach to the diagnosis and treatment of women with acute symptomatic coliform infection of the lower urinary tract. In a more recent study, Hooton et al. [10] confirmed that colony counts of *E. coli* as low as even 10 to 10^2 CFU/mL in midstream urine were sensitive and specific for the presence of *E. coli* in catheter urine in symptomatic women. Therefore, it is not surprising that in the study of Henry et al. [8] of the 469 patients not valid for efficacy, 90% (421) were excluded because no causative organism was isolated in predefined quantity (i.e., $\geq 10^5$ CFU/mL) before treatment. This number was about the same as the 422 patients evaluable for efficacy. This consideration shows that in the past only a highly selected group of patients with acute lower UTI were eligible for clinical studies, although most of the excluded patients may have had about the same symptomatology also caused by acute uncomplicated lower UTI.

Because the traditional diagnostic criterion of $\geq 10^5$ CFU/mL has a very low sensitivity, guidelines by the Infectious Diseases Society of America (IDSA) supported by the U.S. Food and Drug Administration (FDA) recommended to include also patients with a bacteriuria of $\geq 10^3$ CFU/mL of a uropathogen with only little loss of sensitivity (about 80%), but greater specificity (about 90%) as compared to the recommendations of Stamm et al. [9], because routine microbiological techniques can more reliably identify 10^3 CFU/mL than 10^2 CFU/mL [11]. On the other hand, to measure eradication of bacteriuria then became more difficult, because these microbiological techniques have at least an error probability of a decimal power. Therefore, many studies still used the much higher, but easier to handle threshold of 10^5 CFU/mL as demonstrated above [8].

For the clinical inclusion in such a traditional study [8] each patient had to have ≥ 2 signs or symptoms suggestive of an acute uncomplicated UTI (i.e., dysuria, frequency, urgency, suprapubic pain) with an onset of symptoms within 72 h of enrollment. In the study mentioned, the urinary frequency was the most common symptom (97.6%), followed by urgency (95.0%), dysuria (89.6%), and suprapubic pain (89.6%). Most patients in this study reported that the intensity of their symptoms was mild to moderate, although urinary urgency was severe in 37.4% of patients.

Since in actual clinical practice, and also supported by recent guidelines [11–13], culture and susceptibility testing are not often performed in young to middle-aged women with acute uncomplicated UTI, the accurate diagnosis made only by the patient's symptoms has become more important. Therefore the ACSS was developed and validated as a self-reporting questionnaire for diagnosing AC in female patients by assessing typical and differential symptoms, quality of life, and additional health conditions, which may play an important role in such a clinical setting [1,3]. As an optimal threshold to predict AC with 89.3% (95% CI; 81.0–93.7%) sensitivity and 92.5% (95% CI; 86.9–97.0%) specificity, respectively, a total score of 6 points in the domain of typical symptoms could be established in the reevaluated ACSS [3].

Classically clinical outcome is evaluated in such a study [8] on the signs and symptoms of UTI (see above) as *Cure* (disappearance of or improvement in signs and symptoms of the infection such that additional antimicrobial therapy was not required) and *Failure* (no apparent response to therapy, persistence of signs and symptoms of infection, reappearance of signs and symptoms at or before the test-of-cure visit, or use of additional antimicrobial therapy for the current infection). Since in the past clinical outcome was only supportive to the microbiological response, more exact clinical outcome measures were not necessary.

Since even therapeutic strategies of AC are today investigated in controlled randomized trials (RCTs) with only symptomatic versus antibiotic treatment, e.g., ibuprofen versus fosfomycin trometamol [14], reliable measures for the clinical outcome will become critical. The primary aim of such a study is now the patient-reported outcome and not the microbiological response. At least in a pilot study, it has been shown that persistent, but asymptomatic bacteriuria after successful symptomatic therapy does not necessarily trigger early recurrence [15]. In another study on young women with recurrent UTI it also could be established that treatment of asymptomatic bacteriuria between symptomatic episodes may even be harmful and trigger more frequent symptomatic recurrences and as expected is associated with a higher prevalence of antibiotic-resistant strains [16–18]. Therefore patient-reported outcome instruments need to be developed to differentiate more carefully between *Success/Cure* and *Non-success/Failure* to measure benefit or risk in medical product clinical trials as suggested by the FDA [19].

Defining *Success/Cure as* complete disappearance of all signs and symptoms caused by the infection would be ideal, but this cannot realistically be measured. Although the symptoms in the "Typical" domain are of course typical for AC, some patients will have similar symptoms at least of mild severity caused by other reasons. Although it can be assumed, that such kind of symptoms was already present before the onset of infection, reporting of subjective symptoms depends also on cultural behavior and present psychological conditions. Therefore, also in the past disappearance as well as improvement were used to define *Success/Cure*. The question remains how much improvement is necessary to define *Success*.

In the present study 48 female patients diagnosed with AC according to clinical and laboratory assessment and scoring by means of the ACSS (part A) about typical symptoms, differential symptoms, quality of life and additional conditions, were treated and the patient-reported outcome was evaluated with part B of the ACSS.

Considering the results in Table 6 the optimal evaluation would be to define *Success* only in patients with a score of 4 or less in the "Typical" domain (mode Nr. 4) with no specific score >1, which should be confirmed at the same time with a score of 3 or less in the "Quality of Life" domain with no specific score >1 (mode Nr. 7). Such a procedure includes a complete disappearance or at least such an improvement of the typical symptoms, that the interference on the specific items in the two domains is only mild at the same time. If there is an obvious discrepancy between the two domains (typical symptoms and quality of life), patients need to be fully assessed having in mind that (i) these symptoms are in fact typical for acute cystitis, but may also be found at least in part in patients with other diseases; and (ii) quality of life can also be altered not only by the symptoms of acute cystitis but also by underlying conditions of the patient.

The differentiation between *Success* and *Non-success* made only with the scores of the "Main Symptoms" showed that the success rate at a given visit may be overestimated at least in a few patients. Therefore, we recommended to define *Success* by a score of 4 or less in the "Typical" domain or in the "Five Typical Symptoms" domain (mode 3) with no item more than 1 as standard, which then could be also confirmed by the scores obtained in the "Quality of Life" domain as outlined in Table 6. The reason why the same scoring threshold can be used for mode 3 and 4 is explained by the fact, that all patients finally rated as Success had a score of 0 in the subscale "visible blood". This finding may also have clinical significance in that way that a patient at follow-up (e.g., test of cure) with total scores suggesting Success but with a score of ≥ 1 in the subscale "visible blood" should be investigated more thoroughly whether the hematuria might have been caused by other underlying urological or nephrological diseases than by hemorrhagic cystitis.

According to this recommended evaluation, 37 (77.1%) patients would be rated as *Success* and 11 (22.9%) patients as *Non-success* in the present study. At the first glance, such a *Success* rate seems to be lower than reported in most of the clinical trials, but one has to consider that these patients were not treated uniformly according to the most effective strategy and a fixed follow-up visit was not scheduled as part of the study following practice guidelines. Therefore, it can be assumed that many patients treated successfully did not return for a follow-up visit because the purpose of this study was to evaluate the practicability of the ACSS in everyday practice.

The study has also shown that simple overall summary questions like in the "Dynamics" domain and used in many past clinical studies, but never successfully validated, are not sufficient to differentiate between *Success* and *Non-success*. There was, however, a significant correlation with the score reduction in the specific items of the "Typical" and "Quality of Life" domains and the corresponding subscales. Several potential reasons for the lack of clear differentiation between the *Success* and *Non-success* can be discussed. In the present study, the follow-up visit was on average scheduled earlier than the "test-of-cure" visit is usually scheduled, so relapsed patients may not be accounted for and more patients with resolution of symptoms of AC are included in the sample. There were only 10 out of 48 patients with higher values of the scores obtained from the "Dynamics" domain (scores equal to 2 or 3, none for 4), thus, small numbers and an uneven split may have led to the lack of differentiation between *Success* and *Non-Success*. A further reason might be, that the questions in the "Dynamics" domain were not precise enough and need to be improved. To even increase the applicability of the ACSS slight modifications of the questions are suggested as follows:

Score 0: Now I feel back to normal (*All symptoms are gone*);
Score 1: Now I feel much better (*Most of the symptoms are gone*);
Score 2: Now I feel only somewhat better (*Only some of the symptoms are gone*);
Score 3: Now, there are barely any changes (*I have still about the same symptoms*);
Score 4: Now, I feel worse (*My condition is worse*)

Nevertheless, the present ACSS appeared to be a suitable instrument for patient-reported outcome measures because a clear and well-balanced differentiation between *Success* and *Non-success* can be performed. A further advantage of the ACSS would be to use it as patient's diary to measure the time of the symptoms declining or how many patients reach a certain predefined goal. Such an instrument may be especially useful in controlled RCTs to assess not only differences in clinical efficacy at certain predefined visits but to get results almost every day to determine the effectiveness of different therapeutic strategies.

5. Conclusions

The ACSS has proven to be not only a useful instrument to clinically diagnose AC in women by assessing the severity of symptoms and their impact on quality of life as well as to differentiate AC from other urogenital disorders. It is also a suitable instrument for patient-reported outcome measures, with applicability both in daily practice and clinical studies. The results of the study indicate that modifications in the "Dynamics"domain may even increase the applicability.

6. Patents: Copyright and Translations of the ACSS in Other Languages

The ACSS is copyrighted by the Certificate of Deposit of Intellectual Property in Fundamental Library of Academy of Sciences of the Republic of Uzbekistan, Tashkent (Registration number 2463; 26 August 2015) and the Certificate of the International Online Copyright Office, European Depository, Berlin, Germany (Nr. EU-01-000764; 21 October 2015). The Rightholders are Jakhongir Fatikhovich Alidjanov (Uzbekistan), Ozoda Takhirovna Alidjanova (Uzbekistan), Adrian Martin Erich Pilatz (Germany), Kurt Günther Naber (Germany), Florian Martin Erich Wagenlehner (Germany). http://www.avtor-depository.com/index.php?option=com_desposition&task=display _desp_det&id=2612&lang=ru (assessed on 21 May 2018)); http://interoco.com/all-materials/work-of-science/1013-1951954939.html (assessed on 19 February 2018). The e-USQOLAT is copyrighted by the Authorship Certificate of the International Online Copyright Office, European Depository, Berlin, Germany (Nr. EC-01-001179; 18 May 2017). http://inter.interoco.com/copyright-depos itory/computer-programs/1438-2017-05-18-10-59-16.html?path=computer-programs (assessed on 10 February 2018). Translations of the ACSS in other languages are available on the website: http://www.acss.world/downloads.html.

Author Contributions: J.F.A. and K.G.N. conceived and designed the study; J.F.A. and U.A.A. recruited respondents and inputted the data; J.F.A., U.A.A., and K.G.N. analyzed the data; F.M.W., J.F.A., and A.P. contributed analysis tools; K.G.N., J.F.A., and F.M.W. wrote the manuscript.

Funding: Current research received no external funding.

Acknowledgments: The authors would like to express their special gratitude to Dmitrii L. Aroustamov (former director of RSCU) for initiating this study. We thank all the participants of the study for their contribution. The research team acknowledges the staff of the RSCU, Farkhad A. Akilov, and Saidamin A. Makhsudov, for their priceless help with study population and during the decision-making process. J.F. Alidjanov received a 1-year Clinical/Lab Scholarship grant of the European Urological Scholarship Programme (EUSP) of the European Association of Urology (EAU).

References

1. Alidjanov, J.F.; Abdufattaev, U.A.; Makhsudov, S.A.; Pilatz, A.; Akilov, F.A.; Naber, K.G.; Wagenlehner, F.M. New self-reporting questionnaire to assess urinary tract infections and differential diagnosis: Acute cystitis symptom score. *Urol. Int.* **2014**, *92*, 230–236. [CrossRef] [PubMed]

2. Alidjanov, J.F.; Abdufattaev, U.A.; Makhsudov, S.A.; Pilatz, A.; Akilov, F.A.; Naber, K.G.; Wagenlehner, F.M. The acute cystitis symptom score for patient-reported outcome assessment. *Urol. Int.* **2016**, *97*, 402–409. [CrossRef] [PubMed]

3. Alidjanov, J.F.; Naber, K.G.; Abdufattaev, U.A.; Pilatz, A.; Wagenlehner, F.M. Reevaluation of the acute cystitis symptom score, a self-reporting questionnaire. Part, I. Development, diagnosis and differential diagnosis. *Antibiotics* **2018**, *7*, 6. [CrossRef]

4. Cronbach, L.J. Test reliability; Its meaning and determination. *Psychometrika* **1947**, *12*, 1–16. [CrossRef] [PubMed]

5. Wilcoxon, F. Individual comparisons by ranking methods. *Biom. Bull.* **1945**, *1*, 80–83. [CrossRef]

6.   Student. The Probable Error of a Mean. *Biometrika* **1908**, *6*, 1–25. Available online: http://www.jstor.org/st able/2331554 (accessed on 18 May 2018).

7.   Rosenthal, R.; Rosnow, R.L. *Essentials of Behavioral Research: Methods and Data Analysis*; McGraw-Hill: New York, NY, USA, 1984.

8.   Henry, D.C., Jr.; Bettis, R.B.; Riffer, E.; Haverstock, D.C.; Kowalsky, S.F.; Manning, K.; Hamed, K.A. Church DA: Comparison of once-daily extended-release ciprofloxacin and conventional twice-daily ciprofloxacin for the treatment of uncomplicated urinary tract infection in women. *Clin. Ther.* **2002**, *24*, 2088–2104. [CrossRef]

9.   Stamm, W.E.; Counts, G.W.; Running, K.R.; Fihn, S.; Turck, M.; Holmes, K.K. Diagnosis of coliform infection in acutely dysuric women. *N. Engl. J. Med.* **1982**, *307*, 463–468. [CrossRef] [PubMed]

10.   Hooton, T.M.; Roberts, P.L.; Cox, M.E.; Stapleton, A.E. Voided midstream urine culture and acute cystitis in premenopausal women. *N. Engl. J. Med.* **2013**, *369*, 1883–1891. [CrossRef] [PubMed]

11.   Rubin, R.H.; Shapiro, E.D.; Andriole, V.T.; Davis, R.J.; Stamm, W.E. Evaluation of new anti-infective drugs for the treatment of urinary tract infection. Infectious diseases society of America and the food and drug administration. *Clin. Infect. Dis.* **1992**, *15*, S216–S227. [CrossRef] [PubMed]

12.   Gupta, K.; Hooton, T.M.; Naber, K.G.; Wullt, B.; Colgan, R.; Miller, L.G.; Moran, G.J.; Nicolle, L.E.; Raz, R.; Schaeffer, A.J.; et al. Infectious Diseases Society of A, European Society for M, Infectious D: International clinical practice guidelines for the treatment of acute uncomplicated cystitis and pyelonephritis in women: A 2010 update by the infectious diseases society of America and the European society for microbiology and infectious diseases. *Clin. Infect. Dis.* **2011**, *52*, e103–e120. [PubMed]

13.   Grabe, M.; Bartoletti, R.; Bjerklund-Johansen, T.E.; Cai, T.; Çek, M.; Köves, B.; Naber, K.G.; Pickard, R.S.; Tenke, P.; Wagenlehner, F.; et al. Guidelines on Urological Infections; Eau Guidelines, Edition Presented at the 30th EAU Annual Congress. Available online: http://uroweb.org/guideline/urological-infections/ (accessed on 19 December 2015).

14.   Gágyor, I.; Bleidorn, J.; Kochen, M.M.; Schmiemann, G.; Wegscheider, K.; Hummers-Pradier, E. Ibuprofen versus fosfomycin for uncomplicated urinary tract infection in women: Randomised controlled trial. *BMJ* **2015**, *351*, h6544. [CrossRef] [PubMed]

15.   Ivanov, D.; Abramov-Sommariva, D.; Moritz, K.; Eskötter, H.; Kostinenko, T.; Martynyuk, L.; Kolesnik, N.; Naber, K.G. An open label, non-controlled, multicentre, interventional trial to investigate the safety and efficacy of canephron® N in the management of uncomplicated urinary tract infections (uIITs). *Clin. Phytosci.* **2015**, *1*, 1–11. [CrossRef]

16.   Cai, T.; Mazzoli, S.; Mondaini, N.; Meacci, F.; Nesi, G.; D'Elia, C.; Malossini, G.; Boddi, V.; Bartoletti, R. The role of asymptomatic bacteriuria in young women with recurrent urinary tract infections: To treat or not to treat? *Clin. Infect. Dis.* **2012**, *55*, 771–777. [CrossRef] [PubMed]

17.   Wagenlehner, F.M.; Naber, K.G. Editorial commentary: Treatment of asymptomatic bacteriuria might be harmful. *Clin. Infect. Dis.* **2015**, *61*, 1662–1663. [PubMed]

18.   Cai, T.; Nesi, G.; Mazzoli, S.; Meacci, F.; Lanzafame, P.; Caciagli, P.; Mereu, L.; Tateo, S.; Malossini, G.; Selli, C.; et al. Asymptomatic bacteriuria treatment is associated with a higher prevalence of antibiotic resistant strains in women with urinary tract infections. *Clin. Infect. Dis.* **2015**, *61*, 1655–1661. [CrossRef] [PubMed]

19.   U.S. Department of Health and Human Services; Food and Drug Administration. Guidance for Industry. Patient-Reported Outcome Measures: Use in Medical Product Development to Support Labeling Claims. December 2009. Available online: http://www.fda.gov/downloads/Drugs/.../Guidances/UCM193282.pdf (accessed on 20 December 2015).

10

Bacteriophages in the Dairy Environment: From Enemies to Allies

Lucía Fernández *, **Susana Escobedo**, **Diana Gutiérrez**, **Silvia Portilla**, **Beatriz Martínez** ⓘ, **Pilar García** and **Ana Rodríguez**

Instituto de Productos Lácteos de Asturias (IPLA-CSIC), Paseo Río Linares s/n, Villaviciosa, 33300 Asturias, Spain; s.escobedo@ipla.csic.es (S.E.); dianagufer@ipla.csic.es (D.G.); silvia.portilla@ipla.csic.es (S.P.); bmf1@ipla.csic.es (B.M.); pgarcia@ipla.csic.es (P.G.); anarguez@ipla.csic.es (A.R.)

* Correspondence: lucia.fernandez@ipla.csic.es

Academic Editor: Christopher C. Butler

Abstract: The history of dairy farming goes back thousands of years, evolving from a traditional small-scale production to the industrialized manufacturing of fermented dairy products. Commercialization of milk and its derived products has been very important not only as a source of nourishment but also as an economic resource. However, the dairy industry has encountered several problems that have to be overcome to ensure the quality and safety of the final products, as well as to avoid economic losses. Within this context, it is interesting to highlight the role played by bacteriophages, or phages, viruses that infect bacteria. Indeed, bacteriophages were originally regarded as a nuisance, being responsible for fermentation failure and economic losses when infecting lactic acid bacteria, but are now considered promising antimicrobials to fight milk-borne pathogens without contributing to the increase in antibiotic resistance.

Keywords: bacteriophages; dairy industry; pathogens; lactic acid bacteria; fermentation failure; biofilms; antimicrobial resistance

1. Introduction

1.1. Origins and Industrialization of Dairy Production

Archaeological evidence indicates that already in ancient times, the people of Mesopotamia learned to domesticate milk-producing animals, using and preserving milk for nourishment [1]. Thousands of years later, milk is still the most consumed dairy product worldwide, playing a fundamental role in the diet of all populations [2,3]. It is precisely from the exercise of milk extraction by man that the dairy industry was developed [1,4]. Indeed, cheese and yogurt, the first dairy derivatives, were accidentally discovered as a result of the difficulties encountered to transport and preserve milk. From that time to the present, there has been a continuous development of new and improved dairy products. One of the most striking features of the traditional dairy industry is the manner in which chemical, microbiological, physical, and engineering principles were integrated to allow the manufacture of high quality and safe products. This multidisciplinary strategy has led to the wide variety of products available today. Nowadays, aspects like the availability and presentation of products are very important for the consumer. An example of this is the diversification of dairy products by the inclusion of fruits and cereals [3,5,6]. Moreover, the creation of new and sophisticated products that contribute to improving the health of final users, the so-called functional foods, is on high demand [2,5]. Some examples include products with added vitamins and minerals or those supplemented with living beneficial microorganisms (probiotics). Besides dairy products, the technological development of the dairy industry has made it possible to separate solids from milk, and subsequently transform these components into raw material for other food industry sectors [4,7]. It is also worth noting that the diversity of dairy products varies considerably from region to region depending on dietary habits, available milk-making technologies, market demand, and sociocultural circumstances [8].

1.2. Economic Importance of the Dairy Industry in Different Countries

The dairy sector is a dynamic global industry that plays an important economic role in the agricultural sector of most industrialized and developing countries [8,9]. Currently, in the face of rising global demand and imminent industrial globalization, there has been an increase in both the scope and the intensity of world trade of dairy products [8]. Based on data estimates by the Food and Agricultural Organization (FAO), world milk production for 2016 was 817 million tons. In addition, the expected increase in global demand and production of dairy products until 2025 is estimated to be around 6–20 percent [9]. The most important milk producers are Europe, Asia and the Americas. More specifically, the European Union (EU) is the largest producing economic region worldwide, while India is the largest producer as a country [10]. According to the International Dairy Federation [9], milk production has increased by 50 percent in the last three decades, with a total of 150 million smallholders around the world participating in this activity. On the other hand, developed countries account for one-third of the world milk production, while the remaining two-thirds correspond to developing countries. In developing countries, however, growth in the dairy sector is limited by refrigeration, marketing and transportation problems as well as nutritional and zootechnical issues [8]. Thus, smallholders often lack the necessary skills to manage their farms as companies because they have limited access to animal health services, genetic improvement and training of personnel, which results in low yields and poor quality milk. In addition, the economic importance of dairy production both nationally and internationally is directly related to the sustainability of pasture production areas and the size of herds [11]. Other important factors that influence the success of the dairy sector are the degree of government intervention through subsidies and the demand in the export markets. Furthermore, the success of dairy development programs in different countries also depends to a large extent on traditional habits of consumption of dairy products [7,10]. Nonetheless, food safety remains a key global challenge in the dairy industry of any country to prevent economic losses and health concerns. Within this context, bacteriophages (or phages) have consistently played a significant role in the success of the dairy industry. Indeed, bacterial fermentation processes are threatened by contamination of raw milk with phages that infect lactic acid bacteria. This makes necessary the development of techniques to ensure control of the phage load in starting materials and equipment. In contrast, more recently, phages have been proposed as biocontrol agents to eliminate pathogenic or spoilage bacteria in dairy products. This review aims to summarize and discuss both the negative and positive impact of phages in dairy settings, depending on their specific bacterial hosts.

2. Bacteriophages as Unwanted Guests

Phage infection of dairy starter cultures remains the main cause of fermentation failures in the dairy industry. Phage outbreaks can lead to substantial economic losses due to manufacturing delays, waste of ingredients, lower quality product, growth of spoilage and pathogenic microorganisms or even total production loss [12]. Close monitoring of entry routes, quick and effective phage detection methods and control measurements are currently applied to reduce the risk of phage propagation within dairy settings (Figure 1).

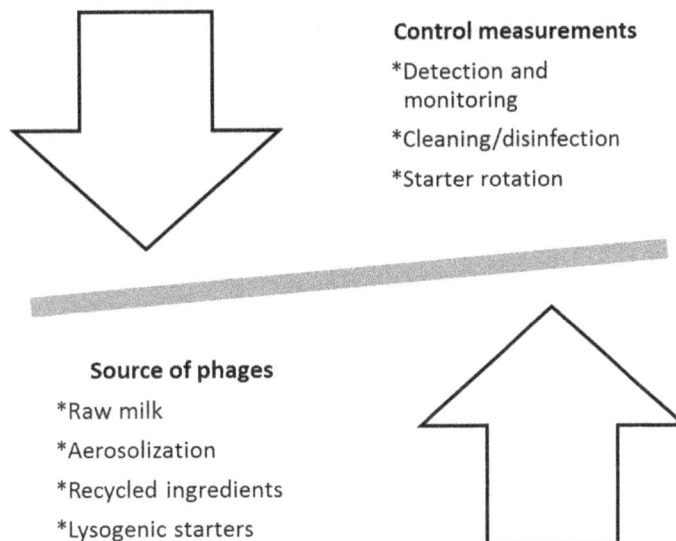

Control measurements

*Detection and
 monitoring

*Cleaning/disinfection

*Starter rotation

Source of phages

*Raw milk

*Aerosolization

*Recycled ingredients

*Lysogenic starters

Figure 1. Factors that contribute to the presence of phages in dairy settings.

2.1. Sources of Contamination

The sources of phage entry into dairy plant facilities and dissemination routes must be identified in order to implement corrective actions to limit their propagation. Due to the wide diversity of phages present in raw milk, either as free virions or as prophages in wild lactic acid bacteria (LAB) strains, milk is considered to be the primary entry route for phages into the dairy environment [13]. As much as 10% of milk samples obtained from different dairies in Spain yielded viable *Lactococcus lactis* phages, while lactococcal and streptococcal phages were detected in 37% of raw milk samples used for yogurt production [14,15].

Personnel and equipment movement, raw materials handling, air displacements around contaminated surfaces and liquid splashes can aerosolize viruses and cause dissemination of phage particles in the air to the entire factory environment [16]. Concentrations ranging from 10^2 PFU/m^3 to 10^8 PFU/m^3 in air have been detected in different areas of a cheese manufacturing plant during the fermentation process [17]. A variety of samplers are now available for viral detection in the air; however, there is no standard sampling procedure [18]. In many cases, these devices may have damaging effects on the virus structure that can lead to false-negative results; that is why analytical methods that are independent of viral infectivity, such as quantitative PCR (qPCR), are more suitable for the analysis of air samples [19]. Other reservoirs of phages include materials and equipment used in the manufacturing process as well as surfaces in dairy facilities. Phages can be found in places where conditions for development of their host are favorable and where cleaning and disinfection are difficult.

A common practice in the manufacturing of yogurt and other fermented products consists in the utilization of reconstituted milk from powder and whey proteins obtained from cheese production to increase the product yield and improve the texture and nutritional value of the final products [20]. However, whey proteins may protect phages during heat; there is a correlation between thermal stability of molecular structures and their ability to protect lactococcal virulent phage P1532 from thermal treatments [21]. In addition, whey protein concentrate often contains high temperature-resistant phages, which are able to survive pasteurization and contaminate starters during the manufacturing process [14]. Furthermore, separation and concentration steps of the whey products, consisting in ultrafiltration and microfiltration, may also increase significantly phage titers in these ingredients [22].

LAB strains used as starter cultures can also be a source of phages since they may contain temperate phages integrated into the bacterial chromosome. Lysogeny is widely distributed among dairy lactococci, lactobacilli and with lower incidence in *Streptococcus thermophilus* strains [23,24]. Prophages may be induced and enter into the lytic life cycle under stress conditions such as heat, salts, bacteriocins, starvation, ultraviolet light or may also occur naturally with a frequency of even up to 9% [25–27].

2.2. Detection and Elimination

Great research efforts have focused on early detection of infective phages in dairy manufacturing. Phage monitoring methods include microbiological and molecular assays designed for rapid, low cost and high sensitive evaluation [28].

One of the most common methods for the detection of phages from industrial dairy plants is the activity test based on the acidification rate of milk that provides a reliable indication of their presence when acid production slows down. Acidification can be evaluated by pH measurements, color change of an indicator compound or variations in the electrical conductance of milk [29]. Another method is the double layer plaque assay, which allows a quantitative analysis of infective phage levels, but requires availability of a sensitive strain [30,31]. Flow cytometry can also be used for detection lysed bacterial cells that are found late in the lytic cycle, allowing an accurate and rapid monitoring of phage contamination [32].

Because microbiological tests are time consuming and mostly rely on the availability of single indicator strains, a number of alternative molecular methods focused on detecting the presence of phage particles or their components (DNA, proteins) have been developed. Immunological assays are based on the use of specific antibodies against principal structural proteins of the virion, while viral DNA can be detected with specific DNA-hybridization probes or by polymerase chain reaction [28]. PCR methods have been successfully adapted to detect and identify phages in different stages of dairy product manufacture. In a single reaction, multiplex PCR test allows the detection of several of the most common phages infecting LAB, such as *L. lactis* phage species P335, 936, and c2 and phages infecting *S. thermophilus* and *Lactobacillus delbrueckii* [15,33]. More sensitive than conventional PCR, real-time qPCR can be used to estimate the copy number of a target gene, allowing quantitative viral contamination diagnosis. By using different fluorogenic reporters in the same reaction it is possible to develop multiplex qPCR to detect different targets [34]. qPCR suppliers constantly offer new solutions to get automated systems adapted to industrial needs. Recently, phage metagenomics studies have been conducted to assess the biodiversity and dynamics of phage populations in dairy settings, providing a rational basis for suitable control strategies [35].

2.3. Control Methods

Significant progress in the control of phage populations within the dairy sector has been made in order to keep these bacterial viruses at bay. Although cleaning of equipment and facilities can remove a large proportion of microorganisms, the presence of residual LAB may increase the risk of phage contamination. The role of disinfection is to kill microorganisms that survived the cleaning procedures, reducing the spread of phages within the facility. Disinfectants active against bacteria are not always efficient to inactivate phages [36]. Several biocides used in the dairy industry as well as cleaning procedures have been tested for viral effectiveness on different phages infecting LAB strains. Peracetic acid and sodium hypochlorite containing products are shown to be the most efficient biocides for inactivation of phage particles, while ethanol and isopropanol were usually not effective [37]. The majority of disinfectants consist of several biocides and they must ensure the lack of negative impact on the final product and be able to degrade into harmless final compounds. Combining biocides and heat or using them at extreme pH conditions have shown to give the best results [38]. Photocatalysis intended to destroy fungi, bacteria and spores in the air has been recently explored for inactivating viruses infecting *Lactobacillus casei*, *Lb. delbrueckii* and *Lactobacillus plantarum* [39]. Photocatalytic reaction has shown to completely eliminate two 936-type phages, CHD and QF9 within 120 and 60 min of exposure; respectively [39]. Of note, UV-A radiation assayed by the authors has the advantage of safe use, thus allowing their application for long periods even in the presence of personnel.

The viral load of the ingredients used in dairy production should be reduced as much as possible. Although heating can reduce the activity of phage particles, many LAB phages are not inactivated by classical pasteurization procedures (63 °C for 30 min or 72 °C for 15 s). Therefore, emerging non-thermal technologies such as pulsed electric field, high hydrostatic pressure and high pressure homogenization as well as the combination with heat are currently being explored for inactivating phages [40]. It is important to take into consideration that phages also react differently to heat depending on the medium. Moreover, protective effects due to the presence of proteins, salt or fat have been reported [21,22].

Phage inhibitory media have been developed for starter propagation in dairy plants. The addition of components that inhibit or delay phage propagation such as chelating agents, sodium tripolyphosphate or purified phage peptides can help protect from further phage infection [41–43].

Rotation of defined phage-free cultures is an efficient phage control method to avoid recontamination by the same phage and the build-up of specific phages. A follow up is necessary in order to detect the emergence of new virulent phages to adjust the strain rotation protocol. Recently, a multiplex PCR method based on the genetic locus of the cell wall polysaccharide that acts as phage receptor for many lactococcal phages has been developed to predict phage susceptibility and aid to design suitable starter rotation schemes [44].

The availability of alternative phage resistant starters is of paramount importance and many efforts are being made to search for potential new starter bacteria with different phage sensitivity profiles or to engineer phage-resistant starters. Bacteria have developed natural defense mechanisms against phage infection based on adsorption inhibition, blockage of phage DNA injection, restriction-modification, abortive infection and CRISPR-Cas systems [45]. Many of these systems are plasmid encoded and can be moved from one strain to another for genetically improving dairy starters. Isolation of spontaneous bacteriophage insensitive mutants (BIMs) is a feasible alternative for bacteria without conjugative plasmids, and involves no genetic manipulation. On the other hand, construction of genetically engineered strains has been intensively studied. Several genetic tools, based in the LAB native phage defense mechanisms as well as phage elements have been designed. Examples of these engineered antiphage approaches include cloning of replication origin, antisense RNA technology, phage triggered suicide systems, overproduction of phage proteins, DARPins and neutralizing antibody fragments [12]. Nevertheless, legislation and consumers' concerns regarding genetically modified organisms (GMOs) makes its application to dairy industry difficult.

3. Problems Associated with Bacterial Contamination

3.1. Foodborne Infectious Diseases in Dairy Products

Ensuring access to safe food products remains one of the major global health challenges. Indeed, foodborne diseases constitute a sanitary and economic burden in countries all over the world. To be effective, food safety measures require the participation of all the different actors along the food supply chain, "from farm to fork", including farmers, manufacturers, vendors and consumers. This has become particularly difficult in our global market economy, as these different actors are often far away from each other, frequently across national borders. In this context, adequate regulatory frameworks need to be in place to ensure that the required safety standards are met throughout the process. Nonetheless, foodborne infections are still a major health care concern, with a total of 600 million people falling ill and 420,000 dying every year from eating contaminated food [46].

Dairy products can get contaminated at different points along the production chain (Figure 2). For instance, raw milk can carry microorganisms from the udder or teat canal, the milking equipment, storage containers, the animal's or handler's skin, etc. [47]. Since some of these microbes can be human pathogens, milk can be a potential source of infections if consumed unpasteurized. These pathogens may even persist in aged products made from raw milk, like some traditionally-manufactured cheeses [48]. Pasteurization, on the other hand, can kill most potentially dangerous microorganisms present in milk [47]. However, outbreaks may still occur due to improper pasteurization or post-pasteurization contamination of the milk. Indeed, proper cleaning and hygiene procedures are essential to prevent milk-borne infections.

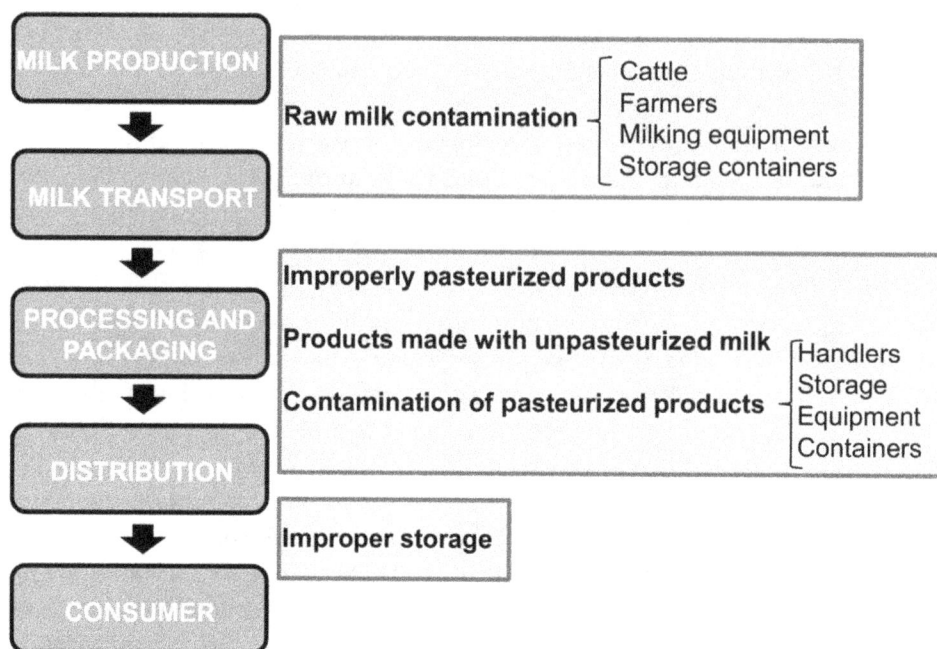

Figure 2. Schematic representation of different points of the dairy supply chain susceptible to microbial contamination.

The pathogens commonly found in the dairy environment include viruses, parasites, fungi and bacteria [49]. Some of the most notorious bacterial pathogens are *Brucella* spp., *Campylobacter jejuni*, *Bacillus cereus*, Shiga toxin-producing *Escherichia coli* (*E. coli* O157:H7), *Staphylococcus aureus*, *Listeria monocytogenes*, *Coxiella burnietti*, *Mycobacterium tuberculosis*, *Mycobacterium bovis*, *Salmonella* spp. and *Yersinia enterocolitica*. Consumption of unpasteurized milk and its derived products is the main source of contamination for most of these pathogens [50–62]. Although unpasteurized milk is not easily available to consumers, it is still consumed by dairy farmers and raw-milk health advocates [51,63]. The human pathogenic bacterium *S. aureus* is one of the microorganisms responsible for mastitis in dairy cows and can also be a source of raw milk contamination [64]. However, this microbe can frequently contaminate food after pasteurization as a result of improper handling during production. *S. aureus* is also problematic due to the production by some strains of heat stable enterotoxins that cannot be easily destroyed by cooking the product [65]. As a result, contaminated products will remain dangerous even after the bacterium has been killed, potentially leading to intoxications.

Taking all of this into account, it is evident that proper hygiene and disinfection measures are essential along the dairy production chain, from the handling of dairy cows to the final product before it reaches the consumer. On top of that, consumers need to be aware that following the instructions for preservation of dairy products and obeying expiry dates are important to ensure their safety.

3.2. Antimicrobial Resistance in the Dairy Environment

Antimicrobials have been overused and misused in human and veterinary medicine ever since their introduction in the clinic. One of the main consequences of this has been the spread of antibiotic resistance determinants amongst microorganisms, including human pathogens, even in environments where antimicrobials themselves were not present [66]. This increase in antibiotic resistance has ultimately led to a decrease in the efficacy of routine disinfection regimes. Indeed, strains belonging to some species have acquired resistance to almost all antibiotics available in the market. The so-called "superbugs" have raised the alarms within the medical and scientific community at large as an indicator that the antibiotic era might be coming to an end. From a less dramatic perspective, perhaps superbugs remind us of the need to understand resistance mechanisms and develop new antimicrobials.

The use of antibiotics in the context of the dairy industry is subject to strict regulations, which are in place to avoid the presence of antibiotic residues in milk aimed for human consumption. For instance, in the US, safety standards for milk are specified in the Grade "A" Pasteurized Milk Ordinance and the Regulation EC 853/2004 defines food safety standards for foodstuffs in the EU [67,68]. In the dairy environment, antimicrobials are used for the treatment of infections in cattle, as growth promoters and as prophylactic agents. The most prevalent infectious illness affecting dairy cattle is mastitis, followed by respiratory infections, lameness, infections of the reproductive system and diarrhea/gastrointestinal tract infections [69]. In many cases, cows require antibiotic treatment with cephalosporins and tetracycline being the most frequently used for mastitis and lameness, respectively [69]. Also, farmers often administer antibiotics to prevent infections, usually penicillin G or dihydrostreptomycin, following the end of the lactation period, the so-called dry cow therapy [69]. The most common routes of antibiotic administration in cows are intramammary and intramuscular [70].

Generalized used of antimicrobials in agriculture and animal farming is considered a potential risk factor for the increased prevalence of antimicrobial resistance in bacteria from food-producing animals [71,72]. Thus, antibiotic pressure would favor the selection and spread of resistance markers by horizontal transfer [73–75]. It must be pointed out, however, that there is no definitive scientific evidence of a direct link between the two. Nevertheless, there have been numerous studies that tried to determine whether antibiotic resistance increased in microorganisms from dairy environments as a result of antimicrobial exposure. However, the results obtained have shown contradictory information. Thus, some studies point that there is an increase in antibiotic resistance over time under antibiotic pressure, while others show no change whatsoever, with differences observed for certain species or antimicrobials [76,77]. Also, some studies have assessed whether there are differences in the amount of antimicrobial resistant organisms in conventional versus organic (antibiotic-free) dairies. For instance, Pol and Ruegg [78] observed that some microorganism-antibiotic combinations were indeed dependent on the farm type while others showed no difference.

Due to the concern regarding antibiotic resistance in pathogenic bacteria, there has been a boom in research regarding the development of novel antimicrobials and new disinfection regimes. Amongst these therapeutic alternatives, phages have been gaining particular attention, as we will discuss below.

4. Bacteriophages as Unexpected Allies

4.1. Phages as Disinfectants and Preservatives in the Dairy Industry

As we mentioned previously, foodborne diseases continue to be a hurdle for human health and those associated to dairy industries are not an exception. Thus, many pathogenic bacteria can spread along the food chain from "farm to fork". In this regard, phages can be used as antimicrobials and biocontrol agents in food industries to prevent and control step by step the pathogenic bacterial contamination during food production (Figure 3). The use of phages has some advantages over conventional disinfectants such as their narrow host range, targeting specifically bacteria from one species or genus, being also effective against bacteria resistant to antibiotics. Moreover, phages have been described as safe for humans, animals, plants and the environment [79]. Besides, they do not cause equipment or surface damage or alter the organoleptic properties of food.

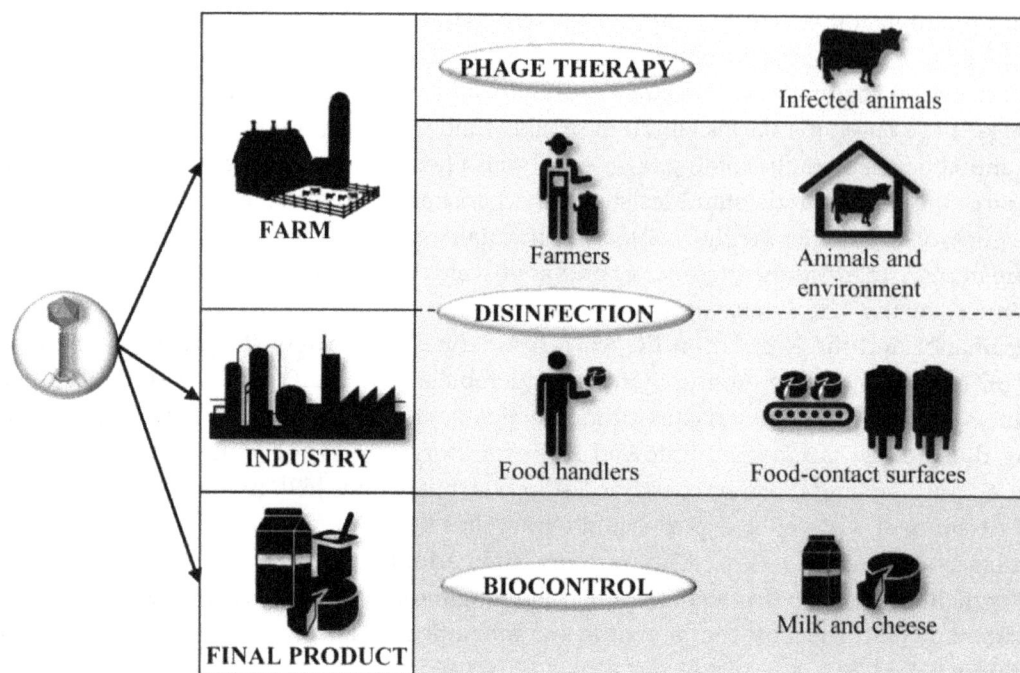

Figure 3. Principal points of disinfection and biocontrol along the dairy chain (from "farm to fork"), where phages can be applied to ensure dairy safety.

The efficacy of phages as an intervention strategy in primary production to reduce bacterial infections in food-producing animals has been widely demonstrated [80]. Nevertheless, data regarding the use of phages in the dairy industry are still scarce. The treatment of subclinical *S. aureus* mastitis in lactating dairy cattle with phage K resulted in a cure rate of 16.7%, although the difference between the treated and non-treated groups was not statistically significant. This can be the consequence of phage inactivation in the udder due to milk proteins and fats [81]. However, utilization of phages as biocontrol agents in milk seems to be a better approach, since the combination of two temperate phages ΦH5 and ΦA72 inhibited the growth of *S. aureus* at 37 °C in ultra-high-temperature (UHT) and traditionally pasteurized whole-fat milk [82]. Moreover, lytic derivatives of these phages, Φ88 and Φ35 were successfully used to completely remove *S. aureus* during curd manufacturing and also during the maturation of fresh and hard-type cheeses [83,84]. Similarly, the application of listeriaphages in combination with a bacteriocin (coagulin C23) to extended shelf life (ESL) milk contaminated with *L. monocytogenes* prevented bacterial growth at 4 °C after 10 days [85].

In the dairy industry, recurrent contamination comes from inadequate cleaning of the equipment and the growth of pathogenic bacteria forming biofilms. Biofilms are structures where bacterial cells are protected by a surrounding matrix, thus becoming difficult to clean and remove. Several studies using biofilms preformed in laboratory conditions (onto polystyrene) have confirmed the potential of phages for staphylococcal biofilm removal. Phage K and a mixture of derivative phages removed biofilms in a time-dependent manner, with the highest reduction occurring after 72 h at 37 °C [86]. The combination of phage K with another staphylococcal phage (DRA88), completely removed biofilms after 48 h at 37 °C [87]. In a similar way, phages phiIPLA-RODI, phiIPLA-C1C, and a mixture of both phages, achieved a reduction of 2 log units after 8 h of treatment at 37 °C [88]. On the other hand, *E. coli* biofilms formed onto materials typically used in food processing surfaces (stainless steel, ceramic tile and high density polyethylene) were removed below the detection level after treatment with a phage mixture named BEC8 [89]. Biofilms formed by *L. monocytogenes* onto stainless steel were reduced up to 5.4 log-units/cm^2 by phage P100 [90]. In this regard, a commercial phage-based product ListShield^{TM}, developed by Intralytix Inc. (Baltimore, MD, USA), has been proposed as a disinfectant for food facilities and also on cheese surfaces [91].

The potential of phages in the food industry is so extensive that several companies have developed phage-based products against important foodborne pathogens that could be used as disinfectants and as food-processing aids. But only Intralytix Inc. (Baltimore, MD, USA) and Micreos BV (Wageningen, The Netherlands) commercialize phage-based products (ListShield™ and PhageGuard Listex, respectively) that can be applied in dairy settings. PhageGuard Listex can be applied as a surface intervention against *Listeria* contamination on cheese by spraying or by immersion, without affecting the color, texture or taste of the product [92]. These phage-based products provide a basis for the future approval of phages as disinfectants and preservatives, overcoming the specific regulatory shortcomings of each country.

4.2. Regulatory Framework for the Application of Phage-Derived Products in the Food Industry

One of the major difficulties for the use of phages as antimicrobial agents is the lack of a proper regulatory framework for their authorization. Moreover, the European Food Safety Authority (EFSA) expressed concerns regarding the efficacy of phages and the danger of recontamination of the food products [93]. In the case of the dairy industry, and food industry at large, phages have great potential for the control of foodborne pathogens. As mentioned previously, phages can be used as food preservatives or for the disinfection of food-contact surfaces, especially against biofilms. However, depending on their intended use and label claims, the procedure for their approval may vary and, in some cases, be time-consuming and costly. Moreover, legislation can differ considerably from country to country.

Probably the easiest route for placing a phage-based product on the market is for application as a food-processing aid. Indeed, several products have been granted clean label processing in the USA, Canada, Israel, Australia, New Zealand, Switzerland, Norway and the EU (The Netherlands). The first product to be approved by the Food and Drug Administration (FDA) and the US Department of Agriculture (USDA) was LISTEX™ P100, now named PhageGuard Listex, in 2007 (EBI Food Safety, Wageningen, The Netherlands). More recently, three phage-based products manufactured by Intralytix Inc. (Baltimore, MD, USA), have also been approved by the FDA for application in food-processing facilities against *L. monocytogenes*, *E. coli* O157:H7, and several *Salmonella* species.

Another potential application of phage-based products is as food additives. So far, only Intralytics has achieved FDA approval for commercializing the phage product ListShield™ as a food additive.

The approval of phage-based products as surface disinfectants for the food industry is proving to be more complicated than the previously discussed applications. Indeed, only one product, ListShield™, produced by Intralytix Inc., has been granted approval by the FDA and the Environmental Protection Agency (EPA) in the United States to be used for disinfection of non-food contact surfaces and equipment in food-processing facilities and food establishments. In the EU, use of these products as disinfectants in food environments requires authorization under the current Biocidal Products Regulation 528/12 [94]. Preparation of a dossier for this purpose can be somewhat complicated and, most especially, very expensive as it requires a number of studies demonstrating the safety for humans and the environment as well as the efficacy of the active substance, in this case phages, and the product itself. Analysis of potential resistance development is also quite frequently requested by the authorities.

Overall, despite the obvious difficulties encountered for marketing phage-based products, the need for alternatives to conventional antimicrobials and disinfectants seems to be encouraging progress in this field. Hopefully, this will only be the first step towards the development of a proper legal framework that allows an easier path to authorization and commercialization of phage-based products.

5. Concluding Remarks

One century after phages were first described, there is no doubt regarding their importance in diverse fields including ecology, biotechnology, medicine and industrial activities. The dairy industry provides a perfect example of the diverse ways in which bacterial viruses can affect human activities.

This review intends to compile these different aspects, both positive and negative, and gives an overview of how phages have in some ways shaped the development of a whole industrial sector. Thus, achieving a good understanding of phages that infect lactic acid bacteria has enabled the development and implementation of strategies to limit the economic losses associated to fermentation failures. On the other hand, phages appear as a viable alternative to conventional disinfectants for application in food industrial surfaces and dairy products themselves. In the midst of a crisis of rising resistance rates to antimicrobials, phages are giving new hope in the fight against bacterial pathogens. Nevertheless, it is still necessary to conduct further research and develop the appropriate regulatory framework in order to ensure that phage disinfection procedures are effective, safe and easily available.

Acknowledgments: Our research was funded by grants AGL2015-65673-R (Ministry of Science and Innovation, Spain), BIO2013-46266-R (MINECO, Spain), EU ANIWHA ERA-NET BLAAT, GRUPIN14-139 (Program of Science, Technology and Innovation 2013–2017 and FEDER EU funds, Principado de Asturias, Spain). L.F. and S.P. were respectively awarded a "Marie Curie Clarin-Cofund" grant and a CONCACYT (Mexico) postdoctoral fellowship. P.G., B.M. and A.R. are members of the bacteriophage network FAGOMA II and the FWO Vlaanderen funded "Phagebiotics" research community (WO.016.14).

Author Contributions: Lucía Fernández, Susana Escobedo, Diana Gutiérrez, Silvia Portilla, Beatriz Martínez, Ana Rodríguez and Pilar García wrote the paper.

References

1. Rodríguez González, A.; Roces Rodríguez, C.; Martínez Fernández, B. Chapter 9: Cultivos Iniciadores en Quesería: Tradición y Modernidad. In *Biocontrol en la Industria Láctea*; Roa, I., Pacheco, M., Tabla, R., Rebollo, J.E., Eds.; Bubok Publishing, S.L.: Madrid, Spain, 2014; pp. 110–125, ISBN 978-84-686-5316-7. (In Spanish)

2. Dugdill, B.; Bennett, A.; Phelan, J.; Scholten, B.A. Chapter 8: Dairy-industry development programmes: Their role in food and nutrition security and poverty reduction. In *Milk and Dairy Products in Human Nutrition*; Muehlhoff, E., Bennett, A., McMahon, D., Eds.; FAO: Rome, Italy, 2013; pp. 313–348, ISBN 978-92-5-107863-1.

3. Kongerslev Thorning, T.; Raben, A.; Tholstrup, T.; Soedamah-Muthu, S.S.; Givens, I.; Astrup, A. Milk and dairy products: Good or bad for human health? An assessment of the totality of scientific evidence. *Food Nutr. Res.* **2016**, *60*. [CrossRef]

4. Chandan, R.C. Dairy Industry: Chapter 2: Production and Consumption Trends. In *Dairy Processing & Quality Assurance*; Chandan, R.C., Kilara, A., Schah, N.P., Eds.; Wiley-Blackwell: Ames, IA, USA, 2008; pp. 41–58, ISBN 978-0813827568.

5. Moncada Jiménez, A.; Pelayo Consuegra, B.H. Chapter 4: El Proceso Industrial de los Productos Lácteos. In *El libro blanco de la Leche y los Productos Lácteos*; Cámara Nacional de Industriales de la Leche: Mexico City, Mexico, 2011; pp. 52–65.

6. Visioli, F.; Strata, A. Milk, dairy products, and their functional effects in humans: A narrative review of recent evidence. *Adv. Nutr.* **2014**, *5*, 131–143. [CrossRef] [PubMed]

7. Chandan, R.C. Chapter 1: Dairy Processing and Quality Assurance: An Overview. In *Dairy Processing & Quality Assurance*; Chandan, R.C., Kilara, A., Schah, N.P., Eds.; Wiley-Blackwell: Ames, IA, USA, 2008; pp. 1–38, ISBN 978-0813827568.

8. OECD/FAO. *OECD-FAO Agricultural Outlook 2016–2025*; OECD Publishing: Paris, France, 2016; ISBN 9789264253223.

9. International Dairy Federation. *The IDF Guide on Biodiversity for the Dairy Sector*; Bulletin of the International Dairy Federation; International Dairy Federation: Schaerbeek, Belgium, 2017; Volume 488.

10. FAO. *Food Outlook Biannual Report on Global Food Markets*; FAO: Rome, Italy, 2016; ISSN 0251-1959.

11. Hemme, T.; Uddin, M.M.; Oghaiki Asaah Ndambi, O.A. Benchmarking cost of milk production in 46 countries. *J. Rev. Glob. Econ.* **2014**, *3*, 254–270.

12. Samson, J.E.; Moineau, S. Bacteriophages in food fermentations: New frontiers in a continuous arms race. *Annu. Rev. Food Sci. Technol.* **2013**, *4*, 347–368. [CrossRef] [PubMed]

13. Kleppen, H.P.; Bang, T.; Nes, I.F.; Holo, H. Bacteriophages in milk fermentations: Diversity fluctuations of normal and failed fermentations. *Int. Dairy J.* **2011**, *21*, 592–600. [CrossRef]

14. Madera, C.; Monjardin, C.; Suarez, J.E. Milk contamination and resistance to processing conditions determine the fate of *Lactococcus lactis* bacteriophages in dairies. *Appl. Environ. Microbiol.* **2004**, *70*, 7365–7371. [CrossRef] [PubMed]

15. Del Rio, B.; Binetti, A.G.; Martin, M.C.; Fernandez, M.; Magadan, A.H.; Alvarez, M.A. Multiplex PCR for the detection and identification of dairy bacteriophages in milk. *Food Microbiol.* **2007**, *24*, 75–81. [CrossRef] [PubMed]

16. Verreault, D.; Moineau, S.; Duchaine, C. Methods for sampling of airborne viruses. *Microbiol. Mol. Biol. Rev.* **2008**, *72*, 413–444. [CrossRef] [PubMed]

17. Neve, H.; Berger, A.; Heller, K.J. A method for detecting and enumerating airborne virulent bacteriophage of dairy starter cultures. *Kieler Milchwirtschaftliche Forschungsberichte* **1995**, *47*, 193–207.

18. Verreault, D.; Gendron, L.; Rousseau, G.M.; Veillette, M.; Masse, D.; Lindsley, W.G.; Moineau, S.; Duchaine, C. Detection of airborne lactococcal bacteriophages in cheese manufacturing plants. *Appl. Environ. Microbiol.* **2011**, *77*, 491–497. [CrossRef] [PubMed]

19. Verreault, D.; Rousseau, G.M.; Gendron, L.; Massé, D.; Moineau, S.; Duchaine, C. Comparison of polycarbonate and polytetrafluoroethylene filters for sampling of airborne bacteriophages. *Aerosol Sci. Technol.* **2010**, *44*, 197–201. [CrossRef]

20. Ipsen, R. Microparticulated whey proteins for improving dairy product texture. *Int. Dairy J.* **2017**, *67*, 73–79. [CrossRef]

21. Geagea, H.; Gomaa, A.I.; Remondetto, G.; Moineau, S.; Subirade, M. Investigation of the protective effect of whey proteins on lactococcal phages during heat treatment at various pH. *Int. J. Food Microbiol.* **2015**, *210*, 33–41. [CrossRef] [PubMed]

22. Atamer, Z.; Samtlebe, M.; Neve, H.; Heller, K.; Hinrichs, J. Review: Elimination of bacteriophages in whey and whey products. *Front. Microbiol.* **2013**, *4*. [CrossRef] [PubMed]

23. Sun, X.; Van Sinderen, D.; Moineau, S.; Heller, K.J. Impact of lysogeny on bacteria with a focus on Lactic Acid Bacteria. In *Contemporary Trends in Bacteriophage Research*; Adams, H.T., Ed.; Nova Science Publishers, Inc.: New York, NY, USA, 2009; pp. 309–336, ISBN 978-1-60692-181-4.

24. Brüssow, H.; Frémont, M.; Bruttin, A.; Sidoti, J.; Constable, A.; Fryder, V. Detection and classification of *Streptococcus thermophilus* bacteriophages isolated from industrial milk fermentation. *Appl. Environ. Microbiol.* **1994**, *60*, 4537–4543. [PubMed]

25. Lunde, M.; Aastveit, A.H.; Blatny, J.M.; Nes, I.F. Effects of diverse environmental conditions on φLC3 prophage stability in *Lactococcus lactis*. *Appl. Environ. Microbiol.* **2005**, *71*, 721–727. [CrossRef] [PubMed]

26. Madera, C.; Garcia, P.; Rodriguez, A.; Suarez, J.E.; Martinez, B. Prophage induction in *Lactococcus lactis* by the bacteriocin Lactococcin 972. *Int. J. Food Microbiol.* **2009**, *129*, 99–102. [CrossRef] [PubMed]

27. Lunde, M.; Blatny, J.M.; Lillehaug, D.; Aastveit, A.H.; Nes, I.F. Use of real-time quantitative PCR for the analysis of φLC3 prophage stability in lactococci. *Appl. Environ. Microbiol.* **2003**, *69*, 41–48. [CrossRef] [PubMed]

28. Magadán, A.H.; Ladero, V.; Martínez, N.; del Río, B.; Martín, M.C.; Alvarez, M.A. Detection of bacteriophages in milk. In *Handbook of Dairy Foods Analysis*; Nollet, L.M.L., Toldrá, F., Eds.; CRC Press, Taylor & Francis Group: Boca Raton, FL, USA, 2009; pp. 469–482, ISBN 978-1-4200-4631-1.

29. Marcó, M.B.; Moineau, S.; Quiberoni, A. Bacteriophages and dairy fermentations. *Bacteriophage* **2012**, *2*, 149–158. [CrossRef] [PubMed]

30. Lillehaug, D. An improved plaque assay for poor plaque-producing temperate lactococcal bacteriophages. *J. Appl. Microbiol.* **1997**, *83*, 85–90. [CrossRef] [PubMed]

31. Cormier, J.; Janes, M. A double layer plaque assay using spread plate technique for enumeration of bacteriophage MS2. *J. Virol. Methods* **2014**, *196*, 86–92. [CrossRef] [PubMed]

32. Michelsen, O.; Cuesta-Dominguez, A.; Albrechtsen, B.; Jensen, P.R. Detection of bacteriophage-infected cells of *Lactococcus lactis* by using flow cytometry. *Appl. Environ. Microbiol.* **2007**, *73*, 7575–7581. [CrossRef] [PubMed]

33. Labrie, S.; Moineau, S. Multiplex PCR for detection and identification of lactococcal bacteriophages. *Appl. Environ. Microbiol.* **2000**, *66*, 987–994. [CrossRef] [PubMed]

34. Del Río, B.; Martín, M.C.; Martínez, N.; Magadán, A.H.; Alvarez, M.A. Multiplex fast real-time polymerase chain reaction for quantitative detection and identification of cos and pac *Streptococcus thermophiles* bacteriophages. *Appl. Environ. Microbiol.* **2008**, *74*, 4779–4781. [CrossRef] [PubMed]

35. Muhammed, M.K.; Kot, W.; Neve, H.; Mahony, J.; Castro-Mejía, J.L.; Krych, L.; Hansen, L.H.; Nielsen, D.S.; Sørensen, S.J.; Heller, K.J.; et al. Metagenomic analysis of dairy bacteriophages: Extraction method and pilot study on whey samples derived from using undefined and defined mesophilic starter cultures. *Appl. Environ. Microbiol.* **2017**, *83*. [CrossRef] [PubMed]

36. Campagna, C.; Villion, M.; Labrie, S.J.; Duchaine, C.; Moineau, S. Inactivation of dairy bacteriophages by commercial sanitizers and disinfectants. *Int. J. Food Microbiol.* **2014**, *171*, 41–47. [CrossRef] [PubMed]

37. Guglielmotti, D.M.; Mercanti, D.J.; Reinheimer, J.A.; Quiberoni, A.L. Review: Efficiency of physical and chemical treatments on the inactivation of dairy bacteriophages. *Front. Microbiol.* **2011**, *2*, 282–297. [CrossRef] [PubMed]

38. Murphy, J.; Mahony, J.; Bonestroo, M.; Nauta, A.; van Sinderen, D. Impact of thermal and biocidal treatments on lactococcal 936-type phages. *Int. Dairy J.* **2014**, *34*, 56–61. [CrossRef]

39. Marcó, M.B.; Quiberoni, A.; Negro, A.C.; Reinheimer, J.A.; Alfano, O.M. Evaluation of the photocatalytic inactivation efficiency of dairy bacteriophages. *Chem. Eng. J.* **2011**, *172*, 987–993. [CrossRef]

40. Capra, M.J.; Patrignani, F.; Guerzoni, M.E.; Lanciotti, R. Non-thermal technologies: Pulsed electric field, high hydrostatic pressure and high pressure homogenization. Application on virus inactivation. In *Bacteriophages in Dairy Processing*; Nova Science Publishers, Inc.: New York, NY, USA, 2012; pp. 215–238, ISBN 978-1-61324-517-0.

41. Mahony, J.; Tremblay, D.M.; Labrie, S.J.; Moineau, S.; van Sinderen, D. Investigating the requirement for calcium during lactococcal phage infection. *Int. J. Food Microbiol.* **2015**, *201*, 47–51. [CrossRef] [PubMed]

42. Carminati, D.; Giraffa, G.; Quiberoni, A.; Binetti, A.; Suárez, V.; Reinheimer, J. Advances and trends in starter cultures for dairy fermentations. In *Biotechnology of Lactic Acid Bacteria: Novel Applications*; Mozzi, F., Raya, R., Vignolo, G., Eds.; Wiley-Blackwell: Ames, IA, USA, 2010; pp. 177–192, ISBN 9781118868409.

43. Hicks, C.L.; Clark-Safko, P.A.; Surjawan, I.; O'Leary, J. Use of bacteriophage derived peptides to delay phage infections. *Food Res. Int.* **2004**, *37*, 115–122. [CrossRef]

44. Mahony, J.; Kot, W.; Murphy, J.; Ainsworth, S.; Neve, H.; Hansen, L.H.; Heller, K.J.; Sørensen, S.J.; Hammer, K.; Cambillau, C.; et al. Investigation of the relationship between lactococcal host cell wall polysaccharide genotype and 936 phage receptor binding protein phylogeny. *Appl. Environ. Microbiol.* **2013**, *79*, 4385–4392. [CrossRef] [PubMed]

45. Labrie, S.J.; Samson, J.E.; Moineau, S. Bacteriophage resistance mechanisms. *Nat. Rev. Microbiol.* **2010**, *8*, 317–327. [CrossRef] [PubMed]

46. World Health Organization. *WHO Estimates of the Global Burden of Foodborne Diseases*; World Health Organization: Geneva, Switzerland, 2015; ISBN 978 92 4 156516 5.

47. Rampling, A. The microbiology of milk and milk products. In *Topley and Wilson's Principles of Bacteriology, Virology, and Immunity*, 8th ed.; Parker, M.T., Collier, L.H., Eds.; B.C. Decker: Philadelphia, PA, USA, 1990; pp. 265–287.

48. Altekruse, S.F.; Timbo, B.B.; Mowbray, J.C.; Bean, N.H.; Potter, M.E. Cheese associated outbreaks of human illness in the United States, 1973 to 1992: Sanitary manufacturing processes protect consumers. *J. Food Prot.* **1998**, *61*, 1405–1407. [CrossRef] [PubMed]

49. Dhanashekar, R.; Akkinepalli, S.; Nellutla, A. Milk-borne infections. An analysis of their potential effect on the milk industry. *Germs* **2012**, *2*, 101–109. [CrossRef] [PubMed]

50. Costard, S.; Espejo, L.; Groenendaal, H.; Zagmutt, F.J. Outbreak-related disease burden associated with consumption of unpasteurized cow's milk and cheese, United States, 2009–2014. *Emerg. Infect. Dis.* **2017**, *23*, 957–964. [CrossRef] [PubMed]

51. Claeys, W.L.; Cardoen, S.; Daube, G.; De Block, J.; Dewettinck, K.; Dierick, K.; De Zutter, L.; Huyghebaert, A.; Imberechts, H.; Thiange, P.; et al. Raw or heated cow milk consumption: Review of risks and benefits. *Food Control* **2013**, *31*, 251–262. [CrossRef]

52. Christidis, T.; Pintar, K.D.; Butler, A.J.; Nesbitt, A.; Thomas, M.K.; Marshall, B.; Pollari, F. *Campylobacter* spp. prevalence and levels in raw milk: A systematic review and meta-analysis. *J. Food Prot.* **2016**, *79*, 1775–1783. [CrossRef] [PubMed]

53. Jamali, H.; Paydar, M.; Radmehr, B.; Ismail, S. Prevalence, characterization, and antimicrobial resistance of *Yersinia* species and *Yersinia enterocolitica* isolated from raw milk in farm bulk tanks. *J. Dairy Sci.* **2015**, *98*, 798–803. [CrossRef] [PubMed]

54. Bernardino-Varo, L.; Quiñones-Ramírez, E.I.; Fernández, F.J.; Vázquez-Salinas, C. Prevalence of *Yersinia enterocolitica* in raw cow's milk collected from stables of Mexico City. *J. Food Prot.* **2013**, *76*, 694–698. [CrossRef] [PubMed]

55. Chmielewski, T.; Tylewska-Wierzbanowska, S. Q fever at the turn of the century. *Pol. J. Microbiol.* **2012**, *61*, 81–93. [PubMed]

56. Mailles, A.; Rautureau, S.; Le Horgne, J.M.; Poignet-Leroux, B.; d'Arnoux, C.; Dennetière, G.; Faure, M.; Lavigne, J.P.; Bru, J.P.; Garin-Bastuji, B. Re-emergence of brucellosis in cattle in France and risk for human health. *Euro Surveill.* **2012**, *17*. [CrossRef]

57. Ning, P.; Guo, M.; Guo, K.; Xu, L.; Ren, M.; Cheng, Y.; Zhang, Y. Identification and effect decomposition of risk factors for *Brucella* contamination of raw whole milk in China. *PLoS ONE* **2013**, *8*. [CrossRef] [PubMed]

58. Pearson, L.J.; Marth, E.H. *Listeria monocytogenes*—Threat to a safe food supply: A review. *J. Dairy Sci.* **1990**, *73*, 912–928. [CrossRef]

59. Swaminathan, B.; Gerner-Smidt, P. The epidemiology of human listeriosis. *Microbes Infect.* **2007**, *9*, 1236–1243. [CrossRef] [PubMed]

60. Bolaños, C.A.D.; Paula, C.L.; Guerra, S.T.; Franco, M.M.J.; Ribeiro, M.G. Diagnosis of mycobacteria in bovine milk: An overview. *Rev. Inst. Med. Trop. Sao Paulo* **2017**, *59*. [CrossRef] [PubMed]

61. Doyle, M.P. *Escherichia coli* O157:H7 and its significance in foods. *Int. J. Food Microbiol.* **1991**, *12*, 289–301. [CrossRef]

62. Honish, L.; Predy, G.; Hislop, N.; Chui, L.; Kowalewska-Grochowska, K.; Trottier, L.; Kreplin, C.; Zazulak, I. An outbreak of *E. coli* O157:H7 hemorrhagic colitis associated with unpasteurized gouda cheese. *Can. J. Public Health* **2005**, *96*, 182–184. [PubMed]

63. Buzby, J.C.; Gould, L.H.; Kendall, M.E.; Jones, T.F.; Robinson, T.; Blayney, D.P. Characteristics of consumers of unpasteurized milk in the United States. *J. Consum. Aff.* **2013**, *47*, 153–166. [CrossRef]

64. Zecconi, A. *Staphylococcus aureus* mastitis: What we need to control them. *Israel J. Vet. Med.* **2010**, *65*, 93–99.

65. Schelin, J.; Wallin-Carlquist, N.; Cohn, M.T.; Lindqvist, R.; Barker, G.C.; Radstrom, P. The formation of *Staphylococcus aureus* enterotoxin in food environments and advances in risk assessment. *Virulence* **2011**, *2*, 580–592. [CrossRef] [PubMed]

66. Martínez, J.L. Natural antibiotic resistance and contamination by antibiotic resistance determinants: The two ages in the evolution of resistance to antimicrobials. *Front. Microbiol.* **2012**, *3*. [CrossRef] [PubMed]

67. United States Food and Drug Administration, Department of Health and Human Services. Grade "A" Pasteurized Milk Ordinance. 2015 Revision. Available online: https://www.fda.gov/downloads/food/guidanceregulation/guidancedocumentsregulatoryinformation/milk/ucm513508.pdf (accessed on 1 October 2017).

68. European Parliament and Council. Regulation EU No 853/2004 laying down specific hygiene rules for on the hygiene of foodstuffs. *Off. J. Eur. Union* **2004**, *139*, 55–205.

69. United States Department of Agriculture, Animal Plant Health Inspection Service National Animal Health Monitoring System. Antibiotic Use on U.S. Dairy Operations, 2002 and 2007. 2008. Available online: https://www.aphis.usda.gov/animal_health/nahms/dairy/downloads/dairy07/Dairy07_is_AntibioticUse.pdf (accessed on 1 October 2017).

70. United States Department of Agriculture, Animal Plant Health Inspection Service National Animal Health Monitoring System. Injection Practices on U.S. Dairy Operations, 2007. 2009. Available online: https://www.aphis.usda.gov/animal_health/nahms/dairy/downloads/dairy07/Dairy07_is_InjectionPrac.pdf (accessed on 1 October 2017).

71. World Health Organization. *WHO Global Principles for the Containment of Antimicrobial Resistance in Animals Intended for Food*; Report of a WHO Consultation, 5–9 June 2000; World Health Organization: Geneva, Switzerland, 2000.

72. World Health Organization. *Monitoring Antimicrobial Usage in Food Animals for the Protection of Human Health*; Report of a WHO Consultation, Oslo, Norway, 10–13 September 2001; World Health Organization: Geneva, Switzerland, 2002.

73. Witte, W. Medical consequences of antimicrobial use in agriculture. *Science* **1998**, *279*, 996–997. [CrossRef] [PubMed]

74. O'Brien, T.F. Emergence, spread, and environmental effect of antimicrobial resistance: How use of an antimicrobial anywhere can increase resistance to any antimicrobial anywhere else. *Clin. Infect. Dis.* **2002**, *34*, S78–S84. [CrossRef] [PubMed]

75. Molbak, K. Spread of resistant bacteria and resistance genes from animals to humans—The public health consequences. *J. Vet. Med. B Infect. Dis. Vet. Public Health* **2004**, *51*, 364–369. [CrossRef] [PubMed]

76. Erskine, R.J.; Walker, R.D.; Bolin, C.A.; Bartlett, P.C.; White, D.G. Trends in antibacterial susceptibility of mastitis pathogens during a seven-year period. *J. Dairy Sci.* **2002**, *85*, 1111–1118. [CrossRef]

77. Rajala-Schultz, P.J.; Smith, K.L.; Hogan, J.S.; Love, B.C. Antimicrobial susceptibility of mastitis pathogens from first lactation and older cows. *Vet. Microbiol.* **2004**, *102*, 33–42. [CrossRef] [PubMed]

78. Pol, M.; Ruegg, P.L. Treatment practices and quantification of antimicrobial drug usage in conventional and organic dairy farms in Wisconsin. *J. Dairy Sci.* **2007**, *90*, 249–261. [CrossRef]

79. Bruttin, A.; Brussow, H. Human volunteers receiving *Escherichia coli* phage T4 orally: A safety test of phage therapy. *Antimicrob. Agents Chemother.* **2005**, *49*, 2874–2878. [CrossRef] [PubMed]

80. Carvalho, C.; Costa, A.R.; Silva, F.; Oliveira, A. Bacteriophages and their derivatives for the treatment and control of food-producing animal infections. *Crit. Rev. Microbiol.* **2017**, *43*, 583–601. [CrossRef] [PubMed]

81. Gill, J.J.; Pacan, J.C.; Carson, M.E.; Leslie, K.E.; Griffiths, M.W.; Sabour, P.M. Efficacy and pharmacokinetics of bacteriophage therapy in treatment of subclinical *Staphylococcus aureus* mastitis in lactating dairy cattle. *Antimicrob. Agents Chemother.* **2006**, *50*, 2912–2918. [CrossRef] [PubMed]

82. García, P.; Madera, C.; Martínez, B.; Rodríguez, A.; Suárez, J.E. Prevalence of bacteriophages infecting *Staphylococcus aureus* in dairy samples and their potential as biocontrol agents. *J. Dairy Sci.* **2009**, *92*, 3019–3026. [CrossRef] [PubMed]

83. García, P.; Madera, C.; Martínez, B.; Rodríguez, A. Biocontrol of *Staphylococcus aureus* in curd manufacturing processes using bacteriophages. *Int. Dairy J.* **2007**, *17*. [CrossRef]

84. Bueno, E.; García, P.; Martínez, B.; Rodríguez, A. Phage inactivation of *Staphylococcus aureus* in fresh and hard-type cheeses. *Int. J. Food Microbiol.* **2012**, *158*, 23–27. [CrossRef] [PubMed]

85. Rodríguez-Rubio, L.; García, P.; Rodríguez, A.; Billington, C.; Hudson, J.A.; Martínez, B. Listeriaphages and coagulin C23 act synergistically to kill *Listeria monocytogenes* in milk under refrigeration conditions. *Int. J. Food Microbiol.* **2015**, *205*, 68–72. [CrossRef] [PubMed]

86. Kelly, D.; McAuliffe, O.; Ross, R.P.; Coffey, A. Prevention of *Staphylococcus aureus* biofilm formation and reduction in established biofilm density using a combination of phage K and modified derivatives. *Lett. Appl. Microbiol.* **2012**, *54*, 286–291. [CrossRef] [PubMed]

87. Alves, D.R.; Gaudion, A.; Bean, J.E.; Perez Esteban, P.; Arnot, T.C.; Harper, D.R.; Kot, W.; Hansen, L.H.; Enright, M.C.; Jenkins, A.T. Combined use of bacteriophage K and a novel bacteriophage to reduce *Staphylococcus aureus* biofilm formation. *Appl. Environ. Microbiol.* **2014**, *80*, 6694–6703. [CrossRef] [PubMed]

88. Gutiérrez, D.; Vandenheuvel, D.; Martínez, B.; Rodríguez, A.; Lavigne, R.; García, P. Two phages, phiIPLA-RODI and phiIPLA-C1C, lyse mono- and dual-species staphylococcal biofilms. *Appl. Environ. Microbiol.* **2015**, *81*, 3336–3348. [CrossRef] [PubMed]

89. Viazis, S.; Akhtar, M.; Feirtag, J.; Diez-Gonzalez, F. Reduction of *Escherichia coli* O157:H7 viability on hard surfaces by treatment with a bacteriophage mixture. *Int. J. Food Microbiol.* **2011**, *145*, 37–42. [CrossRef] [PubMed]

90. Soni, K.A.; Nannapaneni, R. Removal of *Listeria monocytogenes* biofilms with bacteriophage P100. *J. Food Prot.* **2010**, *73*, 1519–1524. [CrossRef] [PubMed]

91. Intralytix Inc. Available online: http://www.intralytix.com (accessed on 1 October 2017).

92. PhageGuard. Available online: https://www.phageguard.com (accessed on 1 October 2017).

93. EFSA. Scientific opinion on the evaluation of the safety and efficacy of Listex™ P100 for the removal of surface contamination of raw fish. *EFSA J.* **2012**, *10*. [CrossRef]

94. European Parliament and Council. Regulation EU No 528/2012 concerning the making available on the market and use of biocidal products. *Off. J. Eur. Union* **2012**, *167*, 1–123.

11

From Erythromycin to Azithromycin and New Potential Ribosome-Binding Antimicrobials

Dubravko Jelić [1] and Roberto Antolović [2],*

[1] Fidelta Ltd., Prilaz baruna Filipovića 29, HR-10000 Zagreb, Croatia; dubravko.jelic@gmail.com
[2] Department of Biotechnology, University of Rijeka, Radmile Matejčić 2, HR-51000 Rijeka, Croatia
*   Correspondence: rantolovic@biotech.uniri.hr

Academic Editor: Claudio O. Gualerzi

Abstract: Macrolides, as a class of natural or semisynthetic products, express their antibacterial activity primarily by reversible binding to the bacterial 50S ribosomal subunits and by blocking nascent proteins' progression through their exit tunnel in bacterial protein biosynthesis. Generally considered to be bacteriostatic, they may also be bactericidal at higher doses. The discovery of azithromycin from the class of macrolides, as one of the most important new drugs of the 20th century, is presented as an example of a rational medicinal chemistry approach to drug design, applying classical structure-activity relationship that will illustrate an impressive drug discovery success story. However, the microorganisms have developed several mechanisms to acquire resistance to antibiotics, including macrolide antibiotics. The primary mechanism for acquiring bacterial resistance to macrolides is a mutation of one or more nucleotides from the binding site. Although azithromycin is reported to show different, two-step process of the inhibition of ribosome function of some species, more detailed elaboration of that specific mode of action is needed. New macrocyclic derivatives, which could be more potent and less prone to escape bacterial resistance mechanisms, are also continuously evaluated. A novel class of antibiotic compounds—macrolones, which are derived from macrolides and comprise macrocyclic moiety, linker, and either free or esterified quinolone 3-carboxylic group, show excellent antibacterial potency towards key erythromycin-resistant Gram-positive and Gram-negative bacterial strains, with possibly decreased potential of bacterial resistance to macrolides.

Keywords: macrocycles; macrolides; quinolones; ribosome binding; dual-binding inhibition; azithromycin; erythromycin

1. Introduction

It is well known that macrocyclic compounds have great potential for broad use in the treatment of different diseases and therefore make very interesting molecules. Most of macrocyclic drugs are predominantly used for the treatment of infectious diseases, but they have also been used in the treatment of cancer, auto-immune, and inflammatory diseases [1–8], since they possess significant anti-inflammatory and immunomodulatory properties [9–13], as well as tuberculostatic, antifungal, antiparasitic, antimalarial, antiviral, and antitumor properties [5–7,14–17]. The best known macrocyclic structures are macrolides, natural compounds produced by *Streptomyces* species that are the most commonly used class of antibiotics, and newly-synthesized macrocycles that also belong to the macrolide or cyclic peptide class. The first 14-membered macrolide, erythromycin A, has been in clinical use since 1952. Erythromycin is active against Gram-positive and some Gram-negative microorganisms and is used in treatment of respiratory, gastrointestinal, and genital tract infections, as well as skin and soft tissue infections [18]. To improve acidic stability and oral bioavailability of erythromycin A, the first generation of natural or semisynthetic macrolides such as spiramycin [19], roxithromycin [20], dirithromycin [21], and clarithromycin [22] were prepared and introduced to medical practice. Discovery of the first 15-membered macrolide—azithromycin, characterized by a basic nitrogen atom inserted into the macrocyclic ring, represented a breakthrough in the macrolide antibiotic era. Azithromycin became one of the best-selling branded antibiotics worldwide.

Structural and biochemical binding information is now available on ribosome-targeting antibiotics in various species, providing insight into principles of targeting and macrolide binding [23,24]. Macrolides, as a class of compounds, express their antibacterial activity by either blocking nascent proteins progression through their exit tunnel, or by paralyzing peptide bond formation at the peptidyl transferase center [23]. Only small macrolides, such as the 12-member macrolactone ring, bind to the peptidyl transferase center. The secondary structure of 23S rRNA is folded due to base pairing and forms six domains, numbered I to VI. The tertiary structure of the rRNA is held together primarily by long-distance RNA-RNA interactions and by proteins [25]. Chemical modifications of the macrolides have a direct influence on the differences in their binding modes as well as the resistances towards the antibiotics. This insight is of fundamental importance for the design of more potent macrolides that could overcome bacterial resistance [26].

A novel class of macrolide antibiotics, named "macrolones", have been derived from azithromycin, and comprising macrocyclic moiety, linker and either free or esterified quinolone 3-carboxylic group [27,28]. They show excellent antibacterial potency towards key erythromycin-resistant Gram-positive and Gram-negative bacterial strains. Compared to azithromycin, most of the new compounds exhibit improved in vitro potency against the key respiratory pathogens [27–29]. These findings create new opportunities for in silico modeling and in vitro optimization work to produce more potent and more selective compounds, which would be less prone to bacterial resistance.

2. Macrolides and Their Mode of Action as Anti-Infectives

The era of modern anti-infective drug discovery started in 1928 when Alexander Fleming discovered (by chance) the first antibiotic from mold: penicillin from *Penicillium notatum*. Together with the discovery of the cephalosporins (from *Cephalosporium acremonium*), the penicillins are part of a large group of beta-lactams, the first generation of antibiotics. Another significant group of antibiotics were the tetracyclines, developed initially from a product of *Streptomyces aureofaciens* (chlorotetracycline). Oxytetracycline, a product of *Streptomyces rimosus*, was discovered in 1950. The macrolides represent a third family of well-known oral antibiotics. Medically-important macrolide antibiotics were originally characterized by a 12-membered (methymycin-like), 14-membered (erythromycin-like), or 16-membered (josamycin-like) lactone ring to which amino and neutral side-sugars are attached A.

Originally applied to compounds originally extracted from natural sources, macrolides, as a broader chemical term, now encompasses all macrocyclic ring lactones varying in size from eight-membered up to 62-membered rings (Figure 1).

Actinomycetes are very effective in production of bioactive compounds, such as macrolides (antibiotics), rapamycin (immunosuppressant) [13], avermectin (antiparastic) [15], nystatin (antifungal) [14], and especially with respect to antitumor compounds (doxorubicin, bleomycin) [16,17]. The importance and use of macrocyclic compounds in immunosuppression, inflammation, cancer, and infection are rapidly growing. The chemical modifications of existing macrocyclic drugs are in progress and their new therapeutic characteristic have improved further. Inflammatory cells bioaccumulate macrolides and transport them to the infected tissues. During the treatment of bacterial infections, macrolide accumulation in inflammatory cells plays an important role, since inflamed tissue releases a whole range of chemoattractant molecules, and polymorphonuclear cells, which are loaded with the antibacterial agent are, therefore, concentrated in the inflamed tissue. Bacterial components activate and degranulate inflammatory cells, and the macrolide is released into the surrounding tissue, contributing to faster clearance of the infectious pathogen [30].

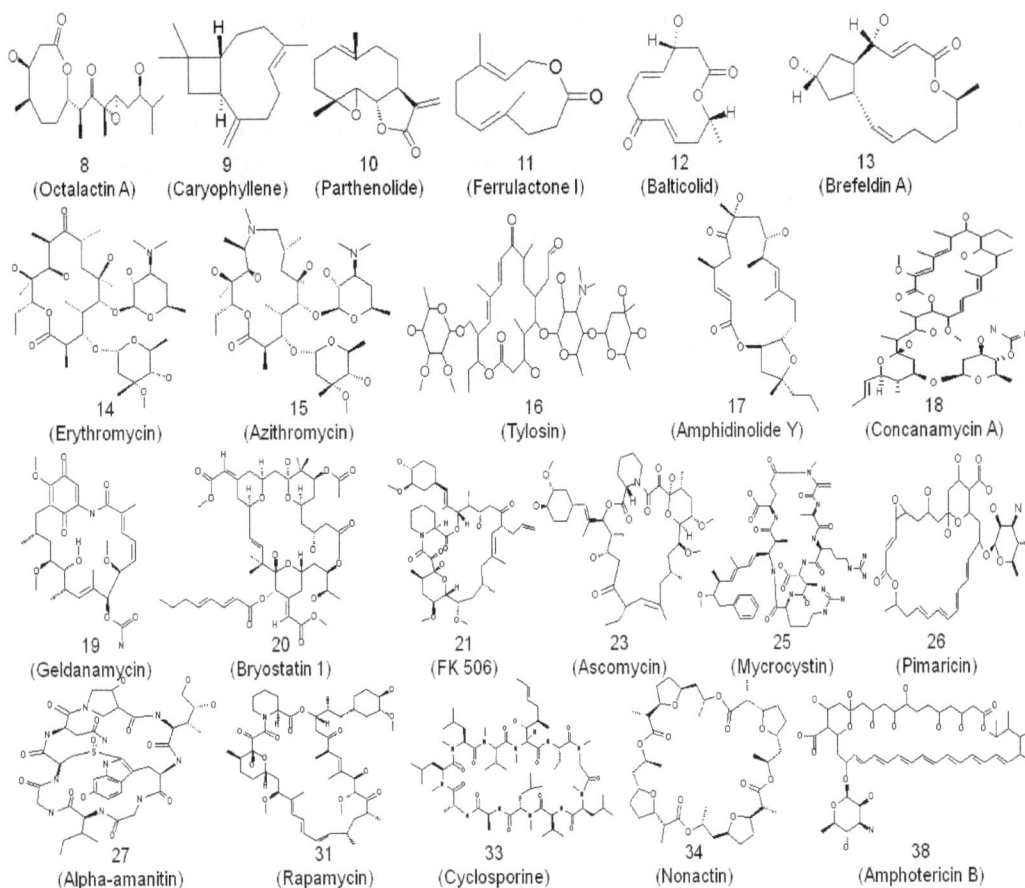

Figure 1. Examples of macrolide diversity [31], where macrocyclic ring lactones vary in size from eight-membered up to 62-membered rings. Numbers indicate the size of the ring.

The medically most important macrolide antibiotics are those structured from 12- to 16-membered large lactone rings with one or more sugar moieties, generally desosamine and cladinose, linked to the macrocyclic core [32]. Macrolides express their antibacterial activity by binding themselves to the bacterial 50S ribosomal subunits and inhibiting protein synthesis. More specifically, they have interactions with the region of the structure of the 50S subunit defining the catalytic core and the ribosomal exit tunnel (peptidyl transferase-associated region) [26]. They bind to the 23S rRNA at the nascent peptide exit tunnel and inhibit the growth of nascent peptides [33].

The ribosome interacts with different molecules in the process of translation, and the global and local structures of ribosome complexes are continuously changed to perform different functions during different stages. The subunit rotations induce conformational change that occurs during elongation, forming a rotated structure [34]. The first high-resolution X-ray crystal structures of a eukaryotic ribosomes was resolved almost two decades ago [35,36], showing ribosomes as interesting biological targets for their complexity and importance in the functioning of the whole cellular machinery. Antibiotics, interfering with ribosomal dynamics and mobility, can facilitate miscoding and influence the protein translation rate, while the degree of attenuation depends on the structure and binding position of antibiotics into the ribosome [37]. The strength of translation attenuation depends on the pause of ribosome function and the degree of ribosome stalling. All the stalling factors induce global conformational changes [38].

The active site of the ribosome is the peptidyl-transferase center in which the peptide bond among amino acids of the newly synthesized protein is formed [39]. Crystal structure of the 50S subunit clearly shows that the environment of the peptidyl transferase center is made of the 23S RNA. The many classes of ribosomal antibiotics (natural or synthesized chemical compounds by its origin) target the peptidyl transferase center [37]. Several antibiotics including the macrolides bind to 23S rRNA close to the pocket in the nascent peptide exit tunnel, approximately 8–10 Å away from the peptidyl transferase center of the 50S subunit. The consequence of that is the bacteriostatic or bactericidal effect of that class of antibiotics [40]. Due to binding closely to the peptidyl transferase center, they effectively block the formation of the peptide bond and extension of the peptide chain leading to dissociation of peptidyl-tRNA [41]. Amino acid and nucleotide identities in the binding pocket determine the binding of antibiotics since mutations in the binding pocket make the bacteria resistant to antibiotics [33]. Macrolide antibiotics, which include the representative drug erythromycin, bind in the exit tunnel near the peptidyl transferase center, contacting RNA (A2058 and A2059) and protein (L4, L22). Variability in macrolide structures has influence on the binding and inhibitory modes. Therefore, extensive efforts in drug discovery and design of new and improved antibacterial macrocyclic agents continue in order to discover new compounds with better profile toward resistant pathogens.

3. From Erythromycin to Azithromycin

The first 14-membered macrolide, erythromycin A, isolated from the actinomycete *Streptomyces erythreus* (*Saccharopolyspora erythraea*), has been in human use since 1952. Erythromycin has an antimicrobial spectrum similar to that of penicillin, and was widely used for patients who are allergic to penicillin. It exerts bacteriostatic and bactericidal properties, depending on the type of microorganism and the antibiotic concentration used. It is most effective against *Staphylococcus aureus* cocci, streptococcal group A, enterococci, and pneumococci. It inhibits the *Neisseriae* strain, and some strains of *Haemophilus influenzae*, *Pasteurellae multocidae*, *Brucellae*, *Rickettsiae*, and *Treponemae*. It is also effective against *Mycoplasma pneumoniae*, *Chlamydiae*, *Legionellae pneumophilae*, and some other atypical mycobacteria. The bioavailability of erythromycin is 30%–65%, and it is distributed in most tissues and body fluids. Plasma protein binding of erythromycin is 70%–90% and it is metabolized in the liver, partly with the formation of inactive metabolites with a $t_{1/2}$ of about 1.4–2 h [42].

Erythromycin, with its ten chiral centers and two sugar substituents (L-cladinose and D-desosamine, Figure 2), was a good starting point for numerous medicinal chemistry efforts for improvement of its biological profile (better activity, higher stability, and improved bioavailability) since the first generation of macrolides, which had low toxicity and good tolerability, were unstable in acidic media, had low toxicity and good tolerability. In the acidic environment of the stomach, erythromycin A is metabolized to its inactive 8,9-anhydroerythromycin-6,9-hemiketal and anhydroerythromycin-6,9:9,12-spiroketal. To improve the acidic stability and oral bioavailability of erythromycin A, the first generation of semisynthetic macrolides were prepared and introduced to medical practice. The main goal was to avoid ketal formation, initially by modifying the keto group or reactive hydroxyl. This approach resulted in various new chemical entities [43–45]. The most important erythromycin derivative from this group of new derivatives was erythromycin A oxime, prepared from erythromycin A and hydroxylamine hydrochloride in the presence of a weak base and buffer (Figure 2) [46–48]. The same was identified by chemists at PLIVA (the largest pharmaceutical company in Croatia and one of the leading companies in Southeast Europe and, today, a member of the Teva Group) and the work continued for the further synthesis of new, more active compounds, such as roxithromycin, dirithromycin, and clarithromycin. The roxithromycin enriched with an N-oxime side chain attached to the macrolactone ring [20], dirithromycin, in which the 9-keto group of the macrolactone ring was converted to an amino group [21], and clarithromycin, in which an additional methyl group in the 6-O-position, in comparison to erythromycin these modifications significantly improved acid-stability [22] (Figure 2).

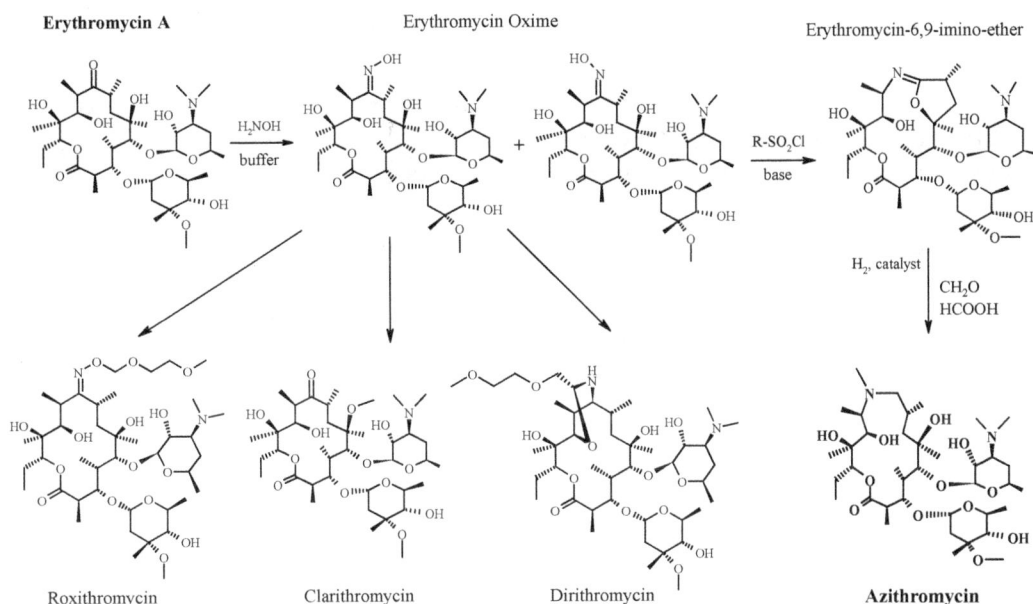

Figure 2. From Erythromycin A to other macrocyclic antibiotics (roxithromycin, dirithromycin, clarithromycin, etc.), including azithromycin, a "blockbuster" anti-infective drug [31].

The first 15-membered macrolide antibiotic on the market—azithromycin (9a-methyl-9-deoxo-9-dihydro-9a-aza-9a-homoerythromycin) (Figure 2), characterized by a basic nitrogen atom inserted into the macrocyclic ring, was synthesized in 1980 by a team of researchers at PLIVA Laboratories [49,50]. Twenty years later, in 2000, for their outstanding contribution to chemistry they received the medal of highest honor, "Heroes of Chemistry", awarded by the American Chemical Society. The discovery of the 15-membered imino-ether, produced by Beckmann's rearrangement of 9(E)-erythromycin A oxime to the amide, led to the production of a qualitatively new group of macrolide antibiotics, named the azalides [50–53]. The key reaction in the formation of azalides was established during the synthesis of O-sulfonyl derivatives of 9(E)-erythromycin A oxime [50,51]. Treatment of 9(E)-erythromycin A oxime with benzenesulfonyl chloride in an acetone-water mixture with sodium bicarbonate yielded an unexpected product, erythromycin-6,9-imino-ether (Figure 2) [51–53]. A breakthrough was the discovery of a way to open the smaller ring by hydration, and it was confirmed that a 15-membered macrocyclic ring with an "incorporated" amino group had been formed [51]. At that moment, the dogma that the macrocyclic erythromycin ring was responsible for antibiotic activity of macrolides was shattered. A new substance had similar activity against Gram-positive bacteria and significantly better activity against Gram-negative bacteria in comparison to erythromycin A [31]. The stability in an acid environment was improved, and acute toxicity decreased, but slightly less than erythromycin. However, this reaction was just one innovative step towards a much more important discovery. Reductive methylation of 9-dihydro-9-deoxo-9a-aza-9a-homoerythromycin A with formaldehyde and formic acid yielded a novel product, a significantly more potent and bioavailable macrolide antibiotic named azithromycin (Figure 2) [51,54]. Its broad spectrum of activity covered all relevant bacteria causing respiratory tract infections, including *Haemophilus influenzae* and *Moraxella catarrhalis*. Azithromycin was up to four times more potent than erythromycin against *Haemophilus influenzae* and *Neisseria gonorrhoeae*, and two-fold more potent against *Branhamella catarrhalis*, *Campylobacter* and *Legionella* sp., and significantly more potent in comparison to many genera of the family *Enterobacteriaceae*. Its minimal inhibitory concentration (MIC) for 90% of strains of *Escherichia*, *Salmonella*, *Shigella*, and *Yersinia* was ≤4 μg/mL, compared with 16 to 128 μg/mL for erythromycin [54]. Tests in animal model has shown that azithromycin treatment is able to clear chlamydial genital infection but is unable to eliminate chlamydial infection in the cecum within the same animal in doses which were effective in clearing the genital infection [55].

The in vivo tests showed that azithromycin is less than half as toxic as erythromycin (erythromycin i.v./p.o. LD50 is 360/4000 mg/kg, while azithromycin i.v./p.o. LD50 is 825/10,000 mg/kg) [52]. Furthermore, in all studies for in vivo efficacy against systemic infections in mice (by *S. aureus*, *S. typhimurium*, *S. pyogenes*, and *S. peneumoniae*), significant superiority of azithromycin was demonstrated, regardless of the administration route (subcutaneous or oral) [52,56]. Pharmacokinetic studies in mice, rats, rabbits, and dogs showed the unique properties of the new molecule, quite different than those of erythromycin. While serum levels of erythromycin oxime and amine, and levels of azithromycin were similar (several times higher than that of erythromycin), retention time was significantly longer, and urine levels were up to a hundred times higher. High and prolonged levels were observed in tissues of some organs, even 24 h after injection (liver, lung, intestine, and kidney). Brain tissue levels were low, indicating that it does not pass the brain-blood barrier [52,57,58]. Chronic toxicity was monitored in rats and dogs after 15 days and after one, three, and six months of daily dosing with 25, 50, 100, and 200 mg/kg azithromycin. Equal or small reversible adverse changes were observed with azithromycin than with erythromycin in animals given the same doses. Mutagenic, carcinogenic, and teratogenic tests were negative [52].

Clinical data exhibited close correspondence with the results obtained in animals. The serum elimination half-life was longer (41 h after oral administration, while for erythromycin it is 2 h), and renal excretion was prolonged, which indicated slow elimination from tissues. Plasma protein binding studies showed that 63% of azithromycin remained unbound in human serum; while in the case of erythromycin the percentage was only 24%, which is in line with the rapid tissue penetration of azithromycin, resulting in high tissue levels, prolonged tissue retention and high oral bioavailability (around 40%) [52]. The pharmacokinetic profile appears to be characterized by rapid and extensive uptake from the circulation into intracellular compartments. Azithromycin is subsequently slowly released, reflecting its long terminal phase elimination half-life relative to that of erythromycin [59]. These factors allowed for a single dose or single daily dose regimen in most infections, with the potential for increased compliance among outpatients for which a more frequent antimicrobial regimen might traditionally be indicated. Such a favorable pharmacokinetic profile was one of the key advantages of azithromycin, compared to the other antibacterials and macrolides [60], evaluated perform on upper respiratory tract infections (throat, sinus, and ear), lower respiratory tract infections (lung), sexually-transmitted diseases (urethritis, gonorrhea), and skin and subcutaneous tissue infections. The antibiotic was very well tolerated, and its antimicrobial spectrum, therapeutic efficacy and pharmacokinetic properties also suggested that a single daily dose of azithromycin could be effective in the treatment of all the above mentioned pathologies, as well as other infections caused by susceptible microorganisms [52,60].

Simultaneously with the testing for anti-infective properties, the physicochemical, pharmacological, and structural properties of azithromycin were investigated [61]. Azithromycin proved to be highly superior to that of erythromycin, relative to stability in acidic conditions [62]. With the determination of the crystal structure of the bacterial ribosome, various scientists tried to prepare binding complexes of ribosome and macrolide antibiotics. Analysis of the crystal structure of the large ribosomal subunit (50S) from *Deinococcus radiodurans*, complexed with azithromycin, showed that azithromycin exerts its antimicrobial activity by blocking the protein exit tunnel [26].

In 1988, azithromycin was introduced to the market by joint collaborative agreement between PLIVA (Sumamed®), and Pfizer (Zithromax®). After the year 2000, azithromycin became the market leader among antibiotics for respiratory tract infections. Pfizer's Zithromax was one of the best-selling branded antibiotics in the United States and worldwide, with total sales peaking at US $2 billion in 2005 before starting to decline with the loss of patent protection in 2006 and the resulting generic competition. Azithromycin, one of the leading drugs of the late 20th century, represents an excellent example of a unique and rational medicinal chemistry and classical structure-activity relationship approach towards drug design. As a result, azithromycin is a drug discovery success story [31]. The discovery of azithromycin was not a typical example of a drug discovery project, since the drug was developed on the basis of its anti-infective activity, and its precise mechanism of action and interaction with the ribosome-RNA complex were only discovered later, subsequent to its successful marketing [63].

4. New Macrocyclic Ribosome Inhibitors as Possible Way to Avoid Resistance Problem

The microorganisms have developed several mechanisms to acquire resistance to antibiotics, including macrolides. One of these mechanisms responsible for the lower binding and deceasing of anti-infective activity of macrolides is the change in the structure of the ribosome target either by methylation or mutation of the 23S rRNA, or mutation and consequent structural changes in the L4 and L22 ribosomal proteins in 50S ribosomal subunit [64]. The resistance to macrolide antibiotics is due to modification of the ribosomal target by methylation or mutation, decreased uptake of the molecules, and active efflux of the drug.

A family of rRNA methyltransferases designated as the Erm enzymes (more than 30 proteins have been reported) in bacteria are responsible for the development of the bacterial resistance to the antibiotics due the methylation of the 23S rRNA, in particular at adenine 2058 [65]. Methylation at A2058 significantly influences the binding of macrolides to the ribosome target and it is responsible for development of a cross-resistance to macrolides [66]. The expression of *erm* genes of bacteria is inducible, regulated by silencing of gene expression and constitutive *erm* gene translation, or constitutive, and it has been reported that the ability of macrolides to induce the expression of the *erm* genes depends on their structure. Macrolides with a 14-member lactone ring are strong inducers of the *erm* genes and these include erythromycin [67]. In addition to the structural changes of the ribosome target in the resistance development, an important role in the resistance development is played by the efflux pumps. For example, the *msrA* gene encodes an ABC transporter in staphylococci and the *mefA* gene encodes the expression of a MFS pump in streptococci [68,69] which transport the antibiotics out of the bacteria.

Azithromycin exerts its antimicrobial activity by blocking the protein exit tunnel, but in contrast to other macrolides, this effect is possibly linked with the distinct binding sites, since an additional binding site has been also recognized within the large ribosomal subunit of *D. radiodurans* [26]. Nitrogen inserted into the lactone ring does not directly contribute to the binding of azithromycin to the ribosome, but this modification alters the conformation of the lactone ring sufficiently to induce novel contacts. One azithromycin molecule interacts with domains IV and V of 23S rRNA, whereas the second azithromycin interacts with two ribosomal proteins L4 and L22 and domain II of 23S rRNA [26], so azithromycin can be considered as a dual-binding ribosome inhibitor. Additionally, in an earlier example of binding of azithromycin on the *Escherichia coli* ribosome, it is shown that azithromycin binds in a two-step process—placing of the drug in a low-affinity site located in the upper part of the exit tunnel, and slow formation of a final complex that is much stronger and more potent in preventing the synthesis of the nascent peptide through the exit tunnel [24].

In order to rationally design better drugs which would be able to overcome the existing resistance mechanisms, new directions in drug discovery have been evaluated, and rational approach to drug design, based on already-known mechanisms of drug actions has been applied. Multiple new macrolides were synthesized with the aim to inhibit the growth or to kill resistant bacterial strains. Concept of combining active macrolide scaffold and (hetero) aromatic unit via a flexible linker resulted with compounds showing remarkable antibacterial activity. This effect was first recognized in the ketolide group of macrolide antibiotics, where the cladinose sugar is substituted with a keto-group, with a cyclic carbamate group attached in the lactone ring, with telithromycin (Figure 3) [29,70–73]. These modifications enable ketolides to become more active on a much broader spectrum than other macrolides [70]. Furthermore, another potential proof of concept (at least in anti-bacterial activity) has been done on azitromycin 4″ derivatives (on cladinose sugar), where quinolone moieties have been linked with macrolactone ring, and activities toward strains which were not sensitive toward classical anti-infective macrolides have been significantly improved (Figure 3) [27].

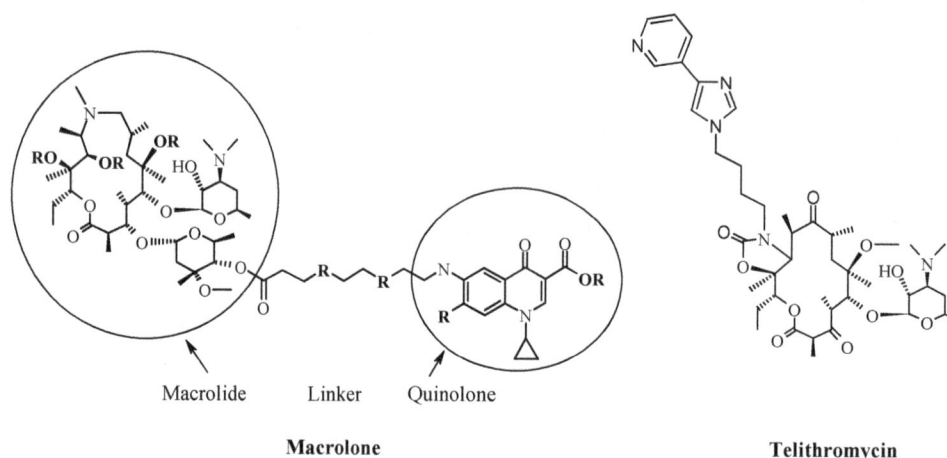

Macrolide   Linker   Quinolone

Macrolone   **Telithromycin**

Figure 3. Schematic presentation of a macrolone molecule with its distinct moieties—macrolide, linker, and quinolone (**left**); and most common chemical modification and variation positions are marked with "R". The structure of telithromycin, the first ketolide antibiotic clinically used to treat community-acquired pneumonia of mild to moderate severity (**right**).

A novel class of macrolide antibiotics—macrolones, which are derived from macrolides are comprised of a macrocyclic moiety, linker and either free or esterified quinolone 3-carboxylic group. Macrolones showed excellent antibacterial potency towards key erythromycin-resistant Gram-positive and Gram-negative bacterial strains. Compared to azithromycin or to quinolones, most of the compounds exhibited improved and superior in vitro potency against the key erythromycin-resistant respiratory pathogens [27–29]. They show activity on eryS- and MLSb-resistant *S. pneumoniae* (ribosome methylation as the major mechanisms of erythromycin resistance) in the murine pneumonia model [74]. For macrolones no demonstration has confirmed yet that their functional target is the ribosome or that they inhibit protein synthesis. However, due to flexibility of their structure, the macrolones are good candidates for possible multiple interactions with the ribosome, and the macrolide part of the macrolone should have a major role in this binding. As is the case with "classical" macrolides, which are known to possess favorable pharmacokinetic properties by accumulating in inflammatory cells, the macrolone class of compounds, with its distinct structural features, shows equal or better accumulation in inflammatory cells [75]. Unlike macrolides and ketolides, macrolones showed rapid bactericidal effects against *H. influenzae*, and they exhibited equal or lower in vitro resistance development potential than azithromycin and telithromycin in *S. pneumoniae, H. influenzae, S. aureus*, and *M. catarrhalis* [74]. Macrolones have a low clearance, large volume of distribution, and long half-life, complying with once-daily dosing potential [74]. However, even after considerable data about its in vitro activity, mode of action, in vivo efficacy, and recognizing macrolones as superior in comparison to the known macrolide antibiotics, true potential of that compound class should still be evaluated after obtaining more detailed structural insight into binding mode to the ribosome. Finally, a full pre-clinical package of ADME/Tox properties (in vitro/in vivo) of this, and similar, classes of conjugates of macrolides and other active moieties, such as quinolones, should be done before we can make a final conclusion about macrolones as a promising new class of compounds.

5. Concluding Remarks

The continuous increase of resistant bacterial strains causes a significant problem in modern health care and drug discovery. Discovery of first macrolide antibiotic erythromycin, and development of semisynthetic macrolides prepared and introduced to medical practice, such as roxithromycin, dirithromycin, spiramycin, clarithromycin, josamycin, and especially azithromycin, significantly changed anti-infective drug picture of 20th century. Azithromycin provided a considerable boost to the worldwide therapy of bacterial infections. Yet now, well into the 21st century, the ketolide group of antibiotics, such as telithromycin and solithromycin as its most important members, together with azithromycin and some of the other macrolide antibiotics, continue to reveal unexpected activities. These factors have maintained the intense research interest and may well spawn new derivatives with therapeutic effects well beyond the field of antibiotics. However, the microorganisms have developed several mechanisms to acquire resistance to all antibiotics, among them also to macrolides. Therefore, in order to design better drugs which would be able to overcome the existing resistance mechanisms, new rational directions in drug discovery and drug design have been and should be evaluated. In addition to the abovementioned ketolides, and azithromycin's possible dual-binding mode of action, where one azithromycin molecule interacts with rRNA domains, and the second azithromycin interacts with two ribosomal proteins (in a two-step process), the concept of combining active macrolide scaffold and (hetero)aromatic unit via a flexible linker has yielded compounds showing remarkable antibacterial activity. The novel class of macrolide antibiotics—macrolones, which are derived from macrolides, and which comprise macrocyclic moiety, linker, and either free or esterified quinolone group, could be great examples of combining excellent antibacterial potency towards key erythromycin-resistant pathogens. The potential novel concept of dual-binding ribosome inhibition is a possible mechanism for preventing growing resistance development.

Acknowledgments: Publishing of this article in open access is supported by the Department of Biotechnology University of Rijeka.

Abbreviations

The following abbreviations are used in this manuscript:

rRNA	ribosomal Ribonucleic acid
tRNA	transfer Ribonucleic acid
MIC	Minimal inhibitory concentration
i.v	Intravenous injection, a route of administration of a drug
p.o	Per oral, a route of administration of a drug
LD50	The median lethal dose
EryS	Erythromycin susceptible
EryR	Erythromycin resistant
MLSb	Macrolide-Lincosamide-Streptogramin b

References

1. Labro, M.T. Anti-inflammatory activity of macrolides: A new therapeutic potential? *J. Antimicrob. Chemother.* **1998**, *41*, 37–46. [CrossRef] [PubMed]
2. Labro, M.T. Macrolide antibiotics: Current and future uses. *Expert Opin. Pharmacother.* **2004**, *5*, 541–550. [CrossRef] [PubMed]
3. Čulić, O.; Eraković, V.; Parnham, M.J. Anti-inflammatory effects of macrolide antibiotics. *Eur. J. Pharmacol.* **2001**, *429*, 209–229. [CrossRef]
4. Amsden, G.W. Anti-inflammatory effects of macrolides—An underappreciated benefit in the treatment of community-acquired respiratory tract infections and chronic inflammatory pulmonary conditions? *J. Antimicrob. Chemother.* **2005**, *55*, 10–21. [CrossRef] [PubMed]
5. Sassa, K.; Mizushima, Y.; Fujishita, T.; Oosaki, R.; Kobayashi, M. Therapeutic effect of clarithromycin on a transplanted tumor in rats. *J. Antimicrob. Chemother.* **1999**, *43*, 67–72.
6. Bukvić Krajačić, M.; Perić, M.; Smith, K.S.; Ivezić Schönfeld, Z.; Žiher, D.; Fajdetić, A.; Kujundžić, N.; Schönfeld, W.; Landek, G.; Padovan, J.; et al. Synthesis, structure-activity relationship, and antimalarial activity of ureas and thioureas of 15-membered azalides. *J. Med. Chem.* **2011**, *54*, 3595–3605. [CrossRef] [PubMed]

7. Perić, M.; Fajdetić, A.; Rupčić, R.; Alihodžić, S.; Žiher, D.; Bukvić Krajačić, M.; Smith, K.S.; Ivezić-Schönfeld, Z.; Padovan, J.; Landek, G.; et al. Antimalarial activity of 9a-N substituted 15-membered azalides with improved in vitro and in vivo activity over azithromycin. *J. Med. Chem.* **2012**, *55*, 1389–1401. [CrossRef] [PubMed]

8. Wolter, J.; Seeney, S.; Bell, S.; Bowler, S.; Masel, P.; McCormack, J. Effect of long term treatment with azithromycin on disease parameters in cystic fibrosis: a randomised trial. *Thorax* **2002**, *57*, 212–216. [CrossRef] [PubMed]

9. Marjanović, N.; Bosnar, M.; Michielin, F.; Willé, D.R.; Anić-Milić, T.; Čulić, O.; Popović-Grle, S.; Bogdan, M.; Parnham, M.J.; Eraković Haber, V. Macrolide antibiotics broadly and distinctively inhibit cytokine and chemokine production by COPD sputum cells in vitro. *Pharmacol. Res.* **2011**, *63*, 389–397. [CrossRef] [PubMed]

10. Piacentini, G.L.; Peroni, D.G.; Bodini, A.; Pigozzi, R.; Costella, S.; Loiacono, A.; Boner, A.L. Azithromycin reduces bronchial hyperresponsiveness and neutrophilic airway inflammation in asthmatic children: A preliminary report. *Allergy Asthma Proc.* **2007**, *28*, 194–198. [CrossRef] [PubMed]

11. Hernando-Sastre, V. Macrolide antibiotics in the treatment of asthma. An update. *Allergol. Immunopathol.* **2010**, *38*, 92–98. [CrossRef] [PubMed]

12. Kino, T.; Hatanaka, H.; Hashimoto, M.; Nishiyama, M.; Goto, T.; Okuhara, M.; Kohsaka, M.; Aoki, H.; Imanaka, H. FK-506, a novel immunosuppressant isolated from a *Streptomyces* I. Fermentation, isolation, and physico-chemical and biological characteristics. *J. Antibiot.* **1987**, *40*, 1249–1255. [CrossRef] [PubMed]

13. Vézina, C.; Kudelski, A.; Sehgal, S.N. Rapamycin (AY-22,989), a new antifungal antibiotic. *J. Antibiot.* **1975**, *28*, 721–726. [CrossRef] [PubMed]

14. Vandeputte, P.; Ferrari, S.; Coste, A.T. Antifungal resistance and new strategies to control fungal infections. *Int. J. Microbiol.* **2012**. [CrossRef] [PubMed]

15. Omura, S.; Shiomi, K. Discovery, chemistry, and chemical biology of microbial products. *Pure Appl. Chem.* **2007**, *79*, 581–591. [CrossRef]

16. Tacar, O.; Sriamornsak, P.; Dass, C.R. Doxorubicin: An update on anticancer molecular action, toxicity and novel drug delivery systems. *J. Pharm. Pharmacol.* **2013**, *65*, 157–170. [CrossRef] [PubMed]

17. Hecht, S.M. Bleomycin: New perspectives on the mechanism of action. *J. Nat. Prod.* **2000**, *63*, 158–168. [CrossRef] [PubMed]

18. Omura, S. *Macrolide Antibiotics. Chemistry, Biology and Practice*; Academic Press Inc.: San Diego, CA, USA, 2002.

19. Kaufman, H.E. Spiramycin. *Arch. Ophthalmol.* **1961**, *66*, 609–610. [CrossRef]

20. Puri, S.K.; Lassman, H.B. Roxithromycin: A pharmacokinetic review of a macrolide. *J. Antimicrob. Chemother.* **1987**, *20*, 89–100. [CrossRef] [PubMed]

21. Fernandes, P.B.; Hardy, D.J. Comparative in vitro potencies of nine new macrolides. *Drugs Exp. Clin. Res.* **1988**, *14*, 445–451. [PubMed]

22. Watanabe, Y.; Morimoto, S.; Adachi, T.; Kashimura, M.; Asaka, T. Selective methylation at the C-6 hydroxyl group of erythromycin A oxime derivatives and preparation of clarithromycin. *J. Antibiot.* **1993**, *46*, 647–660. [CrossRef] [PubMed]

23. Schlünzen, F.; Zarivach, R.; Harms, J.; Bashan, A.; Tocilj, A.; Albrecht, R.; Yonath, A.; Franceschi, F. Structural basis for the interaction of antibiotics with the peptidyl transferase centre in eubacteria. *Nature* **2001**, *413*, 814–821. [CrossRef] [PubMed]

24. Petropoulos, A.D.; Kouvela, E.C.; Starosta, A.L.; Wilson, D.N.; Dinos, G.P. Time-resolved binding of azithromycin to *Excherichia coli* ribosomes. *J. Mol. Biol.* **2009**, *385*, 1179–1192. [CrossRef] [PubMed]

25. Petrov, A.S.; Bernier, C.R.; Hershkovits, E.; Xue, Y.; Waterbury, C.C.; Hsiao, C.; Stepanov, V.G.; Gaucher, E.A.; Grover, M.A.; Harvey, S.C.; et al. Secondary structure and domain architecture of the 23S and 5S rRNAs. *Nucleic Acids Res.* **2013**, *41*, 7522–7535. [CrossRef] [PubMed]

26. Schlünzen, F.; Harms, J.M.; Franceschi, F.; Hansen, A.S.; Bartels, H.; Zarivach, R.; Yonath, A. Structural basis for the antibiotic activity of ketolides and azalides. *Structure* **2003**, *11*, 329–338. [CrossRef]

27. Fajdetić, A.; Cipcić Paljetak, H.; Lazarevski, G.; Hutinec, A.; Alihodžić, S.; Derek, M.; Stimac, V.; Andreotti, D.; Sunjić, V.; Berge, J.M.; et al. 4"-O-(omega-Quinolylamino-alkylamino)propionyl derivatives of selected macrolides with the activity against the key erythromycin resistant respiratory pathogens. *Bioorg. Med. Chem.* **2010**, *18*, 6559–6568. [CrossRef] [PubMed]

28. Fajdetić, A.; Vinter, A.; Paljetak, H.Č.; Padovan, J.; Jakopović, I.P.; Kapić, S.; Alihodžić, S.; Filić, D.; Modrić, M.; Košutić-Hulita, N.; et al. Synthesis, activity and pharmacokinetics of novel antibacterial 15-membered ring macrolones. *Eur. J. Med. Chem.* **2011**, *46*, 3388–3397. [CrossRef] [PubMed]

29. Kapić, S.; Cipčić Paljetak, H.; Palej Jakopović, I.; Fajdetić, A.; Ilijaš, M.; Stimac, V.; Brajša, K.; Holmes, D.J.; Berge, J.; Alihodžić, S. Synthesis of macrolones with central piperazine ring in the linker and its influence on antibacterial activity. *Bioorg. Med. Chem.* **2011**, *19*, 7281–7298. [CrossRef] [PubMed]

30. Amsden, G.W. Advanced-generation macrolides: Tissue-directed antibiotics. *Int. J. Antimicrob. Agents* **2001**, *18*, S11–S15. [CrossRef]

31. Jelić, D.; Mutak, S.; Lazarevski, G. The azithromycin success story. In *Medicinal Chemistry in Drug Discovery. Design, Synthesis and Screening*; Research Signpost: Kerala, India, 2013; pp. 1–16.

32. Gaynor, M.; Mankin, A.S. Macrolide antibiotics: Binding site, mechanism of action, resistance. *Curr. Top. Med. Chem.* **2003**, *3*, 949–961. [CrossRef] [PubMed]

33. Bulkley, D.; Innis, C.A.; Blaha, G.; Steitz, T.A. Revisiting the structures of several antibiotics bound to the bacterial ribosome. *Proc. Natl. Acad. Sci. USA* **2010**, *107*, 17158–17163. [CrossRef] [PubMed]

34. Cornish, P.V.; Ermolenko, D.N.; Noller, H.F.; Ha, T. Spontaneous intersubunit rotation in single ribosomes. *Mol. Cell* **2008**, *30*, 578–588. [CrossRef] [PubMed]

35. Ban, N.; Nissen, P.; Hansen, J.; Moore, P.B.; Steitz, T.A. The complete atomic structure of the large ribosomal subunit at 2.4 A resolution. *Science* **2000**, *289*, 905–920. [CrossRef] [PubMed]

36. Harms, J.; Schluenzen, F.; Zarivach, R.; Bashan, A.; Gat, S.; Agmon, I.; Bartels, H.; Franceschi, F.; Yonath, A. High resolution structure of the large ribosomal subunit from a mesophilic eubacterium. *Cell* **2001**, *107*, 679–688. [CrossRef]

37. Yonath, A. Antibiotics targeting ribosomes: Resistance, selectivity, synergism, and cellular regulation. *Annu. Rev. Biochem.* **2005**, *74*, 649–679. [CrossRef] [PubMed]

38. Yu, D.; Zhang, C.; Qin, P.; Cornish, V.P.; Xu, D. RNA-protein distance patterns in ribosomes reveal the mechanism of translational attenuation. *Sci. China Life Sci.* **2014**, *57*, 1131–1139. [CrossRef] [PubMed]

39. Rodnina, M.V.; Wintermayer, W. Peptide bond formation on the ribosome structure and mechanism. *Curr. Opin. Struct. Biol.* **2003**, *13*, 334–340. [CrossRef]

40. Herman, T. Drugs targeting the ribosome. *Curr. Opin. Struct. Biol.* **2005**, *15*, 335–366. [CrossRef] [PubMed]

41. Leclercq, R. Macrolides, lincosamides, and streptogramins. In *Antibiogram*; Courvalin, P., Leclercq, R., Rice, L., Eds.; ESKA: Portland, OR, USA, 2010; pp. 305–326.

42. Djokić, S.; Kobrehel, G.; Lopotar, N.; Kamenar, B.; Nagl, A.; Mrvos, D. Erythromycin series. Part 13. Synthesis and structure elucidation of 10-dihydro-10-deoxo-11-methyl-11-azaerythromycin A. *J. Chem. Res.* **1988**, *1988*, 152–153. [CrossRef]

43. Kirst, H.A. *Macrolide Antibiotics*; Schoenfeld, W., Kirst, H.A., Eds.; Birkhauser Verlag: Basel, Switzerland, 2002; pp. 1–12.

44. Neu, H.C.; Young, L.S.; Zinner, S.H.; Acar, J.F. *New Macrolides, Azalides and Streptogramins in Clinical Practice*; Dekker, M., Ed.; Marcel Dekker Inc.: New York, NY, USA, 1995.

45. Schoenfeld, W.; Mutak, S. *Macrolide Antibiotics*; Schoenfeld, W., Kirst, H.A., Eds.; Birkhauser Verlag: Basel, Switzerland, 2002; p. 96.

46. Yang, B.V.; Goldsmith, M.; Rizzi, A. A novel product from Beckmann rearrangement of erythromycin A 9(E)-oxime. *Tetrahedron Lett.* **1994**, *55*, 3025–3028. [CrossRef]

47. Fattori, R.; Pelacini, F.; Romagnano, S.; Fronza, G.; Rallo, R. Unusual isoxazoline formation by intramolecular cyclization of (9E)-erythromycin A oxime. *J. Antibiot.* **1996**, *49*, 938–940.

48. Djokić, S.; Tamburasev, Z. 9-Amino-3-O-cladinosyl-6,11,12-trihydroxy 2,4,6,8,10,12-hexamethylpentadecane-13-olide. *Tetrahedron Lett.* **1967**, *17*, 1645–1647. [CrossRef]

49. Kobrehel, G.; Radobolja, G.; Tamburasev, Z.; Djokic, S. 11-Aza-10-Deozo-10-Dihydroerythromycin A and Derivatives Thereof as Well as a Process for their Preparation. U.S. Patent 4,328,334, 4 May 1982.

50. Kobrehel, G.; Djokic, S. 11-Methyl-11-Aza-4-O-Cladinosyl-6-O-Desosaminyl-15-Ethyl-7,13,14-Trihydroxy-3,5,7,9,12,14-Hexamethyloxacyclopentadecane-2-One and Derivatives Thereof. U.S. Patent 4,517,359, 14 May 1985.

51. Djokić, S.; Kobrehel, G.; Lazarevski, G.; Lopotar, N.; Tamburašev, Z.; Kamenar, B.; Nagl, A.; Vicković, I. Ring expansion of erythromycin A oxime by the Beckmann rearrangement. *J. Chem. Soc. Perkin Trans. I* **1986**. [CrossRef]

52. Đokić, S. From erythromycin to azithromycin—From macrolides to azalides. *PLIVA Saopć.* **1988**, *31*, 1–2. (In Croatian)

53. Mutak, S. Azalides from azithromycin to new azalide derivatives. *J. Antibiot.* **2007**, *60*, 85–122. [CrossRef] [PubMed]

54. Retsema, J.; Girard, A.; Schelkly, W.; Manousos, M.; Anderson, M.; Bright, G.; Borovoy, R.; Brenan, L.; Mason, R. Spectrum and mode of action of azithromycin (CP-62,993), a new 15-membered-ring macrolide with improved potency against gram-negative organisms. *Antimicrob. Agents Chemother.* **1987**, *31*, 1939–1947. [CrossRef] [PubMed]

55. Yeruva, L.; Melnyk, S.; Spencer, N.; Bowlin, A.; Rank, R.G. Differential susceptibilities to azithromycin treatment of chlamydial infection in the gastrointestinal tract and cervix. *Antimicrob. Agents Chemother.* **2013**, *57*, 6290–6294. [CrossRef] [PubMed]

56. Bright, G.M.; Nagel, A.A.; Bordner, J.; Desai, K.A.; Dibrino, J.N.; Nowakowska, J.; Vincent, L.; Watrous, R.M.; Sciavolino, F.C.; English, A.R.; et al. Synthesis, in vitro and in vivo activity of novel 9-deoxo-9a-aza-9a-homoerythromycin A derivatives; a new class of macrolide antibiotics, the azalides. *J. Antibiot.* **1988**, *41*, 1029–1047. [CrossRef] [PubMed]

57. Girard, A.E.; Girard, D.; English, A.R.; Gotz, T.D.; Cimochowski, C.R.; Faiella, J.A.; Haskell, S.L.; Retsema, J.A. Pharmacokinetic and in vivo studies with azithromycin (CP-62,993), a new macrolide with an extended half-life and excellent tissue distribution. *Antimicrob. Agent Chemother.* **1987**, *31*, 1948–1954. [CrossRef]

58. Foulds, G.; Shepard, R.M.; Johnson, R.B. The pharmacokinetics of azithromycin in human serum and tissues. *J. Antimicrob. Chemother.* **1990**, *25*, 73–82. [CrossRef] [PubMed]

59. Peters, D.H.; Friedel, H.A.; McTavish, D. Azithromycin. A review of its antimicrobial activity, pharmacokinetic properties and clinical efficacy. *Drugs* **1992**, *44*, 750–799. [CrossRef] [PubMed]

60. Schönwald, S.; Skerk, V.; Petricevic, I.; Car, V.; Majerus-Misic, L.; Gunjaca, M. Comparison of three-day and five-day courses of azithromycin in the treatment of atypical pneumonia. *Eur. J. Clin. Microbiol. Infect. Dis.* **1991**, *10*, 877–880. [CrossRef] [PubMed]

61. Lazarevski, G.; Vinković, M.; Kobrehel, G.; Đokic, S.; Metelko, B.; Vikić-Topić, D. Conformational analysis of azithromycin by nuclear magnetic resonance spectroscopy and molecular modelling. *Tetrahedron* **1993**, *49*, 721–730. [CrossRef]

62. Fiese, E.F.; Steffen, S.H. Comparison of the acid stability of azithromycin and erythromycin A. *J. Antimicrob. Chemother.* **1990**, *25*, 39–47. [CrossRef] [PubMed]

63. Hansen, J.L.; Ippolito, J.A.; Ban, N.; Nissen, P.; Moore, P.B.; Steitz, T.A. The structures of four macrolide antibiotics bound to the large ribosomal subunit. *Mol. Cell* **2002**, *10*, 117–128. [CrossRef]

64. O'Connor, M.; Gregory, S.T.; Dahlberg, A.E. Multiple defects in translation associated with altered ribosomal protein L4. *Nucleic Acids Res.* **2004**, *32*, 5750–5756. [CrossRef] [PubMed]

65. Bailey, M.; Chettiath, T.; Mankin, A.S. Induction of *erm*(C) expression by noninducing antibiotics. *Antimicrob. Agents Chemother.* **2008**, *52*, 866–874. [CrossRef] [PubMed]

66. Maravić, G. Macrolide resistance based on the Erm-mediated rRNA methylation. *Curr. Drug Targets Infect. Disord.* **2004**, *4*, 193–202. [CrossRef] [PubMed]

67. Leclercq, R.; Courvalin, P. Resistance to macrolides and related antibiotics in *Streptococcus pneumonia*. *Antimicrob. Agents Chemother.* **2002**, *46*, 2727–2734. [CrossRef] [PubMed]

68. Cai, Y.; Kong, F.; Gilbert, G.L. Three new macrolide efflux (*mef*) gene variants in *Streptococcus agalactiae*. *J. Clin. Microbiol.* **2007**, *45*, 2754–2755. [CrossRef] [PubMed]

69. Burnie, J.P.; Matthews, R.C.; Carter, T.; Beaulieu, E.; Donohoe, M.; Chapman, C.; Williamson, P.; Hodgetts, S.J. Identification of an immunodominant ABC transporter in methicillin-resistant *Staphylococcus aureus* infections. *Infect. Immun.* **2000**, *68*, 3200–3209. [CrossRef] [PubMed]

70. Scheinfeld, N. Telithromycin: A brief review of a new ketolide antibiotic. *J. Drugs Dermatol.* **2004**, *3*, 409–413. [PubMed]

71. Agouridas, C.; Denis, A.; Auger, J.M.; Benedetti, Y.; Bonnefoy, A.; Bretin, F.; Chantot, J.F.; Dussarat, A.; Fromentin, C.; D'Ambrières, S.G.; et al. Synthesis and antibacterial activity of ketolides (6-O-methyl-3-oxoerythromycin derivatives): A new class of antibacterials highly potent against macrolide-resistant and -susceptible respiratory pathogens. *J. Med. Chem.* **1998**, *41*, 4080–4100. [CrossRef] [PubMed]

72. Evrard-Tedeschi, N.; Gharbi-Benarous, J.; Gaillet, C.; Verdier, L.; Bertho, G.; Lange, C.; Parent, A.; Girault, J.-P. Conformations in solution and bound to bacterial ribosomes of ketolides, HMR 3647 (telithromycin) and RU 72366: A new class of highly potent antibacterials. *Bioorg. Med. Chem.* **2000**, *8*, 1579–1597. [CrossRef]

73. Bukvić Krajačić, M.; Novak, P.; Cindrić, M.; Brajša, K.; Dumić, M.; Kujundžić, N. Azithromycin-sulfonamide conjugates as inhibitors of resistant *Streptococcus pyogenes* strains. *Eur. J. Med. Chem.* **2007**, *42*, 138–145. [CrossRef] [PubMed]

74. Cipcic Paljetak, H.; Banjanac, M.; Ergovic, G; Peric, M.; Padovan, J.; Dominis-Kramaric, M.; Kelneric, Z.; Verbanac, D.; Holmes, D.J.; Erakovic Haber, V. Macrolones—Novel class of macrolide antibiotics active against key resistant respiratory pathogens. In Proceedings of the 53rd ICAAC Meeting, Denver, CO, USA, 10–13 September 2013.

75. Munić Kos, V.; Koštrun, S.; Fajdetić, A.; Bosnar, M.; Kelnerić, Ž.; Stepanić, V.; Eraković Haber, V. Structure-property relationship for cellular accumulation of macrolones in human polymorphonuclear leukocytes (PMNs). *Eur. J. Pharm. Sci.* **2013**, *49*, 206–219. [CrossRef] [PubMed]

12

Novel Polyethers from Screening *Actinoallomurus* spp.

Marianna Iorio [1], **Arianna Tocchetti** [1], **Joao Carlos Santos Cruz** [2], **Giancarlo Del Gatto** [1], **Cristina Brunati** [2], **Sonia Ilaria Maffioli** [1], **Margherita Sosio** [1,2] **and Stefano Donadio** [1,2,*]

[1] NAICONS Srl, Viale Ortles 22/4, 20139 Milano, Italy; miorio@naicons.com (M.I.);
atocchetti@naicons.com (A.T.); giancarlo_delgatto@hotmail.it (G.D.G.);
smaffioli@naicons.com (S.I.M.); msosio@naicons.com (M.S.)
[2] KtedoGen Srl, Viale Ortles 22/4, 20139 Milano, Italy; maildocruz@gmail.com (J.C.S.C.);
cbrunati@naicons.com (C.B.)
* Correspondence: sdonadio@naicons.com

Abstract: In screening for novel antibiotics, an attractive element of novelty can be represented by screening previously underexplored groups of microorganisms. We report the results of screening 200 strains belonging to the actinobacterial genus *Actinoallomurus* for their production of antibacterial compounds. When grown under just one condition, about half of the strains produced an extract that was able to inhibit growth of *Staphylococcus aureus*. We report here on the metabolites produced by 37 strains. In addition to previously reported aminocoumarins, lantibiotics and aromatic polyketides, we described two novel and structurally unrelated polyethers, designated α-770 and α-823. While we identified only one producer strain of the former polyether, 10 independent *Actinoallomurus* isolates were found to produce α-823, with the same molecule as main congener. Remarkably, production of α-823 was associated with a common lineage within *Actinoallomurus*, which includes *A. fulvus* and *A. amamiensis*. All polyether producers were isolated from soil samples collected in tropical parts of the world.

Keywords: *Actinoallomurus*; antibiotics polyethers; screening

1. Introduction

Antimicrobial resistance among bacterial pathogens is becoming a major threat to human health and well-being. While different approaches can be deployed to mitigate and delay the insurgence and spread of antibiotic resistance, it is also clear that we will need a constant supply of new antibiotics, especially new chemical classes not affected by current resistance mechanisms. However, new chemical classes of antibiotics have been extremely difficult to discover from combinatorial and chemical libraries and microbial products still represent a major source of drug leads as antibiotics [1].

One of the main issues with antibiotic discovery based on microbial products is the probability of rediscovering known metabolites. This requires introducing one or more elements of novelty in the screening with respect to past efforts [2,3]. An attractive element of novelty can be represented by using novel strains, for example a taxonomic group that has not witnessed extensive analyses of its secondary metabolites, since taxonomic diversity can be seen as a surrogate for chemical diversity [4]. The main idea behind this concept is that organisms that have been subjected to different evolutionary pressures have developed unique biology to survive and, for some taxa, secondary metabolites are an important part of their biology. However, since production of secondary metabolites is not distributed equally among all species, it is important to select a taxon with a high potential to produce bioactive compounds in order to increase the probability of finding new compounds with a reasonable screening effort. Following this rationale, we initiated over a decade ago a project aimed at finding taxonomically divergent filamentous *Actinobacteria*, which led to the discovery of several novel taxa, including new suborders, families and genera [5–8]. One of the new taxa, originally designated as "alpha" [5], turned out to coincide with the genus *Actinoallomurus* (family *Thermomonosporaceae*), formally described in 2009 [9] with new entries added since [10–15]. With proper isolation methods, strains belonging to the genus *Actinoallomurus* could be effectively retrieved from a variety of soil samples, enabling the creation of a consistent collection of about 1000 isolates [2,12].

Strains belonging to the genus *Actinoallomurus* have been shown to produce a variety of metabolites [12,15–19] originating from different biosynthetic pathways. In this study, we explored 200 randomly picked *Actinoallomurus* isolates from the NAICONS strain collection. Together with the metabolites previously described [16–19], we analyzed the antibacterial compounds produced by 37 strains. This set of compounds includes two novel polyethers, as described here.

2. Results and Discussion

2.1. The Screened Set

The selected *Actinoallomurus* strains were isolated from a variety of samples collected in different continents, and representing diverse environments such as densely vegetated areas, sulfur-enriched craters of volcanic origin, and plant rhizosphere. The geographic distribution of the screened strains is listed in Table 1.

Table 1. Geographic origin of the analyzed strains.

Continent	Analyzed Strains	Active Strains	Active (%)
Europe	124	59	48%
Africa [a]	24	17	71%
Asia [a]	12	3	25%
Americas [b]	40	25	62%

[a] All from tropical countries; [b] All from tropical countries, except four strains from continental USA.

Three extract types were prepared from the strains—see Material and Methods—and evaluated for their ability to inhibit growth of *Staphylococcus aureus* and of a ΔtolC mutant of *Escherichia coli*. Overall, 104 and 17 strains produced at least one extract with activity against *S. aureus* and *E. coli*, respectively. All extracts with activity against *E. coli* were also active against *S. aureus*. The highest activity was observed in the mycelium and the ethyl acetate extracts at comparable frequency (57 and 46, respectively), and only in one case was the ethyl acetate exhaust extract more active. Except perhaps for an under-representation of active strains isolated from Asian samples, there was no apparent effect of the continent of origin on the frequency of anti-staphylococcal activity (Table 1). Positive extracts were analyzed as described under Material and Methods, leading to preliminary information on the chemical identity of the identified compounds. We report below the characterization of the molecules identified from 37 of the active strains.

2.2. Coumermycins, Spirotetronates, Lantibiotics and Diketopiperazines

Coumarin antibiotics target bacterial DNA gyrase and one member of this family, novobiocin, has been used to treat bacterial infections in humans caused by Gram-positive bacteria [20]. Coumermycins are other member of this family with higher antibacterial activity than novobiocin [20]. We have previously reported that the *Actinoallomurus* sp. K275, belonging to the Alp18 phylotype, produced several members of the coumermycin complex [12]. In the course of screening the 200 strains, two additional coumermycin producers were identified: strains ID145250 and ID145519, belonging to the Alp22 phylotype. The main coumermycin congeners produced by these three strains were A2, D1 and A1, respectively. Relevant data are shown in Supplementary Materials Figure S1. Coumermycins have been reported mostly from *Streptomyces* spp. [20].

Tetronate-containing polyketide natural products represent a large and diversified family of microbial metabolites with different bioactivities [21]. Halogenated spirotetronates designated NAI-414

A and B were previously described as the main products of *Actinoallomurus* sp. ID145414 [16]. During our screening, two strains (ID145260 and ID145814) were found to produce a molecule with *m/z* [M−H]⁻ 839, an isotopic pattern compatible with the presence of two chlorines and a UV spectrum with maxima at 228 and 268 nm (see Supplementary Materials Figure S2). These properties closely resemble those reported for NAI-414 and actually match those reported for pyrrolosporin, a compound structurally related to NAI-414 but containing an additional unsaturation in the polyketide backbone. Pyrrolosporin was previously reported as a metabolite from a *Micromonospora* sp. [22,23].

Ribosomally synthesized and post-translationally modified peptides represent a rapidly expanding family of microbial metabolites, with lantibiotics as one of better known representatives [24]. *Actinoallomurus* sp. ID145699 was previously reported to produce the chlorinated lantibiotic NAI-107 and its brominated variant in Br-supplemented medium [19]. In the course of our screening, we identified strain ID145640 as an additional NAI-107 producer, with the known variations at Trp4 (hydrogen or chlorine) but just zero or one hydroxylation at Pro14 (Supplementary Materials Figures S3 and S4). Previously, NAI-107 was reported as the product of two independent *Microbispora* isolates [25,26].

Diketopiperazines represent a broad family of cyclized dipeptides produced by a large variety of microorganisms [27]. It is thus no surprise that one of the strains in the present work, *Actinoallomurus* sp. ID145219, produced two compounds with activity against *S. aureus* that were identified as cyclo-Phe-Leu and cyclo-Phe-Phe (see Supplementary Materials Figure S5). The structures of the metabolites mentioned in Section 2.2 are illustrated in Figure 1.

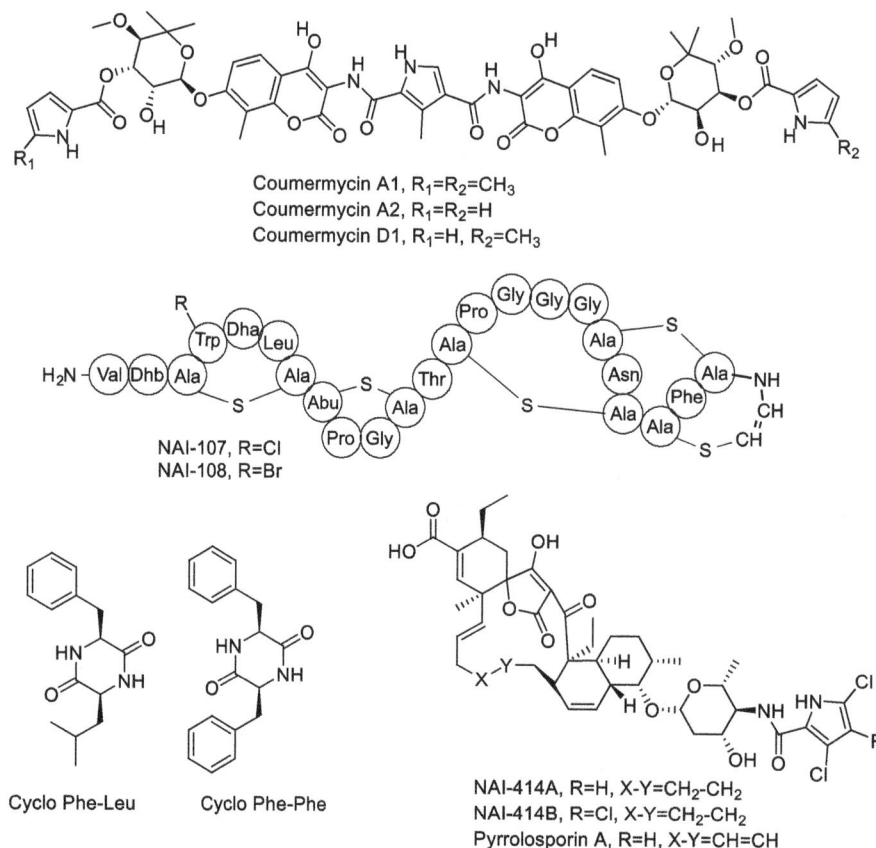

Coumermycin A1, $R_1=R_2=CH_3$
Coumermycin A2, $R_1=R_2=H$
Coumermycin D1, $R_1=H, R_2=CH_3$

NAI-107, R=Cl
NAI-108, R=Br

Cyclo Phe-Leu   Cyclo Phe-Phe

NAI-414A, R=H, X-Y=CH₂-CH₂
NAI-414B, R=Cl, X-Y=CH₂-CH₂
Pyrrolosporin A, R=H, X-Y=CH=CH

Figure 1. Chemical structures of molecules produced by *Actinoallomurus* and described in Section 2.2.

2.3. Aromatic Polyketides

During the course of our screening, we frequently encountered strains producing aromatic polyketides. Identified products included the allocyclinones, hyper-halogenated angucyclinones detected from twelve independent strains belonging to three different phylotypes [17]; the paramagnetoquinones, highly paramagnetic tetracenes produced by three independent strains belonging to three different phylotypes [18]; three producers of the related dihydrobenzo-(alpha)-naphthacenequinones pradimicin (strains ID145114 and ID145318) and benanomicin (strain ID145226) (see Supplementary Materials Figure S6). Pradimicin and benanomicin present a common polyketide core decorated with a disaccharide unit and differ for the presence/absence of an *N*-methyl on the aminated-sugar. Both compounds were previously reported as products of *Actinomadura* spp., with pradimicin produced by a confirmed species of the genus, *Actinomadura hibisca* [28]. Benanomicin had already been reported as a metabolite of *Actinoallomurus* strain K15 [12].

Overall, this brief survey of aromatic polyketides indicates that *Actinoallomurus* spp. are capable of producing decaketides (i.e., paramagnetoquinones), undecaketides (i.e., allocyclinones, presumably undergoing oxidative ring cleavage after polyketide formation) and dodecaketides (i.e., pradimicin and benanomicin). The structures of these metabolites are shown in Figure 2.

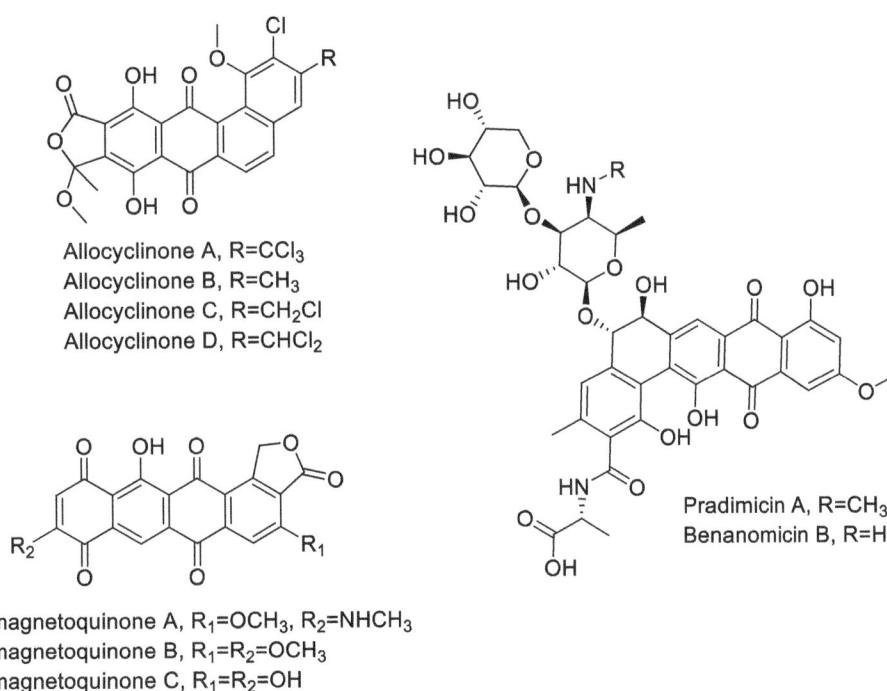

Allocyclinone A, R=CCl$_3$
Allocyclinone B, R=CH$_3$
Allocyclinone C, R=CH$_2$Cl
Allocyclinone D, R=CHCl$_2$

Paramagnetoquinone A, R$_1$=OCH$_3$, R$_2$=NHCH$_3$
Paramagnetoquinone B, R$_1$=R$_2$=OCH$_3$
Paramagnetoquinone C, R$_1$=R$_2$=OH

Pradimicin A, R=CH$_3$
Benanomicin B, R=H

Figure 2. Chemical structures of aromatic polyketides produced by *Actinoallomurus* and described in Section 2.3.

2.4. Polyethers

The extracts from several strains presented large inhibition halos against *S. aureus* but little or no activity against the *E. coli* Δ*tolC* strain. Upon resolution by high performance liquid chromatography (HPLC), the active fractions showed a retention time of 5–11 min and, with one exception, had no ultraviolet (UV) absorption. Mass spectrometry (MS) analysis indicated the presence of *m/z* signals consistent with the formation NH$_4^+$ and Na$^+$ adducts but with no detectable H$^+$ adducts. It should be noted that the extraction procedure and the liquid chromatography (LC)-MS eluent do not contain ammonium or sodium ions. Hence, the observation of NH$_4^+$ and Na$^+$ adducts suggests a high cation-binding ability of the active molecules. Moreover, the fragmentation pattern showed losses of 44 amu (free carboxylic acid) and 62 amu (decarboxylation and dehydratation). As demonstrated below, we identified three distinct polyether families within twelve strains: one new compounds, designated α-823, produced by ten independent isolates; an additional new polyether, designated α-770, and the previously reported octacyclomycin, produced by one strain each. Table 2 lists the identified polyether-producing *Actinoallomurus* isolates, along with their origins, accession number of the 16S rRNA gene sequences and the *m/z* value of the most abundant congener.

Table 2. Polyether-producing *Actinoallomurus* strains.

Strain	Origin	Accession Number [a]	*m/z* [M—Na]$^+$	Compound
ID145265	soil, Nicaragua	MH3933000	937	α-823
ID145554	soil, Mauritius	MH3933001	937	α-823
ID145603	soil, Brazil	MH3933002	937	α-823
ID145770	soil, Niger	MH3933011	857	α-770
ID145802	soil, Nicaragua	MH3933003	937	α-823
ID145804	soil, Cameroon	MH3933004	937	α-823
ID145811	soil, Cameroon	MH3933005	937	α-823
ID145816	soil, Cameroon	MH3933006	937	α-823
ID145817	soil, Cameroon	MH3933010	1039	octacyclomycin
ID145823	soil, Venezuela	MH3933007	937	α-823
ID145828	soil, Nicaragua	MH3933008	937	α-823
ID145830	soil, Nicaragua	MH3933009	937	α-823

[a] On the basis of the 16S rRNA gene sequence.

Several strains produced a likely polyether with major *m/z* signals [M+NH$_4$]$^+$ 932 and [M+Na]$^+$ 937 (see Figure 4a,b for representative example). The metabolite produced by all these strains appeared identical (Table 2) and those from strain ID145823 were analyzed in detail. The strain produced a complex of related molecules (Figure 4a; Supplementary Materials Table S1) with similar HPLC retention times (they all eluted at ≥90% acetonitrile; see Supplementary Materials Figure S7), appearing as both [M+NH$_4$]$^+$ and [M+Na]$^+$ adducts, and with similar fragmentation patterns (Supplementary Materials Figure S7). The deduced molecular formulae indicate that the congeners varied in methyl group(s) and oxygen(s) (Supplementary Materials Table S1). The structure of the major congener, designated α-823, was elucidated by a combination of NMR (Supplementary Materials Figures S8–S13) and HR-ESI-MS (Figure S14) and MS/MS analyses. The molecular formula was defined as C$_{48}$H$_{82}$O$_{16}$Na (calculated 937.5495 [M+Na]$^+$, found 937.5510 [M+Na]$^+$). The analysis of ^{1}H-monodimentional spectrum revealed the presence of four singlet and six doublet methyl signals, along with four methoxy groups. Moreover, several diastereotopic methylene signals were observed using 2D-HSQC (bi-dimensional Heteronuclear Single Quantum Coherence) experiments, indicating CH$_2$ inserted into rigid structures or close to stereocenters. COSY (COrrelated SpectroscopY) and TOCSY (TOtal Correlated SpectroscopY) analyses, along with HMBC (Heteronuclear Multiple Bond Correlation, resulted in the structure shown in Figure 3. α-823 consists of a C$_{30}$ chain with three substituted tetrahydrofuranes and three substituted tetrahydropyranes. Tetrahydrofurane C carries a deoxysugar (Figure 4). Structurally, α-823 closely resembles the polyether SF-2361, produced by an *Actinomadura* sp. [29,30]. Despite an identical molecular formula, α-823 carries a methyl at C-6, while a methyl group in SF-2361 has been assigned to C-2. Indeed, in the α-823 spectrum C-2 is a free methylene with δ$_H$ signal at 2.18–2.54 ppm and δ$_C$ at 44.7 ppm (due to the proximity to a hemiacetal and a carboxylic acid), while C-6 carries no proton (δ$_C$ at 78.6 ppm) and shows HMBC correlations with a methoxy at 3.38 ppm and a singlet methyl at 1.16 ppm.

Strain ID145817 was found to produce a bioactive compound eluting at 9.0 min with no UV adsorption. Upon MS analysis, it showed *m/z* signals [M+NH$_4$]$^+$ 1034 and [M+Na]$^+$ 1039, corresponding to the NH$_4^+$ and Na$^+$ adduct of a molecule of 1016 amu, with major fragments at 990–995 and 972–977 (Supplementary Materials Figure S15). Additionally, a Δ*m/z* of 129 suggested the elimination of a deoxysugar. All these properties are consistent with the metabolite produced by strain ID145817 being identical to octacyclomycin, a di-glycosylated polyether previously reported from a *Streptomyces* sp. [31]. NMR analysis of the purified compound confirmed this hypothesis showing signals identical to those reported in literature for octacyclomycin (data not shown). The structure of octacyclomycin is reported in Figure 4. Octacyclomycin, SF-2361 and α-823 derive from a C$_{30}$ chain with identical sequence of tetrahydrofuranes and tetrahydropyranes, but differ for the number and position of methyls, oxygens and glycosyl moieties.

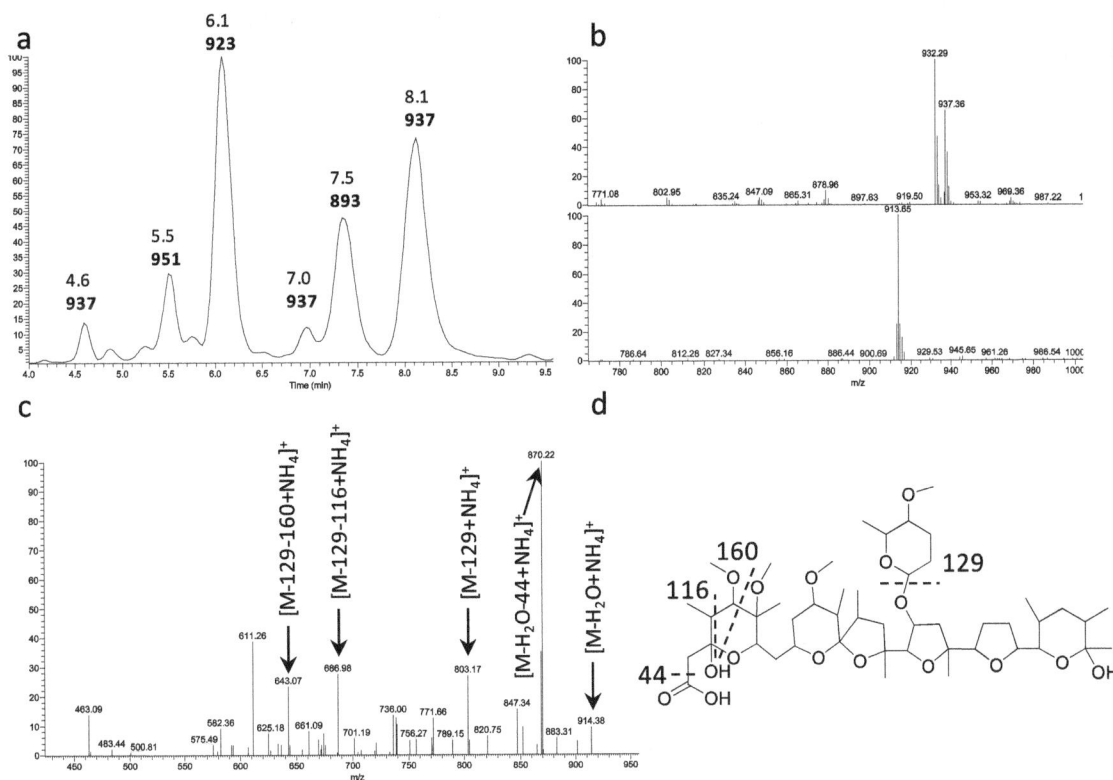

Figure 3. Analysis of α-823. (**a**) Base peak chromatogram of the 4.0–10.0 min portion with retention times and m/z $[M+MH4]^+$ values. Data obtained with a partially purified extract of *Actinoallomurus* sp. ID145823 (see Table S1 and Figure S7 for the congeners comparison); (**b**) mass spectrometry (MS) at 8.1 min in positive (above) and negative (below) ionization mode; (**c**) MS^2 analysis of m/z $[M+NH_4]^+$ 932; (**d**) putative fragmentation pathway for α-823.

Strain ID145770 was found to produce an active peak eluting at 6.9 min and showing the polyether-diagnostic m/z signals $[M+NH_4]^+$ 852 and $[M+Na]^+$ 857, corresponding to a molecule of 834 amu (Figure 5a,b). Unlike the other polyethers, however, this peak showed a UV signal with maximum at 314 nm (Figure 5a) and a $\Delta m/z$ 135 upon MS fragmentation, consistent with presence of a methylsalicylate moiety (Figure 5c), a chromophore previously found in the polyether cationomycin [32]. The active molecule was produced along with a related, $\Delta m/z$ +14 species, consistent with the presence of an extra methyl group atom, as listed in Table S3 and shown in Figure S16. The structure of the major congener α-770 was elucidated by a combination of NMR (Figures S17–S22), HR-ESI-MS (Figure S23) and MS/MS analyses (Figure 5). The molecular formula was defined as $C_{45}H_{70}O_{14}Na$ (calculated 857.4658 $[M+Na]^+$, found 857.4695 $[M+Na]^+$). The analysis of ^{1}H- and HSQC spectra revealed the presence of 2 methoxy along with 10 methyl groups, with four of them devoid of multiplicity. Moreover, several diastereotopic methylene signals were observed, indicating CH_2 inserted into rigid structures or close to stereocenters. The 2D-NMR-experiments allowed assigning the carbons in a structure consisting four substituted tetrahydrofuranes and one substituted tetrahydropyran, as shown in Figure 4. The overall structure of α-770 is similar to that of cationomycin, produced by an *Actinomadura* sp. [32]. Both polyethers consists of a C_{27} chain with identical positioning of the methyl groups, suggesting they a common origin from incorporation of the same sequence of propionate and acetate precursors [33]; and both polyethers carry a 6-methylsalicylate moiety linked in an ester bond the C-3 hydroxyl. However, despite these similarities and the small mass difference (16 amu), α-770 and cationomycin differ significantly in the hydroxyl and methoxy decorations. Indeed, 2D-HMBC correlations established that α-770 lacks the hydroxyls at positions 15 and 5′, which are present as methoxy groups in cationomycin, as well as the hydroxyl at position 3. In contrast, α-770 carries methoxys at positions 11 and 21, while cationomycin has no hydroxyls at those positions.

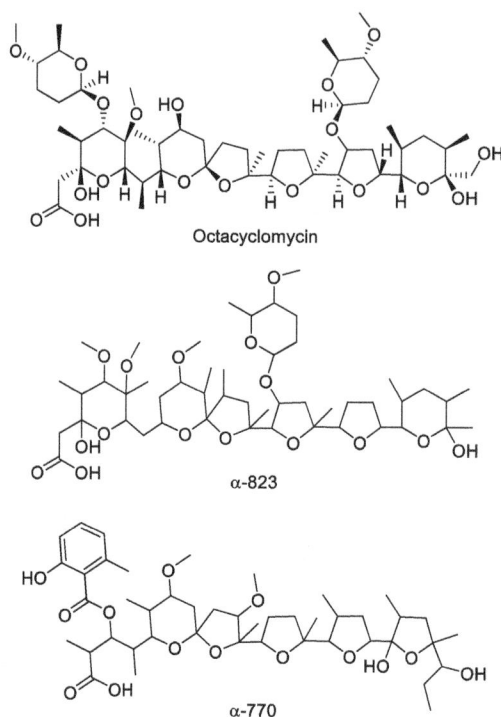

Figure 4. Chemical structure of polyethers produced by *Actinoallomurus* and described in Section 2.4.

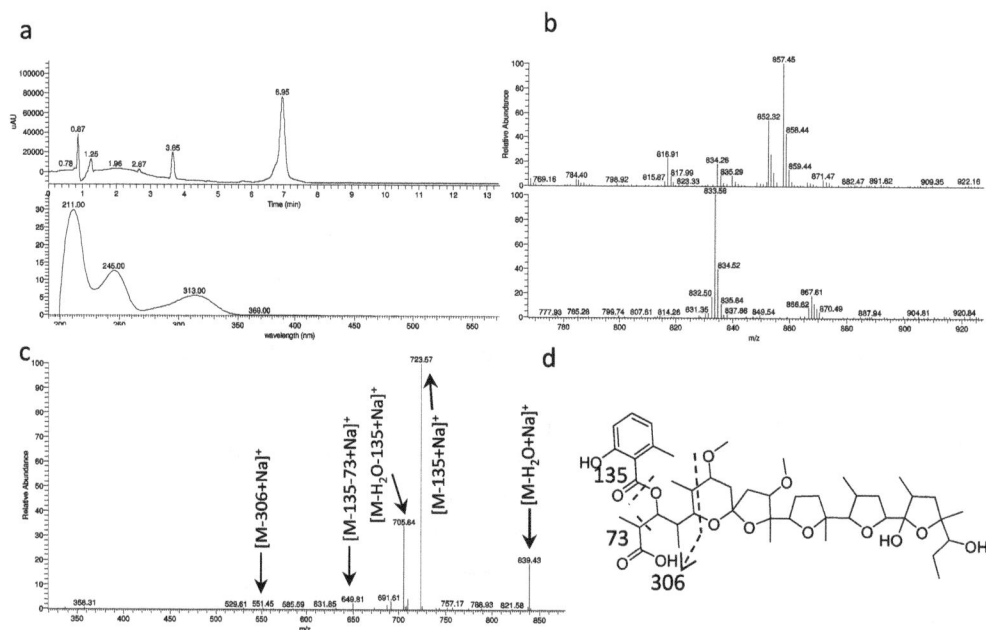

Figure 5. Analysis of α-770. (**a**) UV chromatogram at 230 nm and UV spectrum of 6.9-min peak. Data obtained with a partially purified extract of *Actinoallomurus* sp. ID145770; (**b**) MS at 6.9 min in positive (above) and negative (below) ionization mode; (**c**) MS² of m/z [M+NH₄]⁺ 852; (**d**) putative fragmentation pathway for α-770.

The carbon chain of polyethers is assembled by type I PKSs, followed by ring formation by dedicated epoxidases [33]. The carbon chains of α-770 and α-823 are likely to derive from trideca- and pentadeca-ketide precursors, respectively. In addition, the 6-methylsalicylate unit of cationomycin has been show to result from acetate incorporation [34], consistent with the involvement of a type III PKS system.

The antimicrobial activity of polyethers is strictly connected to their ability to insert into cellular membranes and alter transport of metal cations, which leads to changes in the osmotic pressure inside the cytoplasm and cell death [30,35]. However, polyethers generally lack cellular selectivity. The antibacterial activities of α-823 and α-770 are reported in Table 3. They show potent activities against most Gram-positive bacteria, with minimal inhibitory concentrations (MICs) well below 1 μg/mL for α-770, the most active of the three compounds, with 2–4 times lower MICs than salinomycin against most of the tested strains. The polyether α-823 was generally 4–16 times less active than α-770, except for an increased activity against *Mycobacterium smegmatis*. No activities were detected against Gram-negative strains (not shown), except for *Moraxella catarrhalis*.

Table 3. MICs (Minimal Inhibitory Concentrations) of α-770 and α-823 in comparison with salinomycin.

Microorganism [a]	Code	MIC (μg/mL)		
		α-770	α-823	Salinomycin
Staphylococcus aureus (MSSA)	ATCC 6538P	0.125	0.5	0.25
S. aureus (MRSA)	L1400	0.125	2	0.5
S. aureus (GISA)	L3797	0.125	1	0.125
Streptococcus pyogenes	L49	≤0.03	≤0.03	≤0.03
S. pneumoniae	L44	≤0.03	0.125	0.125
S. haemolyticus	L1730	0.125	1	0.5
S. epidermidis	ATCC 12228	0.125	1	0.5
Enterococcus faecalis	L559	≤0.03	0.25	≤0.03
E. faecium	L568	0.25	1	1
Bacillus subtilis	ATCC 6633	≤0.03	0.125	0.125
Micrococcus luteus	ATCC 10240	0.125	0.5	0.5
Mycobacterium smegmatis	mc^2 155	16	2	64
Moraxella catarrhalis	L3292	2	8	16
Clostridium difficile	L4013	0.5	0.125	0.25
Candida albicans	L145	>64	>64	>64

[a] abbreviations: MRSA, methicillin-resistant *Staphylococcus aureus*; MSSA, methicillin-sensitive *Staphylococcus aureus*; GISA, glycopeptide-intermediate *Staphylococcus aureus*.

Some polyethers (e.g., salinomycin, monensin) are commercially used as coccidiostatic agents and salinomycin has also been evaluated as anticancer agents [36]. Recently, salinomycin and other ionophores have been shown to have transmission blocking activity against the etiological agent of malaria [37]. When tested against one chloroquine-sensitive and one chloroquine-resistant strain of *Plasmodium falciparum*, α-770 and α-823 showed inhibitory activity in the 2–10 nM range comparable to those of salinomycin [37]. It should be noted that, although there are over 120 reported polyethers in the literature, their mechanism of action has been studied on a limited number of molecules [30] and we are not aware of studies aimed at making polyethers selective towards a particular cell type.

The 16S rRNA gene sequences of the polyether-producing *Actinoallomurus* strains of Table 2 were determined and compared to those of all described *Actinoallomurus* species. The results are shown in Figure 6. All the ten α-823 producers cluster together in a compact branch that includes the type strains *Actinoallomurus fulvus* and *A. amamiensis*: specifically, the identical 16S rRNA gene sequences from strains ID145265, -145554, -145603 and -145830 are 100% identical to that from *A. fulvus*; the 16S rRNA genes sequences from ID145802 and -145828 are 99.9% and 100% identical, respectively, to that from *A. amamiensis*; while the identical 16S rRNA gene sequences from strains ID145804, -145811 and -145816 and that from strain ID145823 are less related to those of described species (Figure 6). The octacyclomycin producer ID145817 is less closely related (≤99.1% identity) to *A. bryophytorum* and *A. yoronensis*, although all these strains belong to a related phylogenetic branch. The α-770 producer, instead, is distantly related to *A. spadix* (98.7% identity) and belongs to an unrelated branch that includes, among others, strain ID145113, the producer of the aromatic polyketide paramagnetoquinone [18]. Remarkably, all polyether-producing *Actinoallomurus* strains were isolated from soil samples of tropical origin (Table 2), notwithstanding that 64% of the screened strains were of non-tropical origin (mostly from Europe; see Table 1). These observations suggest that the branch including *A. fulvus*, *A. amamiensis* and the α-823 producers might consist of cosmopolitan strains and that polyether production might be mostly associated with *Actinoallomurus* strains from tropical environment. Previous studies have established a correlation between different classes of secondary metabolites and geographic origin [38,39], although we are unaware of previous reports on biogeography of polyether production.

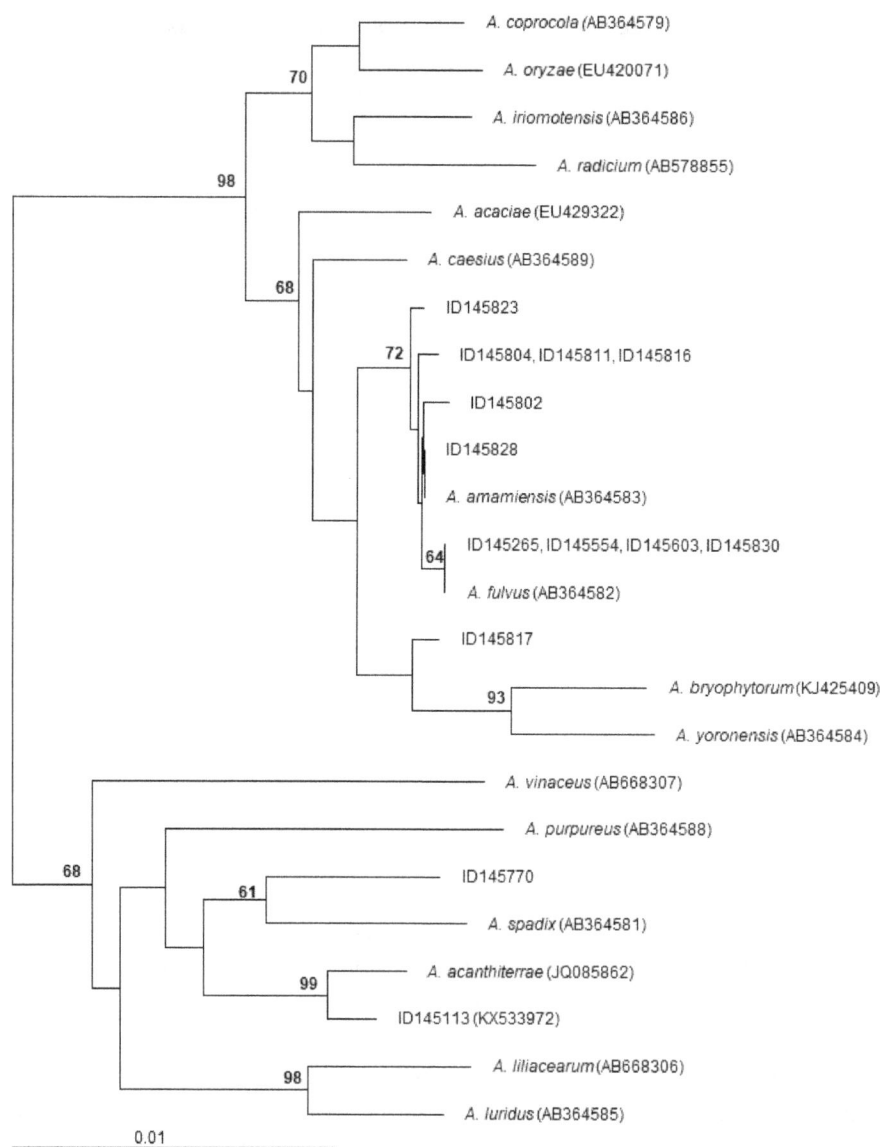

Figure 6.   Neighbor-joining tree showing the phylogenetic position of polyether-producing *Actinoallomurus* strains. Type-strains of all described *Actinoallomurus* species are included. The sequence of the paramagnetoquinone producer *Actinoallomurus* sp. ID145113 is also included. The tree is based on 1309 unambiguously aligned positions in the 16S rRNA gene sequences. Numbers at the nodes are bootstrap values based on 100 resamplings; only values higher than 60 are shown. Scale bar represents 1 inferred substitutions per 100 nucleotides. The tree was rooted using *Streptosporangium roseum* 16S rRNA gene sequence (X89947) as outgroup.

3. Materials and Methods

3.1. Bacterial Strains and Media

Actinoallomurus strains are from the NAICONS strain library. Each strain was propagated on S1-5.5 plates (60 g/L oatmeal, 18 g/L agar, 1 mL/L Trace Elements Solution) at 30 °C for two to three weeks. From these plates, the grown mycelium was used to inoculate AF-A medium (10 g/L dextrose monohydrate, 4 g/L soybean meal, 1 g/L yeast extract, 0.5 g/L NaCl, 1.5 g/L 2-(*N*-morpholino) ethanesulfonic acid, pH adjusted to 5.6) in shake-flasks. After 8 days in a rotatory shaker (200 rpm) at 30 °C, cultures were harvested and extracted (see Section 3.2).

PCR amplifications with the eubacterial primers F27 and R1492 and phylogenetic analyses of the 16S rRNA gene sequences were performed as previously described [40]. The 16S rRNA gene sequences have been deposited in GenBank, as listed in Table 2.

3.2. Preparation of Extracts

Three different extracts were prepared from each culture. The culture was centrifuged at 16,000 rcf for 5 min and the resulting pellet was resuspended in 0.4 vol ethanol, while the supernatant was used for ethyl acetate extraction (see below). After shaking 1 h at 55 °C, the suspension was centrifuged once more (16,000 rcf, 5 min) and the supernatant transferred to a new tube, dried under vacuum and resuspended in 10% DMSO at 0.2× the original culture volume. This extract was designated as the mycelium extract.

The supernatant from the first centrifugation step above was extracted with 0.5 vol ethyl acetate. After mixing and phase separation, the organic phase was transferred to a new tube and the aqueous phase extracted again with further 0.5 vol ethyl acetate. The two organic phases were combined, dried and resuspended at 5× the original concentration in 10% DMSO. This extract was designated as EtAc extract. The exhausted aqueous phase was also retained and tested as such.

3.3. Antibacterial Assays

The screening was performed by agar diffusion, using plates containing 15 mL of Müller-Hinton Agar and inoculated with 5×10^5 CFU/mL of the indicator strain. Strains used in this assay were *Staphylococcus aureus* ATCC 6538P and *Escherichia coli* L4242, a Δ*tolC* derivative of MG1061. After spotting 20 µL of the resuspended extract, plates were incubated 18–20 h at 37 °C. After HPLC fractionation, bioactive fractions were identified using the same methodology.

MIC determinations of purified compounds were performed by broth micro dilution in sterile 96-well polystyrene microtiter plates according to CLSI guidelines, using Müller Hinton broth (Difco Laboratories) containing 20 mg/L CaCl$_2$ and 10 mg/L MgCl$_2$ for all strains except for *Streptococcus* spp., which were grown in Todd Hewitt broth. Strains were inoculated at 5×10^5 CFU/mL and incubated at 37 °C for 20−24 h. Strain with an L prefix are from the NAICONS pathogens library.

3.4. Analytical Procedures

For monitoring metabolites production analytical HPLC was performed on Shimadzu Series 10 spectrophotometer (Kyoto, Japan), equipped with a reverse-phase column, LiChrospher RP-18, 5 µm, 4.6 × 125 mm (Merck, Darmstadt, Germany). Phase A was 0.1% trifluoroacetic acid (TFA), phase B acetonitrile, and the flow rate was 1 mL/min. Resolution was achieved with a linear gradient from 10% to 36% phase B in 5 min; from 36% to 50% phase B in 7 min; and from 50% to 80% phase B in 1 min; followed by a 4-min isocratic step at 80% phase B and column re-equilibration. UV detection was at 230 and 270 nm. LC-MS analyses were performed on a Dionex UltiMate 3000 coupled with an LCQ Fleet (Thermo scientific) mass spectrometer equipped with an electrospray interface (ESI) and a tridimensional ion trap. The column was an Atlantis T3 C18 5 µm × 4.6 mm × 50 mm maintained at 40 °C at a flow rate of 0.8 mL/min. Phases A and B were 0.05% TFA in water and acetonitrile, respectively. The elution was with a 14-min multistep program that consisted of 10, 10, 95, 95, 10 and

10% phase B at 0, 1, 7, 12, 12.5 and 14 min, respectively. UV-VIS signals (190–600 nm) were acquired using the diode array detector. The m/z range was 110–2000 and the ESI conditions were as follows: spray voltage of 3500 V, capillary temperature of 275 °C, sheath gas flow rate at 35 units and auxiliary gas flow rate at 15 units.

High resolution MS spectra were recorded at Unitech OMICs (University of Milano, Italy) using a Triple TOF® 6600 (Sciex) equipped with an ESI source. The experiments were carried out by direct infusion in positive ionization mode. The ESI parameters were the following: curtain gas 25 units, ion spray voltage floating 5500 v, temperature 50 °C, ion source gas1 10 units, ion source gas2 0 units, declustering potential 80 v, syringe flow rate 10 μL/min, accumulation time 1 s.

Mono- and bi-dimensional NMR spectra were measured in CDCl$_3$ at 298K using an AMX 400 MHz spectrometer. Chemical shifts are reported relative to CDCl$_3$ (δ 7.26 ppm).

3.5. Purification of Polyethers

α-823: Nine parallel 100-mL cultures of *Actinoallomurus* sp. ID145823 in AF-A medium were harvested at seven days and filtered through paper under reduced pressure to separate the mycelium from the clear broth. The latter (860 mL) was extracted three times with 450 mL ethyl acetate while the mycelium was treated with 100 mL acetone, kept on a rotary shaker 1 h and centrifuged. The combined organic phases were dried under reduced pressure and dissolved in 2 mL dichloromethane. The sample was resolved on a 12 g direct-phase Flash column RediSep RF (Teledyne Isco) by using a CombiFlash RF Teledyne Isco medium-pressure chromatography system. The column was previously conditioned at 100% dichloromethane and then eluted at 15 mL/min with a 20-min linear gradient from 0 to 10% methanol. Fractions were analyzed by LC-MS and those with the highest purity were pooled and dried, obtaining 14 mg of purified α-823. Five mg were dissolved in CDCl$_3$ for NMR analysis.

Octacyclomycin: Two parallel 100-mL cultures of *Actinoallomurus* sp. ID145817 in AF-A medium were harvested at seven days and filtered through paper under reduced pressure to separate the mycelium from the clear broth. The latter (170 mL) was extracted three times with 80 mL ethyl acetate while the mycelium was treated with 100 mL ethanol, kept 1 h on a rotary shaker and centrifuged. The combined organic phases were dried under reduced pressure and dissolved in 2 mL dichloromethane. The sample was resolved by medium-pressure chromatography as described above for α-823. Fractions were analyzed by LC-MS and processed as above. Four mg of purified octacyclomycin were obtained.

α-770: Two parallel 100-mL cultures of *Actinoallomurus* sp. ID145770 in medium M8 [41] were harvested at seven days. Mycelium was harvested by centrifugation (10 min at 4000 rpm), treated with 20 mL ethanol, kept 1 h on a rotary shaker and centrifuged. The organic phase was recovered, dried under reduced pressure, dissolved in 2 mL dichloromethane and resolved by medium-pressure chromatography as described for α-823, except that the flow rate was set at 30 mL/min. Fractions 11–14, which showed activity against *S. aureus*, were analyzed by LC-MS and the ones containing similar signals were pooled, dried and dissolved in dichloromethane. A further purification step was performed by preparative thin layer chromatography on silica gel (Analtech Preparative Silica Gel GF with UV254 2000 μm; Sigma-Aldrich, St Louis, MO, USA) in dichloromethane:methanol 9:1. The spot at R$_f$ 0.9 was dried and dissolved in CDCl$_3$ for NMR analysis. Four mg of purified α-770 were obtained.

4. Conclusions

When grown under one routine condition in shake-flasks and only looking at metabolites with growth inhibitory activity towards *S. aureus*, we have been able to show that *Actinoallomurus* strains can express several types of biosynthetic pathways: type I (for making polyethers and spirotetronates), type II (for aromatic polyketides) and type III (for the 6-methylsalicylate moiety of the polyether α-770) polyketide synthases; ribosomally synthesized and post-translationally modified peptides (lantibiotic); aminocoumarins; and short non-ribosomal peptide synthase derived products (diketopiperazines).

Some of the observed metabolites, e.g., the previously reported aromatic polyketide allocyclinones [17] and the polyether α-823, seem to be relatively frequent metabolites in the screened *Actinoallomurus* strains. Other metabolites represent rarer discovery events, with identical or close matches in several *Actinobacteria* genera. Indeed, the genus *Actinoallomurus* resulted from a reclassification of *Actinomadura* spp. within the family *Thermomonosporaceae*, order *Streptosporangiales* [9]. Some of the compounds described here (e.g., pradimicin and benanomicin) and the α-770- and α-823-related polyethers cationomycin and SF-2361, respectively, were previously reported from *Actinomadura* spp. Others of the described metabolites are produced by distantly related taxa, such as NAI-107 by *Microbispora* spp. (family *Streptosporangiaceae*, order *Streptosporangiales*), pyrrolosporin by a *Micromonospora* sp. (order *Micromonosporales*), in addition to the *Streptomyces*-produced coumermycin and octacyclomycin.

Supplementary Materials: The following are available online at http://www.mdpi.com/2079-6382/7/2/47/s1, Figure S1: LC-MS, UV analysis of ethyl acetate extract of *Actinoallomurus* sp. ID145519, Figure S2: LC-MS, UV analysis of ethyl acetate extract of *Actinoallomurus* sp. ID145814, Figure S3: LC-MS, UV analysis of mycelium extract of *Actinoallomurus* sp. ID145640, Figure S4: Comparison between mycelium extract of *Actinoallomurus* sp. ID145640 and NAI-107 standard, Figure S5: LC-MS, UV analysis of ethyl acetate extract of *Actinoallomurus* sp. ID145219, Figure S6: LC-MS, UV analysis of ethyl acetate extract of *Actinoallomurus* sp. ID145114, Figure S7: Fragmentation patterns of the eight different congeners of α-823, Figure S8: 1H-NMR spectrum of α-823, Figure S9: 1H-COSY NMR spectrum of α-823, Figure S10: 1H-TOCSY NMR spectrum of α-823, Figure S11: 1H-13C HSQC NMR spectrum of α-823, Figure S12: 1H-13C HMBC NMR spectrum of α-823, Figure S13: Major COSY and HMBC correlations of α-823, Figure S14: HRESI-MS spectrum of α-823, Figure S15: LC-MS, UV analysis of mycelium extract of *Actinoallomurus* sp. ID145817, Figure S16: Fragmentation patters of the two different congeners of α-770, Figure S17: 1H NMR spectrum of α-770, Figure S18: 1H-COSY NMR spectrum of α-770, Figure S19: 1H-TOCSY NMR spectrum of α-770, Figure S20: 1H-13C HSQC NMR spectrum of α-770, Figure S21: 1H-13C HMBC NMR spectrum of α-770, Figure S22: Major COSY and HMBC correlations of α-770, Figure S23: HRESI-MS spectrum of α-770, Table S1: Different α-823 congeners detected in the extract from *Actinoallomurus* sp. ID145823, Table S2: 1H and 13C NMR data for α-823 in CDCl3, Table S3: α-770 congeners detected in the extract from *Actinoallomurus* sp. ID145770, Table S4: 1H and 13C NMR data for α-770 in CDCl3.

Author Contributions: M.S. and S.D. conceived and designed the experiments; M.I., A.T., J.C.S.C., G.D.G., C.B. and S.I.M. performed the experiments; M.I., A.T., J.C.S.C., G.D.G., C.B., S.I.M., M.S. and S.D. analyzed the data; M.I., A.T. and S.D. wrote the paper.

Acknowledgments: Portion of this work was part of a PhD dissertation of J.C.S.C. at the University of Warwick, UK. This work was partially supported by the European Community's Seventh Framework Programme (FP7/2007-2013) under grant agreement 289285 and by grants from Regione Lombardia. We are grateful to Carlo Mazzetti, Mirko Ornaghi, Roberta Pozzi and Matteo Simone for their early contributions to this project, and to Donatella Taramelli and Silvia Parapini for the anti-plasmodium activity tests. We also thank the Unitech OMICs platform at the University of Milano for HRMS analyses.

References

1. Genilloud, O. Actinomycetes: Still a source of novel antibiotics. *Nat. Prod. Rep.* **2017**, *34*, 1203–1232. [CrossRef] [PubMed]

2. Monciardini, P.; Iorio, M.; Maffioli, S.; Sosio, M.; Donadio, S. Discovering new bioactive molecules from microbial sources. *Microb. Biotechnol.* **2014**, *7*, 209–220. [CrossRef] [PubMed]

3. Wright, G.D. Opportunities for natural products in 21st century antibiotic discovery. *Nat. Prod. Rep.* **2017**, *34*, 694–701. [CrossRef] [PubMed]

4. Jaspars, M.; Challis, G. Microbiology: A talented genus. *Nature* **2014**, *506*, 38–39. [CrossRef] [PubMed]

5. Donadio, S.; Busti, E.; Monciardini, P.; Bamonte, R.; Mazza, P.; Sosio, M.; Cavaletti, L. Sources of polyketides and non-ribosomal peptides. *Ernst Schering Res. Found. Workshop* **2005**, *51*, 19–41.

6. Busti, E.; Cavaletti, L.; Monciardini, P.; Schumann, P.; Rohde, M.; Sosio, M.; Donadio, S. *Catenulispora acidiphila* gen. nov., sp. nov., a novel, mycelium-forming actinomycete, and proposal of *Catenulisporaceae* fam. nov. *Int. J. Syst. Evol. Microbiol.* **2006**, *56*, 1741–1746. [CrossRef] [PubMed]

7. Cavaletti, L.; Monciardini, P.; Schumann, P.; Rohde, M.; Bamonte, R.; Busti, E.; Sosio, M.; Donadio, S. *Actinospica robiniae* gen. nov., sp. nov. and *Actinospica acidiphila* sp. nov.: Proposal for *Actinospicaceae* fam.

nov. and *Catenulisporinae* subord. nov. in the order *Actinomycetales*. *Int. J. Syst. Evol. Microbiol.* **2006**, *56*, 1747–1753. [CrossRef] [PubMed]

8. Monciardini, P.; Cavaletti, L.; Ranghetti, A.; Schumann, P.; Rohde, M.; Bamonte, R.; Sosio, M.; Mezzelani, A.; Donadio, S. Novel members of the family *Micromonosporaceae*, *Rugosimonospora acidiphila* gen. nov., sp. nov. and *Rugosimonospora africana* sp. nov. *Int. J. Syst. Evol. Microbiol.* **2009**, *59*, 2752–2758. [CrossRef] [PubMed]

9. Tamura, T.; Ishida, Y.; Nozawa, Y.; Otoguro, M.; Suzuki, K. Transfer of *Actinomadura spadix* Nonomura and Ohara 1971 to *Actinoallomurus spadix* gen. nov., comb. nov., and description of *Actinoallomurus amamiensis* sp. nov., *Actinoallomurus caesius* sp. nov., *Actinoallomurus coprocola* sp. nov., *Actinoallomurus fulvus* sp. nov., *Actinoallomurus iriomotensis* sp. nov., *Actinoallomurus luridus* sp. nov., *Actinoallomurus purpureus* sp. nov. and *Actinoallomurus yoronensis* sp. nov. *Int. J. Syst. Evol. Microbiol.* **2009**, *59*, 1867–1874. [PubMed]

10. Thamchaipenet, A.; Indananda, C.; Bunyoo, C.; Duangmal, K.; Matsumoto, A.; Takahashi, Y. *Actinoallomurus acaciae* sp. nov., an endophytic actinomycete isolated from *Acacia auriculiformis* A. Cunn. ex Benth. *Int. J. Syst. Evol. Microbiol.* **2010**, *60*, 554–559. [CrossRef] [PubMed]

11. Indananda, C.; Thamchaipenet, A.; Matsumoto, A.; Inahashi, Y.; Duangmal, K.; Takahashi, Y. *Actinoallomurus oryzae* sp. nov., an endophytic actinomycete isolated from roots of a Thai jasmine rice plant. *Int. J. Syst. Evol. Microbiol.* **2011**, *61*, 737–741. [CrossRef] [PubMed]

12. Pozzi, R.; Simone, M.; Mazzetti, C.; Maffioli, S.; Monciardini, P.; Cavaletti, L.; Bamonte, R.; Sosio, M.; Donadio, S. The genus *Actinoallomurus* and some of its metabolites. *J. Antibiot.* **2011**, *64*, 133–139. [CrossRef] [PubMed]

13. Koyama, R.; Matsumoto, A.; Inahashi, Y.; Omura, S.; Takahashi, Y. Isolation of actinomycetes from the root of the plant, *Ophiopogon japonicus*, and proposal of two new species, *Actinoallomurus liliacearum* sp. nov. and *Actinoallomurus vinaceus* sp. nov. *J. Antibiot.* **2012**, *65*, 335–340. [CrossRef] [PubMed]

14. Matsumoto, A.; Fukuda, A.; Inahashi, Y.; Omura, S.; Takahashi, Y. *Actinoallomurus radicium* sp. nov., isolated from the roots of two plant species. *Int. J. Syst. Evol. Microbiol.* **2012**, *62*, 295–298. [CrossRef] [PubMed]

15. Inahashi, Y.; Iwatsuki, M.; Ishiyama, A.; Matsumoto, A.; Hirose, T.; Oshita, J.; Sunazuka, T.; Panbangred, W.; Takahashi, Y.; Kaiser, M.; et al. Actinoallolides A-E, new anti-trypanosomal macrolides, produced by an endophytic actinomycete, *Actinoallomurus fulvus* MK10-036. *Org. Lett.* **2015**, *17*, 864–867. [CrossRef] [PubMed]

16. Mazzetti, C.; Ornaghi, M.; Gaspari, E.; Parapini, S.; Maffioli, S.; Sosio, M.; Donadio, S. Halogenated spirotetronates from *Actinoallomurus*. *J. Nat. Prod.* **2012**, *75*, 1044–1050. [CrossRef] [PubMed]

17. Cruz, J.C.S.; Maffioli, S.; Bernasconi, A.; Brunati, C.; Gaspari, E.; Sosio, M.; Wellington, E.; Donadio, S. Allocyclinones, hyperchlorinated angucyclinones and common metabolites from *Actinoallomurus*. *J. Antibiot.* **2017**, *70*, 73–78. [CrossRef] [PubMed]

18. Iorio, M.; Cruz, J.; Simone, M.; Bernasconi, A.; Brunati, C.; Sosio, M.; Donadio, S.; Maffioli, S.I. Antibacterial paramagnetic quinones from *Actinoallomurus*. *J. Nat. Prod.* **2017**, *80*, 819–827. [CrossRef] [PubMed]

19. Cruz, J.C.S.; Iorio, M.; Monciardini, P.; Simone, M.; Brunati, C.; Gaspari, E.; Maffioli, S.I.; Wellington, E.; Sosio, M.; Donadio, S. Brominated variant of the lantibiotic NAI-107 with enhanced antibacterial potency. *J. Nat. Prod.* **2015**, *78*, 2642–2647. [CrossRef] [PubMed]

20. Kammerer, B.; Kahlich, R.; Laufer, S.; Li, S.M.; Heide, L.; Gleiter, C.H. Mass spectrometric pathway monitoring of secondary metabolites: Systematic analysis of culture extracts of *Streptomyces* species. *Anal. Biochem.* **2004**, *335*, 17–29. [CrossRef] [PubMed]

21. Vieweg, L.; Reichau, S.; Schobert, R.; Leadlay, P.F.; Süssmuth, R.D. Recent advances in the field of bioactive tetronates. *Nat. Prod. Rep.* **2014**, *31*, 1554–1584. [CrossRef] [PubMed]

22. Lam, K.S.; Hesler, G.A.; Gustavson, D.R.; Berry, R.L.; Tomita, K.; MacBeth, J.L.; Ross, J.; Miller, D.; Forenza, S. Pyrrolosporin A, a new antitumor antibiotic from *Micromonospora* sp. C39217-R109-7. I. Taxonomy of producing organism, fermentation and biological activity. *J. Antibiot.* **1996**, *49*, 860–864. [CrossRef] [PubMed]

23. Schroeder, D.R.; Colson, K.L.; Klohr, S.E.; Lee, M.S.; Matson, J.A.; Brinen, L.S.; Clardy, J. Pyrrolosporin A, a new antitumor antibiotic from *Micromonospora* sp. C39217-R109-7. II. Isolation, physic-chemical properties, spectroscopic study and X-ray analysis. *J. Antibiot.* **1996**, *9*, 865–872. [CrossRef]

24. Arnison, P.G.; Bibb, M.J.; Bierbaum, G.; Bowers, A.A.; Bugni, T.S.; Bulaj, G.; Camarero, J.A.; Campopiano, D.J.; Challis, G.L.; Clardy, J.; et al. Ribosomally synthesized and post-translationally modified peptide natural products: Overview and recommendations for a universal nomenclature. *Nat. Prod. Rep.* **2013**, *30*, 108–160. [CrossRef] [PubMed]

25. Lee, M.D. Antibiotics from Microbispora. U.S. Patent 6,551,591, 22 April 2003.

26. Lazzarini, A.; Gastaldo, L.; Candiani, G.; Ciciliato, I.; Losi, D.; Marinelli, F.; Selva, E.; Parenti, F. Antibiotic 107891, Its Factors A1 and A2, Pharmaceutically Acceptable Salts and Compositions, and Use Thereof. U.S. Patent 7,351,687, 1 April 2008.

27. Belin, P.; Moutiez, M.; Lautru, S.; Seguin, J.; Pernodet, J.L.; Gondry, M. The nonribosomal synthesis of diketopiperazines in tRNA-dependent cyclodipeptide synthase pathways. *Nat. Prod. Rep.* **2012**, *29*, 961–979. [CrossRef] [PubMed]

28. Oki, T.; Kinoshi, M.; Tomatsu, K.; Tomita, K.; Saitoh, K.; Tsunakawa, M.; Nishio, M.; Miyaki, T.; Kawaguchi, H. Pradimicin, a novel class of potent antifungal antibiotics. *J. Antibiot.* **1999**, *11*, 1701–1704. [CrossRef]

29. Tadashi, N.; Yukio, T.; Yuko, K.; Mamoru, I.; Taneto, T.; Shinji, M.; Masaji, S.; Michio, K. Novel antibiotic substance SF-2361, production and used thereof. Japan Patent 61260888, 19 November 1986.

30. Kevin, D.A., II; Meujo, D.A.F.; Hamann, M.T. Polyether ionophores: Broad-spectrum and promising biologically active molecules for the control of drug-resistant bacteria and parasites. *Expert Opin. Drug Discov.* **2009**, *4*, 109–146. [CrossRef] [PubMed]

31. Funayama, S.; Nozoe, S.; Tronquet, C.; Anraku, Y.; Komiyama, K.; Omura, S. Isolation and structure of a new polyether antibiotic, octacyclomycin. *J. Antibiot.* **1992**, *45*, 1686–1691. [CrossRef] [PubMed]

32. Nakamura, G.; Kobayashi, K.; Sakurai, T.; Isono, K. Cationomycin, a new polyether ionophore antibiotic produced by *Actinomadura* nov. sp. *J. Antibiot.* **1981**, *34*, 1513–1514. [CrossRef] [PubMed]

33. Minami, A.; Oguri, H.; Watanabe, K.; Oikawa, H. Biosynthetic machinery of ionophore polyether lasalocid: Enzymatic construction of polyether skeleton. *Curr. Opin. Chem. Biol.* **2013**, *17*, 555–561. [CrossRef] [PubMed]

34. Ubukata, M.; Uzawa, J.; Isono, K. Biosynthesis of cationomycin: Direct and indirect incorporation of 13C-acetate and application of homoscalar correlated 2-D carbon-13 NMR and double quantum coherence. *J. Am. Chem. Soc.* **1984**, *106*, 2213–2214. [CrossRef]

35. Rutkowski, J.; Brzezinski, B. Structures and properties of naturally occurring polyether antibiotics. *BioMed Res. Int.* **2013**, *2013*, 162513. [CrossRef] [PubMed]

36. Zhou, S.; Wang, F.; Wong, E.T.; Fonkem, E.; Hsieh, T.C.; Wu, JM.; Wu, E. Salinomycin: A novel anti-cancer agent with known anti-coccidial activities. *Curr. Med. Chem.* **2013**, *20*, 4095–4101. [CrossRef] [PubMed]

37. D'Alessandro, S.; Corbett, Y.; Ilboudo, D.P.; Misiano, P.; Dahiya, N.; Abay, S.M.; Habluetzel, A.; Grande, R.; Gismondo, M.R.; Dechering, K.J.; et al. Salinomycin and other ionophores as a new class of antimalarial drugs with transmission-blocking activity. *Antimicrob. Agents Chemother.* **2015**, *59*, 5135–5144. [CrossRef] [PubMed]

38. Charlop-Powers, Z.; Owen, J.G.; Reddy, B.V.B.; Ternei, M.A.; Brady, S.F. Chemical-biogeographic survey of secondary metabolism in soil. *Proc. Natl. Acad. Sci. USA* **2014**, *111*, 3757–3762. [CrossRef] [PubMed]

39. Charlop-Powers, Z.; Pregitzer, C.C.; Lemetre, C.; Ternei, M.A.; Maniko, J.; Hover, B.M.; Calle, P.Y.; McGuire, K.L.; Garbarino, J.; Forgione, H.M.; et al. Urban park soil microbiomes are a rich reservoir of natural product biosynthetic diversity. *Proc. Natl. Acad. Sci. USA* **2016**, *113*, 14811–14816. [CrossRef] [PubMed]

40. Monciardini, P.; Sosio, M.; Cavaletti, L.; Chiocchini, C.; Donadio, S. New PCR primers for the selective amplifcation of 16S rDNA from different groups of actinomycetes. *FEMS Microbiol. Ecol.* **2002**, *42*, 419–429. [PubMed]

41. Donadio, S.; Monciardini, P.; Sosio, M. Chapter 1. Approaches to discovering novel antibacterial and antifungal agents. *Methods Enzymol.* **2009**, *458*, 3–28. [PubMed]

13

Antimicrobial Activity of Bee Venom and Melittin against *Borrelia burgdorferi*

Kayla M. Socarras ⓘ, Priyanka A. S. Theophilus, Jason P. Torres, Khusali Gupta and Eva Sapi *

Lyme Disease Research Group, Department of Biology and Environmental Science, University of New Haven, West Haven, CT 06519, USA; kmsocarras@gmail.com (K.M.S.); priyankaannabel@gmail.com (P.A.S.T.); jtorr3@unh.newhaven.edu (J.P.T.); kgupt2@unh.newhaven.edu (K.G.)
* Correspondence: Esapi@newhaven.edu

Academic Editor: Christopher C. Butler

Abstract: Lyme disease is a tick-borne, multi-systemic disease, caused by the bacterium *Borrelia burgdorferi*. Though antibiotics are used as a primary treatment, relapse often occurs after the discontinuation of antimicrobial agents. The reason for relapse remains unknown, however previous studies suggest the possible presence of antibiotic resistant Borrelia round bodies, persisters and attached biofilm forms. Thus, there is an urgent need to find antimicrobial agents suitable to eliminate all known forms of *B. burgdorferi*. In this study, natural antimicrobial agents such as *Apis mellifera* venom and a known component, melittin, were tested using SYBR Green I/PI, direct cell counting, biofilm assays combined with LIVE/DEAD and atomic force microscopy methods. The obtained results were compared to standalone and combinations of antibiotics such as Doxycycline, Cefoperazone, Daptomycin, which were recently found to be effective against Borrelia persisters. Our findings showed that both bee venom and melittin had significant effects on all the tested forms of *B. burgdorferi*. In contrast, the control antibiotics when used individually or even in combinations had limited effects on the attached biofilm form. These findings strongly suggest that whole bee venom or melittin could be effective antimicrobial agents for *B. burgdorferi*; however, further research is necessary to evaluate their effectiveness in vivo, as well as their safe and effective delivery method for their therapeutic use.

Keywords: Lyme disease; bee venom; melittin; biofilms; persisters; antibiotic resistance

1. Introduction

Through the years, the severity of infectious diseases and the inability to effectively treat them with antibiotics have become a rapidly growing epidemic. One such disease that has spread across the United States, Europe, Asia, Australia and in some parts of Africa is Lyme borreliosis, alternatively known as Lyme disease [1,2]. The known causative agent of Lyme disease is *Borrelia burgdorferi*, which is transmitted primarily through Ixodid ticks [1,3]. According to the Center of Disease Control, the United States has approximately 300,000 newly reported Lyme disease cases every year [4]. Successfully diagnosed individuals are often prescribed antibiotics such as Doxycycline, Amoxicillin and Ceftriaxone; however, recent studies demonstrated that these antibiotics are insufficient in eliminating certain forms of *Borrelia* spp. in vitro and in vivo [5–13].

Borrelia spp., by its traditional definition, is a spirochetal bacterium with internalized flagella [14,15], however, other morphological forms were also identified such as round bodies, stationary phase persisters and biofilm forms [16–22]. *B. burgdorferi* can transform between these morphologies depending on its environment [23]. Some factors that cause these different forms are certain unfavorable conditions such as changes in pH, nutrient starvation, host immune system attacks, or even antibiotics could promote these morphological changes [16,17,20,22,24]. These defensive forms were reported to have high resistance to the antimicrobials agents that are currently used to treat Lyme disease (7, 21, 22). For example, while Doxycycline is very effective eliminating spirochetes in vitro, it did not reduce antibiotic resilient persisters and/or biofilms [6,7,22,25]. Furthermore, it was demonstrated that none of the antibiotics currently used to treat Lyme disease effective against the "persister" and attached biofilm forms of *Borrelia* [7–10,22,25,26]. It was also reported that several antibiotics (Cefoperazone, Daptomycin) might have potential in effectively eliminating *Borrelia* persisters especially when in combination with Doxycycline [8,10]. Unfortunately, attached *Borrelia* biofilms, which were recently proven to be present in infected human skin tissues, did not respond well to these new antibiotic combinations [26].

Considering the limiting effects that standard antibiotics may have on the Borrelial morphologies, our research group began searching for potential alternative antimicrobials. In a recent study, *Stevia rebaudiana* leaf extract was found to be very effective in eliminating all known Borrelia morphological forms including attached biofilms [26]. Based on these findings, we looked for additional alternative agents that may also have similar effect. One alternative agent is apotoxin—also known as bee venom—derived from the insect *Apis mellifera* better known as the honeybee. The use of this venom has been documented for its medicinal purposes for approximately 6000 years ago and several studies have proven its antimicrobial effects [27,28]. In a previous study, bee venom's component melittin was shown to have significant effects on *Borrelia* spirochetes at MIC concentrations of 100 μg/mL [29]. Recent data shows similar MIC values for melittin when used to treat several other gram-negative microorganisms such as *Salmonella enterica* and *Yersinia kristensenii* [30]. In this report, we expanded these findings by testing the sensitivity of different forms of *B. burgdorferi* to bee venom and its component melittin in comparison to antibiotics recently found effective against Borrelia persister forms [7–10]. To assess antimicrobial sensitivity of bee venom and melittin, previously published methods such as SYBR Green I/PI assay combined with total direct live cell counting were used for log phase spirochetes and stationary phase persisters [6,31], while attached biofilms were analyzed by crystal violet and LIVE/DEAD staining techniques [6]. Fluorescent and atomic force microscopy methods were also employed to further visualize the effect of these antimicrobial agents on Borrelia.

2. Results

Prior to testing the potential antimicrobial effect of bee venom on *B. burgdorferi* using SYBR Green I/PI assay, bee venom, melittin and all the antibiotics used in this study were analyzed for auto fluorescence due to reported findings of potential auto-fluorescence issues of certain antimicrobials in previous studies [24,29,31]. Values from auto fluorescence detected from any of the antimicrobials were deducted from future experiments. However, due to reports of cellular auto fluorescence from antibiotic treated bacterial cells following intracellular damage [32] all results from the SYBR Green I/PI were confirmed using the direct counting method of live/dead cells using the Live/Dead assay [6–10,26,31].

In the first set of experiments, antibiotics recently reported to be effective for several *Borrelia* forms were tested to confirm the previous findings [31]. Doxycycline, Cefoperazone, Daptomycin, as well as the combination of the three-antibiotics (D + C + D), were used in concentrations reported effective on both logarithmic phase (spirochetes) and stationary phase (persisters) cells of *B. burgdorferi*. To determine the long-term effects of all antimicrobials, recovery cultures were used in which treated cells were further cultured in antibiotic free media for 7 days as described previously [7–10,26,31]. Furthermore, because our previous research shows that the free floating and surface bound aggregate forms could have different antibiotic sensitivity [6,26], we separately studied the effect of bee venom and melittin on the surface attached biofilm form as well as the free-floating aggregates. As a negative control, appropriate amounts of sterile PBS buffer were used in all experiments. To determine the effectiveness of the different antimicrobials, SYBR Green I/PI assay and direct counting methods were used in parallel and results are depicted in Figure 1A,B respectively. Data generated from both methods were in good agreement to previously reported data for all the antibiotics tested [31], i.e., Doxycycline significantly reduced the number of spirochetes but not the persisters (Figure 1A). In contrast, Cefoperazone, Daptomycin and the three-antibiotic combination (D + C + D) significantly reduced viable spirochetes and persisters (Figure 1A). However, results from SYBR Green I/PI assay and direct counting were significantly different. The direct counting method indicated a higher cell death rate for Daptomycin and the three-antibiotic combination (D + C + D) treatments (Figure 1A,B respectively).

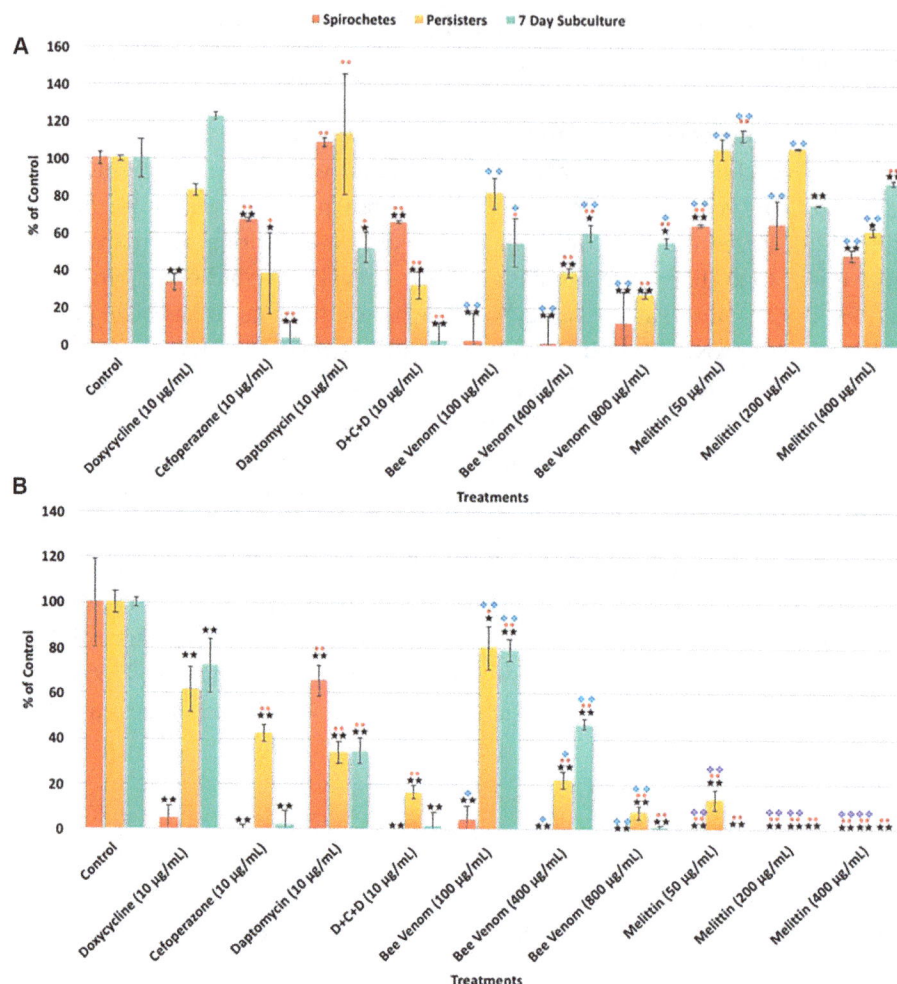

Figure 1. The effects of various antimicrobial agents on *B. burgdorferi* as determined by SYBR Green I/PI assay Panel (**A**) or direct counting assay Panel (**B**). Doxycycline, Cefoperazone, Daptomycin and their combination (D + C + D) as well as different concentrations of bee venom and melittin were tested on *B. burgdorferi* logarithmic phase (spirochetes) culture and stationary phase (persisters) cultures as well as in 7-day recovery subculture as described previously [6–8]. Significance against sterile PBS buffer (control vehicle) with the *p* value of <0.05 and <0.01 are indicated in * and ** respectively. Significance against Doxycycline with the *p* value of <0.05 and <0.01 are indicated in ♦ and ♦♦ respectively. Significance against the three-antibiotic combination (D + C + D) with the *p* value of <0.05 and <0.01 are indicated in ❖ and ❖❖ respectively. *n* = 9.

Furthermore, due to the unknown half-life of the potentially active components in bee venom on Borrelia, we compared the effect of bee venom administered in both a single treatment and daily regimens for 3 days (Figure 1 and Figures S1–S4, Table S1 in Supplementary Materials). The daily treatment protocol was found to be significantly more effective and is shown in Figure 1 and used in future experiments.

When SYBR Green I/PI assay was used, bee venom data showed that the number of viable logarithmic phase spirochetes were significantly lower at all concentrations (*p* value ≤ 0.01) than the

PBS treated negative control or any of the antibiotic treated cultures except Doxycycline (p value $\leq$ 0.01) (Figure 1A). When bee venom was used at a concentration above 100 µg/mL, bee venom, the results demonstrated a greater reduction in spirochetes than the Doxycycline treated cultures. Stationary phase persisters treated with bee venom concentrations above 100 µg/mL were significantly reduced compared to the negative control and Doxycycline (p value $\leq$ 0.01) (Figure 1A). In addition, the effect of bee venom treatment was comparable to Cefoperazone and the three antibiotics combination (D + C + D) at concentrations at greater than or equal to 400 µg/mL (Figure 1A). In the 7-day subculture experiments testing for cells, which were able to recover after antimicrobial treatments, there was a significant decrease (p value $\leq$ 0.01) in the number of viable cells compared to the negative control and Doxycycline (p value $\leq$ 0.01).

In parallel experiments, one of the major antimicrobial components of bee venom, melittin, was tested first using SYBR Green I/PI assay (Figure 1A). Bee venom is comprised of 50% melittin, therefore the concentrations used for testing melittin were 50% less than when whole bee venom was used. Melittin was administered daily at concentrations shown previously to have significant effect on Borrelia spirochetes [29]. Results from this study showed that melittin could significantly decrease the numbers of persisters (p value $\leq$ 0.05) compared to the negative control (Figure 1A). Melittin, at concentrations below 400 µg/mL however, showed significantly higher viable spirochete numbers (p value $\leq$ 0.05) than Doxycycline (p value $\leq$ 0.01). In the 7-day recovery subculture there were significantly fewer cells (p value $\leq$ 0.01) when concentrations above 200 µg/mL of melittin were used compared to the negative control and Doxycycline (Figure 1A). Melittin was significantly less effective on recovered subculture cells (p value $\leq$ 0.01) in comparison to the three-antibiotic combination treatment (D + C + D).

To confirm *B. burgdorferi* viability after bee venom and melittin treatment, all SYBR Green I/PI assay results were confirmed via a total viability direct counting method as described previously [6–8,26]. In these experiments, a significant reduction of viable cells was found when exposed to whole bee venom at all concentrations compared to the negative control and Daptomycin (p value $\leq$ 0.01) (Figure 1B). Similarly, exposure with concentrations >100 µg/mL of whole bee venom resulted in significantly fewer persisters in comparison to the negative control, Doxycycline and Cefoperazone (p value $\leq$ 0.01) in a dose-dependent manner (Figure 1B). The 7-day subculture experiments showed that doses above 400 µg/mL of bee venom effectively eliminated live cells similarly to Cefoperazone and to the three-antibiotic combinations (D + C + D) (Figure 1B).

When the effectiveness of melittin on *B. burgdorferi* was tested using a direct counting approach, there was again a significant difference between the results from the SYBR Green I/PI assay and total direct counting method (Figure 1B). Results showed that melittin significantly reduced the numbers spirochetes (p value $\leq$ 0.01) at all concentrations compared to the negative control and Doxycycline (p value $\leq$ 0.01) (Figure 1B). Persisters treated with melittin showed significant reduction at all concentrations (p value $\leq$ 0.01) compared to the negative control, Doxycycline and the three-antibiotic combination (D + C + D) (Figure 1B). The 7-day recovery subcultures exposed to all concentrations of melittin were also significantly reduced (p value $\leq$ 0.01) compared to the negative control, bee venom and all used antibiotics (Figure 1B). In summary, we concluded that the MIC concentration of bee venom on Borrelial spirochetes is 200 µg/mL and the MIC for melittin is 100 ug/mL.

To further verify the effectiveness of all antimicrobial agents, the viability of the different morphological forms and cultures of *B. burgdorferi* were evaluated by a LIVE/DEAD staining method combined with fluorescent microscopy imaging. Representative images visualize the effects of these treatments on spirochetes (Figure 2), persister cells (Figure 3) and 7-day recovery subcultures (Figure 4). Panel As in Figures 2–4 depict the negative control (PBS control), while positive controls (antibiotics and antibiotic combinations) were shown in panels (B–F) in Figures 2–4. For the individual antibiotics and the antibiotic combination, the obtained images were in agreement with the direct counting data. For example, Cefoperazone and three-antibiotics combination (D + C + D) were very effective in eliminating spirochetes, a data which was found by the direct counting data but not with SYBR Green I/PI method (Figure 1A,B).

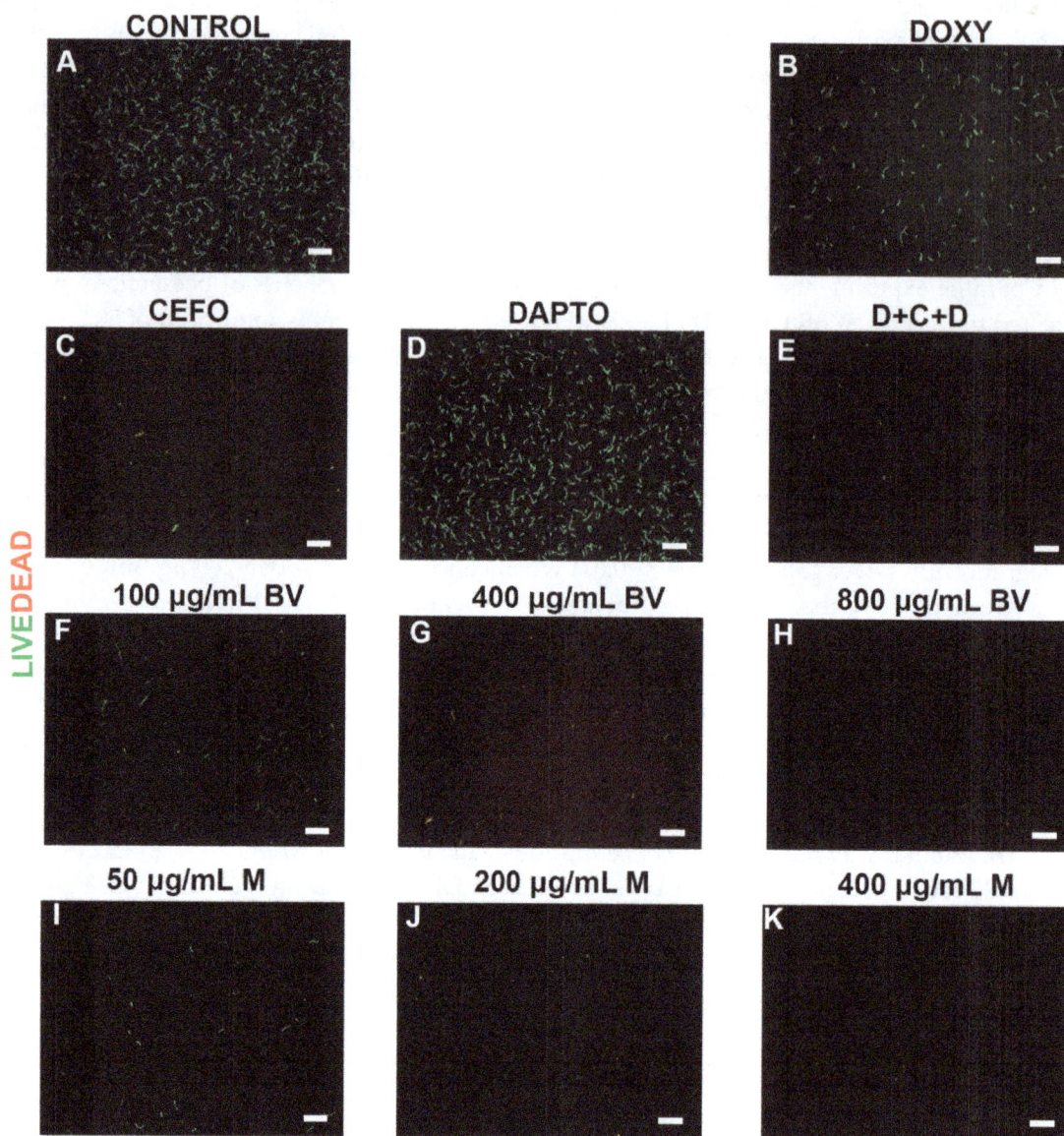

Figure 2. Representative Live/Dead staining images of *B. burgdorferi* log phase spirochetal cultures treated with different antimicrobial agents. Cells were stained with SYBR Green I/PI as outlined in the Methods and representative images were taken at 100× magnification. Panel (**A**) Borrelia culture treated only with PBS was used as a negative control. Panel (**B**) Doxycycline (DOXY) treated; Panel (**C**) Cefoperazone (CEFO) treated; Panel (**D**) Daptomycin (DAPTO) treated and Panel (**E**) Three-antibiotic combination (D + C + D). Panels (**F–H**) Bee venom (BV) was used in increasing concentrations while Panels (**I–K**) depicts melittin (M) treated cells. Live cells are stained with green color while dead cells are stained red. Scale bar: 100 μm.

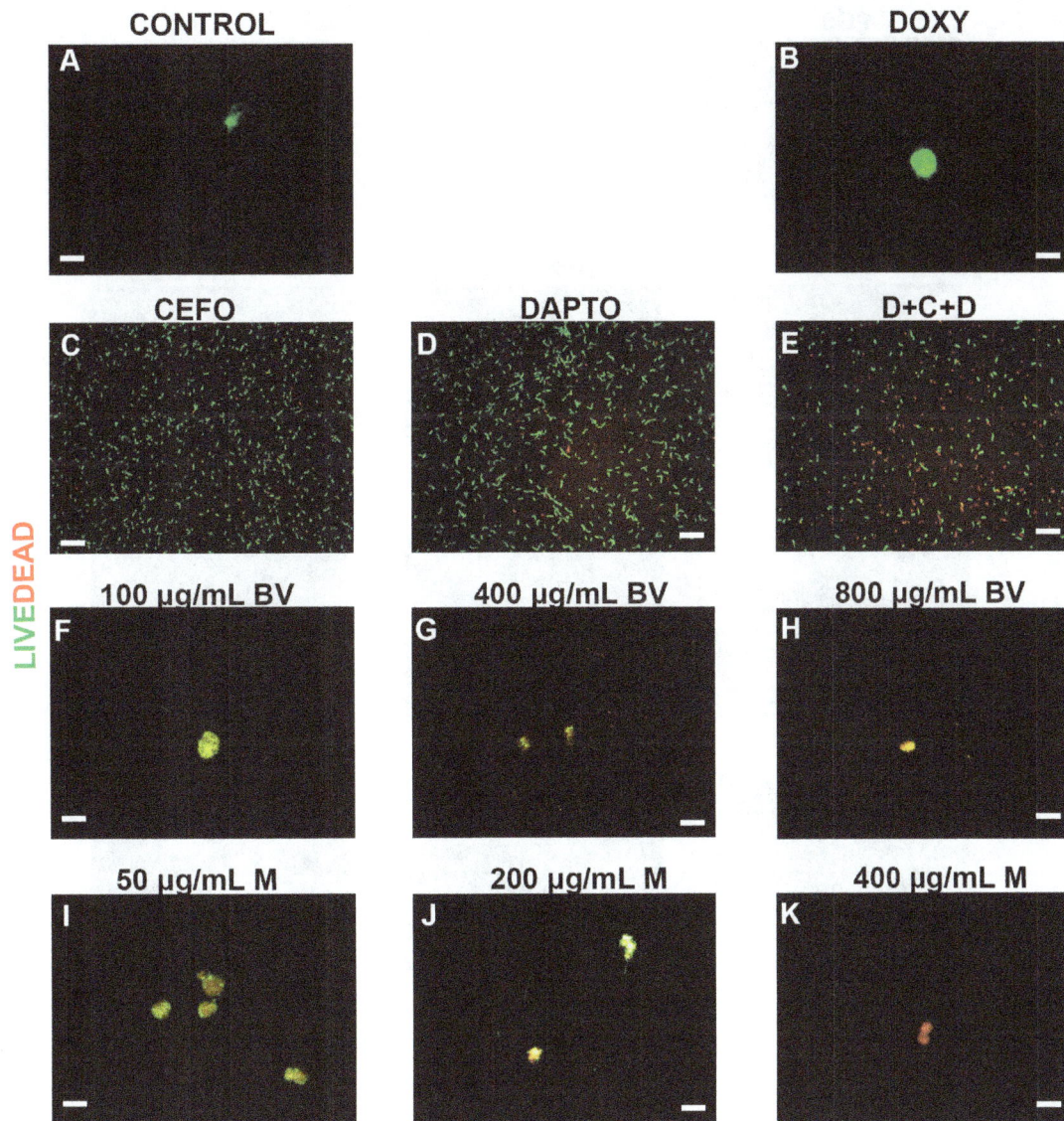

Figure 3. Representative Live/Dead staining images of *B. burgdorferi* stationary phase persister cultures following treatment with different antimicrobial agents. Cells were stained with SYBR Green I/PI as outlined in the Methods and representative images were taken at 100× magnification. Panel (**A**) Borrelia culture treated only with PBS was used as a negative control. Panel (**B**) Doxycycline (DOXY) treated, Panel (**C**) Cefoperazone (CEFO) treated, Panel (**D**) Daptomycin (DAPTO) treated and Panel (**E**) Three-antibiotic combination (D + C + D). Panels (**F–H**) Bee venom (BV) was used in increasing concentrations while Panels (**I–K**) depicts melittin (M) treated cells. Live cells are stained with green color while dead cells are stained red. Scale bar: 100 μm.

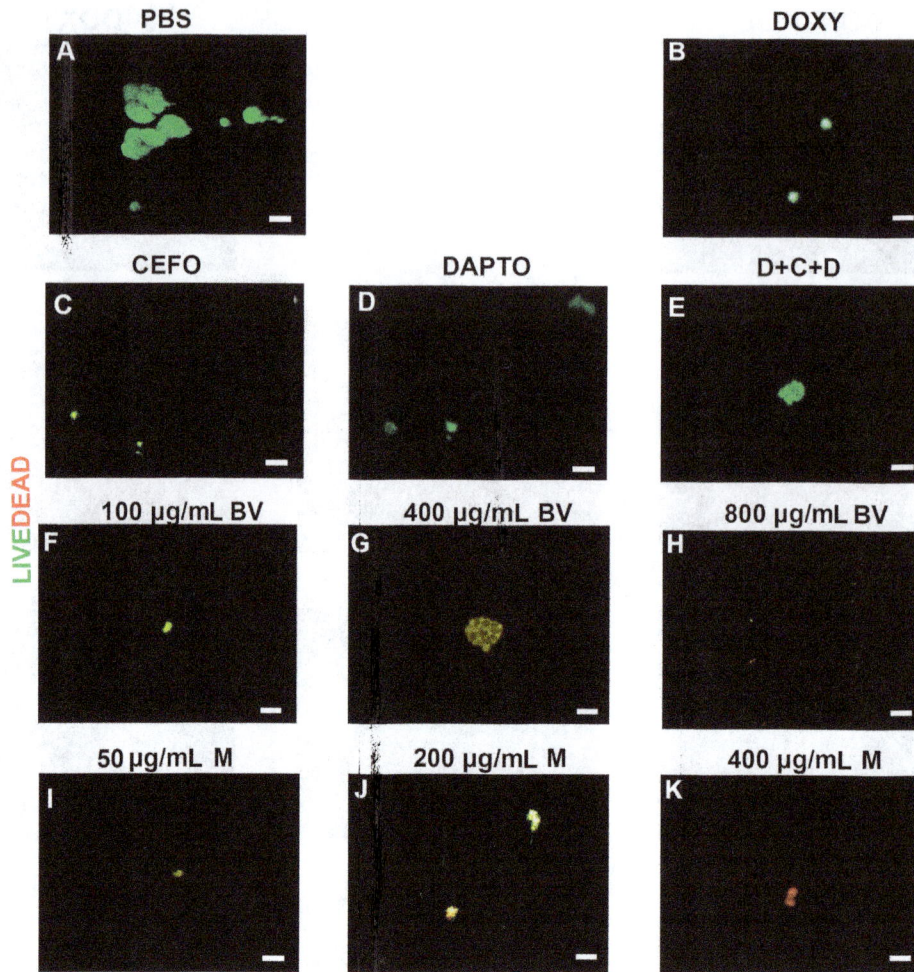

Figure 4. Representative Live/Dead staining images of *B. burgdorferi* 7-day recovery cultures following treatment with different antimicrobial agents. Cells were stained with SYBR Green I/PI as outlined in the Material and Methods and representative images were taken at 100× magnification. Panel (**A**) Borrelia culture treated only with PBS was used as a negative control. Panel (**B**) Doxycycline (DOXY) treated, Panel (**C**) Cefoperazone (CEFO) treated, Panel (**D**) Daptomycin (DAPTO) treated and Panel (**E**) Three-antibiotic combination (D + C + D). Panels (**F–H**) Bee venom (BV) was used in increasing concentrations while Panels (**I–K**) depict melittin (M) treated cells at different concentrations. Live cells are stained with green color while dead cells are stained red. Scale bar: 100 μm.

B. burgdorferi cultures treated with various concentrations of bee venom were shown in the subsequent panels (G–I) (Figures 2–4), while cultures treated with melittin were shown in panels (J–L) (Figures 2–4). As previously mentioned, results from these images supported the total direct count numerical data but not the SYBR Green I/PI assay. For example, bee venom exposure showed a significant decrease in the number of spirochetes, persisters, as well as 7-day recovery subculture in comparison to the negative and positive controls (Panels (G–I) in Figures 2–4). Similarly, melittin treatment demonstrated a dramatically significant decrease in live cell numbers for both log phase, stationary phase and recovery cultures, which agreed with the direct counting data (Panels (J–L), Figures 2–4). Table 1 summarizes the effects of various antimicrobial agents on *B. burgdorferi* as determined by SYBR Green I/PI (Panel (A)) or direct counting assays (Panel (B)).

Table 1. The effects of various antimicrobial agents on *B. burgdorferi* as determined by SYBR Green I/PI assay (Panel (A)) or direct counting assay (Panel (B)). Doxycycline, Cefoperazone, Daptomycin and their combination (D + C + D) as well as different concentration of bee venom and melittin were tested on *B. burgdorferi* logarithmic phase (spirochetes) culture and stationary phase (persisters) cultures as well as in 7-day recovery subculture as described previously [6–8,26]. n = 9.

A. SYBR Green I/PI Assay

Treatments	Spirochetes			Persisters			7 Day Subculture		
	% Control	% SD	% Median	% Control	% SD	% Median	% Control	% SD	% Median
Control	100	11	100	100	12	100	100	16	100
Doxycycline (10 µg/mL)	33	4	33	83	3	86	122	2	83
Cefoperazone (10 µg/mL)	67	1	66	38	22	41	4	9	3
Daptomycin (10 µg/mL)	108	2	107	113	32	120	52	8	43
D + C + D (10 µg/mL)	66	1	65	32	7	34	3	9	2
Bee venom (100 µg/mL)	61	11	63	62	7	74	88	29	141
Bee venom (400 µg/mL)	45	11	37	44	25	43	59	19	115
Bee venom (800 µg/mL)	33	8	32	32	2	35	95	31	55
Melittin (50 µg/mL)	65	1	67	105	6	91	113	3	103
Melittin (200 µg/mL)	65	24	67	106	0	94	75	0	69
Melittin (400 µg/mL)	49	6	54	61	2	57	87	1	80

B. Direct Counting Assay

Treatments	Spirochetes			Persisters			7 Day Subculture		
	% Control	% SD	% Median	% Control	% SD	% Median	% Control	% SD	% Median
Control	100	19	100	100	5	100	100	8	100
Doxycycline (10 µg/mL)	5	6	5	62	10	67	72	12	60
Cefoperazone (10 µg/mL)	1	1	0	43	4	43	2	6	2
Daptomycin (10 µg/mL)	65	7	73	34	5	36	35	6	175
D + C + D (10 µg/mL)	0	0	0	17	3	17	2	6	0
Bee venom (100 µg/mL)	5	6	4	80	10	79	79	5	65
Bee venom (400 µg/mL)	0	0	0	22	4	21	47	2	29
Bee venom (800 µg/mL)	0	0	0	8	3	7	1	1	0
Melittin (50 µg/mL)	0	0	0	13	5	13	0	0	0
Melittin (200 µg/mL)	0	0	0	0	0	0	0	0	0
Melittin (400 µg/mL)	0	0	0	0	0	0	0	0	0

In the past several years, a novel aggregate form, called biofilm, was found for Borrelia and was shown to be very antimicrobial resistant vitro and in vivo especially in attached forms [6,22,25,26,33]. Therefore, in subsequent experiments we tested all antimicrobials for effectiveness in eliminating the attached biofilm form. To evaluate the effect of antimicrobial agents on the attached Borrelia biofilms, first we used crystal violet quantitative biofilm assay as described previously [6,26]. As negative control, the appropriate amounts of PBS were used (control vehicle) and all presented data were normalized to the negative control. Bee venom exposure at >100 μg/mL but none of the antibiotics or their combination (D + C + D), significantly reduced Borrelia biofilm mass (p value ≤ 0.01) in comparison to the negative control (Figure 5). Melittin also reduced Borrelia biofilm mass at different concentrations compared to the negative control (p value ≤ 0.05), or Doxycycline (p value ≤ 0.01), or the three-antibiotic combination (D + C + D; p value ≤ 0.01) but were found less effective than whole bee venom at >100 μg/mL (Figure 5). To verify these findings, LIVE/DEAD staining method combined with fluorescent microscopy imaging was used. Representative microscopy images confirmed the decreased size of Borrelia biofilm with the bee venom (Figure 6, panels (F–H)) and melittin treatment (Figure 6, panels (J–L)). Interestingly, melittin also significantly reduced biofilm viability (red stain Figure 6, panels (I–K)). Some of the antibiotics (Cefoperazone and Daptomycin and the three antibiotic combination (D + C + D); Figure 6, panels (C–E) respectively) also showed some reduction in biofilm sizes, which were not detected with the crystal violet assay; however, those remaining biofilms were stained green suggesting that they are viable (Figure 6, panels (A–J)).

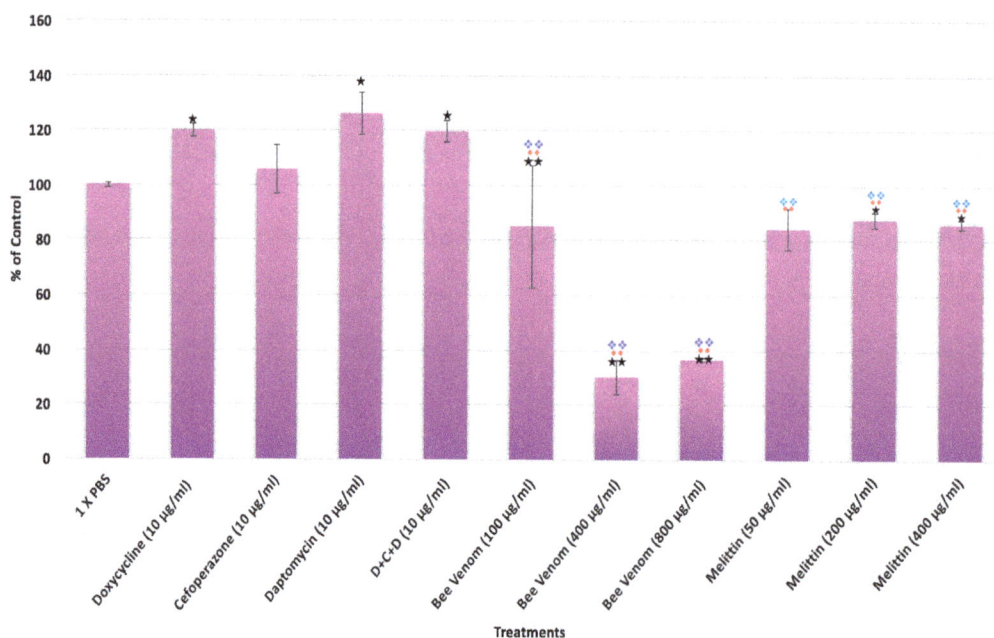

Figure 5. Effect of different antimicrobial agents on attached *B. burgdorferi* biofilms. Susceptibility of attached *B. burgdorferi* biofilms to antimicrobial agents after a three-day treatment was analyzed by crystal violet method as described in Material and Methods. Doxycycline, Cefoperazone, Daptomycin and their combination (D + C + D) as well as different concentration of bee venom and melittin were tested on attached Borrelia biofilms. Significance against PBS buffer (negative control vehicle) with the p value of <0.05 and <0.01 are indicated in * and ** respectively. Significance against Doxycycline with the p value of <0.05 and <0.01 are respectively indicated in ♦ and ♦♦ Significance against the three-antibiotic combination (D + C + D) with the p-value of <0.05 and <0.01 are indicated in ❖ and ❖❖ respectively. $n = 9$.

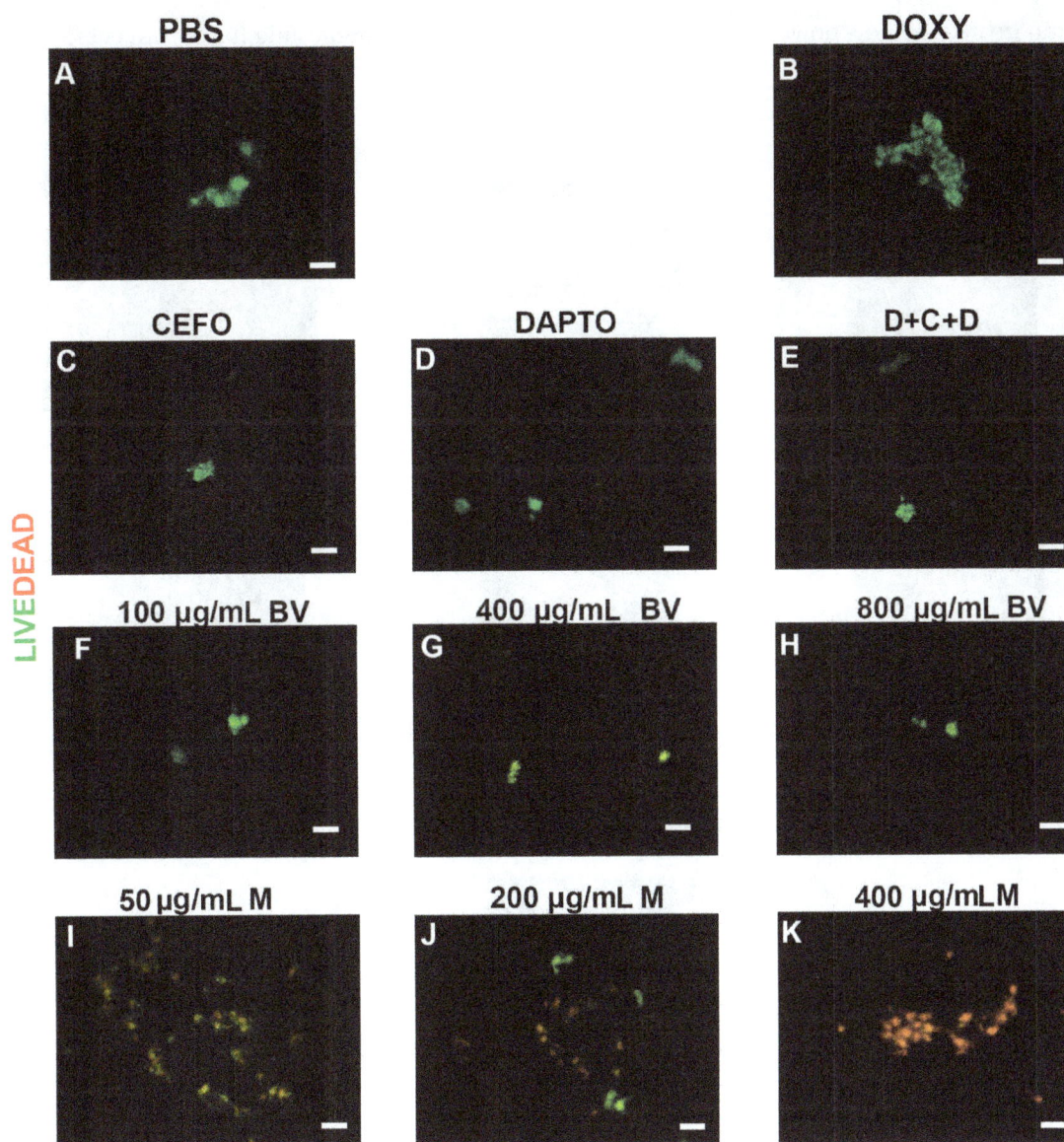

Figure 6. Representative Live/Dead images of the viability of attached Borrelia biofilms following treatment with different antimicrobial agents. Biofilms were stained with SYBR Green I and PI as outlined in the Material and Methods and representative images were taken at 100× magnification. Panel (**A**) Borrelia culture treated only with PBS was used as a negative control. Panel (**B**) Doxycycline (DOXY) treated, Panel (**C**) Cefoperazone (CEFO) treated, Panel (**D**) Daptomycin (DAPTO) treated and Panel (**E**) Three-antibiotic combination (D + C + D). Panels (**F–H**) Bee venom (BV) was used in increasing concentrations while Panels (**I–K**) depict melittin treated cells at different concentration. Live cells are stained with green color while dead cells are stained red. Scale bar: 100 μm.

Finally, the ultrastructure of attached *B. burgdorferi* biofilms treated with different antimicrobials were studied using atomic force microscopy. In these experiments, attached Borrelia biofilms were exposed to the different antimicrobials as described above then analyzed for changes in topography and size (Figure 7). The atomic force microscopic images are 3D rendered and digitally colored for improved visualization (Figure 7). The negative control was shown in Figure 7 Panel (A) followed by the positive controls in Panels (B–E). Subsequently, the effects of bee venom and melittin were shown in Panels (F) and (G) respectively. The drug-free control had a very compact and rigid structure (Figure 7, Panel (A)) similarly to the biofilms treated with Doxycycline, Cefoperazone, Daptomycin and three-antibiotic combination (D + C + C) respectively (Figure 7, Panels (B–E)). Bee venom and melittin treated biofilms however, revealed a very loose structure suggesting the effectiveness of those agents against biofilm structure (Figure 7, Panel (F,G)).

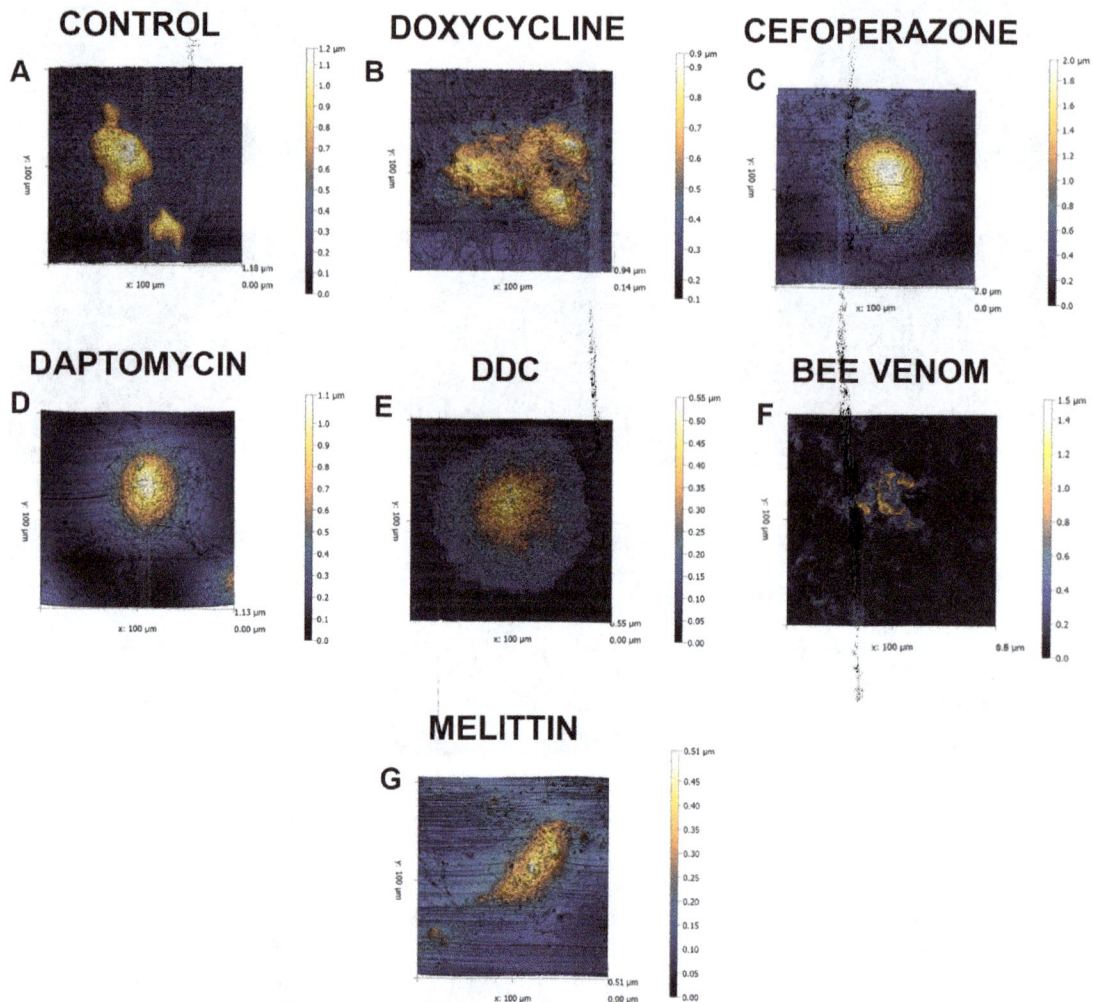

Figure 7. Representative atomic force microscopy images showing the ultrastructural details of Borrelia biofilm before and after treatment with antimicrobial agents. The preparations of *B. burgdorferi* strain B31 biofilms on chamber slides are described in Methods section. All biofilms were scanned at 0.4 Hz using contact mode and the individual Z ranges (height) are indicated next to each panel by means of a scale. The images were scanned using the Nanosurf Easyscan 2 software and the images were processed using Gwyddion software. Scale bar located on the side of corresponding AFM scan indicate the height changes of the topography of the biofilm. Darker colors (black and blue) indicate the surface of the slide while lighter colors (yellow to white) indicate high points of attached biofilms. Attached Borrelia biofilms treated with Panel (**A**) PBS (control), Panel (**B**) Doxycycline (10 µg/mL), Panel (**C**) Cefoperazone (10 µg/mL), Panel (**D**) Daptomycin (10 µg/mL), Panel (**E**) Three antibiotic combination: Doxycycline + Daptomycin + Cefoperazone (DCC, 10 µg/mL/each), Panel (**F**) Bee venom (400 µg/mL) and Panel (**G**) Melittin (200 µg/mL).

3. Discussion

The spirochetal bacterium *B. burgdorferi* sensu lato is the main pathological agent of Lyme disease in North America and Europe [1,2]. While this infectious disease may be treated with antibiotics, there has been a rise in antibiotic resistance in recent years [34]. Therefore, extensive effort has been made in finding novel antimicrobial compounds that can assist in the treatment of Lyme disease. In this study, whole bee venom, as well as its component, melittin, were tested on different forms of

Borrelia. This idea was based on a promising earlier study, which showed that melittin significantly affected *B. burgdorferi* sensu stricto spirochetes by decreasing the bacterium's motility as well as its growth [29]. The effects of bee venom and melittin were compared against antibiotics from a study that used the FDA drug library to find highly effective agents for *B. burgdorferi* [7]. The study also confirmed several previous findings that not all antibiotics being used for Lyme disease treatment are effective on all morphological forms of *B. burgdorferi* [6–8,26]. A later study showed that newly discovered antibiotic combinations that were effective for Borrelia persisters [7–10] had limited effect on attached Borrelia biofilms [26]. Therefore, our study aimed to evaluate whether bee venom and melittin could be effective for all morphological forms of Borrelia.

We utilized several different methods to evaluate the effect of all antibiotics and antimicrobials and found that certain techniques such as SYBR Green I/PI needed to be confirmed by additional assays. A potential explanation for the findings is that the SYBR Green I/PI assay could be affected by auto fluorescent components of the dying cells as previously reported for *Escherichia coli* treated with antibiotics [32]. It was suggested that cell death could trigger changes in intrinsic cellular constituents and produce fluorescent chemical compounds [35].

Based on findings from different techniques, we concluded that both whole bee venom and melittin could have significant effects on all Borrelia morphological forms including inhibiting the recovery of spirochetal cells and persisters as evidenced by recovery cultures in antimicrobial free media. Whole bee venom and melittin also significantly reduced the number and/or viability of attached biofilms, which based on previous research, is the most antibiotic resistant form of *B. burgdorferi* [6,25,26]. The MIC concentration values for melittin, for example, were in good agreement with previous studies that evaluated melittin on Borrelia spirochetes [29] and on several other gram-negative microorganisms such as *S. enterica* and *Y. kristensenii* [30].

Comparison of the observed effects of whole bee venom and melittin on Borrelia showed some differences, however. For example, ultrastructure analyses using atomic force microscopy revealed that whole bee venom treatment had more of an effect on the morphology and size of the biofilms than its viability, suggesting the complexity of biofilm responsiveness to antimicrobial agents, which requires further investigation. Differences in bee venom and melittin effectiveness on *B. burgdorferi* suggest that there may be other components within the whole bee venom, that also have an effect on Borrelia biofilms. Similar findings were reported by a recent study testing different whole leaf Stevia extracts on *B. burgdorferi* [26], which found that while whole Stevia leaf extracts were effective, its known component stevioside was not. The results suggested that other components within the whole Stevia leaf extract might affect Borrelia either individually or in a potentially synergistic capacity with stevioside. In addition, the standard antibiotics used in this study had little or no effect on attached biofilm forms of *B. burgdorferi*. Similar findings were observed in previous studies on *Pseudomonas aeruginosa* and *Staphylococcus aureus*, which found that antibiotics could not eliminate the biofilm form and in some cases, could even increase its size [36–39]. In our study, a similar result was found for Doxycycline; it actually increased the attached Borrelia biofilm mass, an observation that agreed to previously published findings [6,25,26].

Bee venom has been shown in past studies to have a wide range of applications in reducing or even eliminating ailments [28,40–44] which can be explained by the multitude of components of bee venom that give it its properties. One type of component, called antimicrobial peptides, could not just eliminate pathogens but could also affect inflammation, enhanced would healing and even had anti-biofilm behavior on different microorganisms [30,42,45–49]. Furthermore, these specific peptides could also affect the bacteria's ability to create fully functional biofilms [50]. Thus, it is vital to understand the components used within the study to comprehend its significance as an antimicrobial treatment.

Melittin is a small, amphipathic α–helical antimicrobial peptide of 26 amino acids and comprises approximately 50% of the whole bee venom used within our study [40,41,43,44,51]. The antimicrobial peptides in bee venom, including melittin and phospholipase A_2, have been a topic of interest within the scientific community, due to the versatility in its function in innate immunity, as well as minimizing chances of adverse immunological reactions when used in combination with other compounds. In this study, Phospholipase A_2 was also tested at different concentrations but did not show any significant effect on any of the morphological forms of *Borrelia* (data not shown).

In recent years, there has been a focus on melittin and its mechanism of action for targeting different microbes [27,42]. This antimicrobial peptide, similar to most of its kind, is amphipathic. This allows for melittin integration into target phospholipid bilayers in low concentrations, while in high concentrations it homodimerizes to form pores, releasing Ca^{2+} ions or disrupting phospholipid head groups [27,38,52–54]. In *B. burgdorferi*, the Ca^{2+} ions are used for the development of a protective outer shell for mature biofilms, for the evasion of potential host resistance [22,25]. The specific mechanism of action of melittin, much like other antimicrobial peptides, are dependent on the target bacteria's phospholipid bilayer composition, as well as evasion of common antimicrobial treatments which could affect the binding locations of peptides to the cell membrane [45,54,55].

Antimicrobial peptides are well known to have very high activity towards microbial membranes with low antimicrobial resistance development [48,56–58]. One of the important reasons that biofilm structure could provide high resistance to antibiotics is mainly due to the presence of dormant microbial populations (sleepers) inside the biofilms. These biofilms are very difficult to kill with standard antibiotics, which often relies on actively growing cells [59]. The use of certain antimicrobial peptides such as mellittin could eliminate this problem by permeabilizing microbial membranes, which results in membrane disruption and cell death even for those dormant cells in the center of the biofilm [48,49]. Interestingly, however, recent findings indicate that antimicrobial peptides can also have intracellular targeting that affects nucleic acid and/or protein synthesis even protein foldings [60]. However future studies are necessary to evaluate whether this is true for melittin.

Another focus in recent publications on bee venom or melittin is the clinical effectiveness of these natural antimicrobials on different diseases. Melittin, for example, was shown to have a very strong immunoregulatory activity, anticancer effect and even shows promise as chemotherapy of human immunodeficiency virus (HIV) infection [41,43,61,62]. Unfortunately, several issues were raised as to the safe administration of melittin in the clinical setting, due its cytotoxicity to human cells; for example, it has the ability to lyse human erythrocytes, exhibits necrotic activity against gastrointestinal and vaginal epithelial cells and can trigger severe allergic reactions [43,63–65]. To reduce it cytotoxic affects, recent studies showed that melittin could be paired with various pharmaceutical agents to specifically eliminate cancer cells, which led to further promising clinical trials [51,66]. In another effort of reducing melittin cytotoxicity, melittin was bound to a nanoparticle, which protected normal human cells while it efficiently attacks HIV infected cells (Hood et al., 2013). The findings from these studies could help promote the design of a novel approach for the successful application of bee venom or melittin in the treatment against *B. burgdorferi,* as well as other pathogenic microbes.

4. Materials and Methods

4.1. Bacterial Culture

Borrelia burgdorferi strain B31 was obtained via American Type Culture Collection (ATCC, #35210). Bacteria were maintained at low passage isolates ($\leq$4) in Barbour-Stoner-Kelly H (BSK-H) media (Sigma, St. Louis, MO, USA) supplemented with 6% rabbit serum (Pel-Freez Biologicals, Rogers, AR, USA) free from antibiotics in sterile glass 15 mL tubes and incubated at 33 °C with 5% CO_2.

4.2. Antimicrobial Agent Preparation

Apis mellifera venom for in vitro testing and prepared using sterile 1× phosphate buffer saline pH 7.4 (PBS) (Fisher, Waltham, MA, USA). Natural melittin extracted from bee venom was purchased (Sigma, St. Louis, MO, USA) and prepared for testing as directed by the manufacturer. The antibiotics (Doxycycline, Cefoperazone, Daptomycin) were purchased from Sigma and prepared at 10 mg/mL stock per manufacturer's instructions. In addition, Doxycycline, Cefoperazone and Daptomycin were also combined (D + C + D) to test on *B. burgdorferi* for the treatment of persister cells. All antimicrobial agents were sterilized using a 0.1 μm filter unit (Millipore, Billercia, MA, USA), aliquoted and stored at −20 °C before further use.

4.3. Antimicrobial Testing

4.3.1. Bacterial Preparation

Antimicrobial treatment effectiveness was tested on logarithmic phase and stationary phase of *B. burgdorferi* spirochetes using SYBR Green I/PI assay and direct counting method [6,26,31]. Spirochetes in logarithmic phase were seeded at 1×10^5 cells/mL on 96-well sterile tissue culture plates (BD Falcon, Frankline Lakes, NJ, USA) then incubated for 48 h prior to antimicrobial treatment. Stationary phase cultures were seeded at 5×10^6 cells/mL in a 96-well sterile tissue culture plate for 5 days prior to treatment. Spirochetes for surface attached biofilms were seeded at 5×10^6 cells/mL in 4-well Permanox chamber slides (Thermo Scientific, Waltham, MA, USA) for 5 days to establish biofilm form. Floating spirochete cells and aggregates from the supernatant were removed to ensure only surface attached biofilms will be analyzed.

4.3.2. Subculture Experiments

Experiments were prepared with a 1:75 dilution of antimicrobial treated stationary culture placed into antimicrobial agent free media and incubated for 7 days using standard culture conditions. Following incubation, the viability was assessed using the SYBR Green I/PI assay and direct counting method as described below.

4.3.3. SYBR Green I/Propidium Iodide Assay

To analyze antimicrobial agent effectiveness, a standard SYBR Green I/Propidium Iodide assay (SYBR Green I/PI) was performed as previously described [26,31]. Staining mixture was prepared using sterile nuclease free water (Fisher, Waltham, MA, USA), SYBR Green I (10,000× stock, Invitrogen, Grand Island, NY, USA) and propidium iodide (20 mM, Thermo Scientific) before being used on *B. burgdorferi* samples. Stained culture was incubated in the dark for 15 min on a rocking platform before being measured on a fluorescent reader (BioTek FL×800) at 485 nm (setting excitation), the absorbance wavelength at 535 nm (green emission) and 635 nm (red emission). Standard curves were generated for spirochetes, persisters and 7-day subculture cells by preparing live:dead samples. Dead cells were prepared by adding 70% isopropyl alcohol for 15 min (Fisher Scientific, Waltham, MA, USA) while live cells were left untreated. To generate a standard curve, different ratios of live and dead cell suspensions (live:dead ratios = 0:10, 2:8, 5:5, 8:2, 10:0) were added to the wells of the 96-well plate and stained as aforementioned. Using least square fitting analysis, the regression equation was calculated between the percentage of live bacteria and green/red fluorescence ratios. The regression equation was used to calculate the percentage of live cells in each sample of the screening plate. Also, images of the treated sample were taken using fluorescent microscopy (Leica DM2500, Leica Microsystems, Inc. Buffalo Grove, IL, USA) at 100× magnification.

4.3.4. Direct Viable Cell Counts of *B. burgdorferi*

As a confirmation test, the SYBR Green/PI stained cultures were assessed for cell growth by directly counting live and dead bacteria using a bacterial counting chamber (Hausser Scientific, Horsham, PA, USA) using fluorescent microscopy (Leica DM2500). As above, using least square fitting analysis the regression equation was calculated and used to calculate the percentage of live cells in each sample.

4.3.5. Autofluorescence of Antimicrobials

All antimicrobial agents were tested for auto fluorescence due to previously reported issues in SYBR Green I/PI assay for detection potential auto fluorescence of the agents [7,26]. In a 96-well plate, antimicrobials were tested in 100 µL of BSK-H media using the SYBR Green I/PI assay and the obtained auto fluorescence values were subtracted from the obtained experimental values.

4.3.6. Quantitative Assay for Attached Biofilms.

The efficacy of antimicrobial agents on attached biofilms were quantified by measuring the total biomass using crystal violet staining before and after antimicrobial treatments. All centrifugation steps were performed at $12,000 \times g$ at room temperature for 5 min. At the end of the treatment regimen, culture media was discarded and attached biofilms were collected by adding 500 µL of 1× PBS before being pelleted. Supernatant was discarded and 50 µL of (0.01% w/v) crystal violet (Sigma, St. Louis, MO, USA) was added to biofilms prior to a 10-min incubation at room temperature. Unbound stain was removed by centrifugation before the biofilm pellet was washed with non-sterile 1× PBS and re-centrifuged. The resulting supernatant was discarded and 200 µL of 10% acetic acid (Sigma, St. Louis, MO, USA) was added to the pellet to release and dissolve excess crystal violet stain during a 15-min incubation period at room temperature. Following incubation, the biofilms were centrifuged and the remaining crystal violet staining was extracted, transferred to a 96-well plate and read at 595 nm using a BioTek Spectrophotometer (BioTek, Winooski, VA, USA).

4.4. Atomic Force Microscopy

Further visualization of Borrelia biofilm structure after antimicrobial treatments (Thermos Scientific, Waltham, MA, USA) were performed using atomic force microscopy. BSK-H media was removed immediately before biofilms were analyzed. All scans were conducted using contact mode AFM imaging in air using the Nanosurf Easyscan 2 AFM (Nanosurf, Woburn, MA, USA) using SHOCONG probes (AppNANO, Mountain View, CA, USA) Images were processed using Gwyddion software (Department of Nanometrology, Czech Metrology Institute. Brno, Czech Republic) [67].

4.5. Statistical Analysis

Quantitative results were analyzed using the median value of all the readings from antimicrobial screen in addition to a two-tailed Student's t-test (Microsoft Excel, Redmond, WA, USA) as well as graphed using Microsoft Excel software. All experiments were performed a minimum of four independent times with at least three samples per experiment. Data represents the mean $\pm$ SD.

5. Conclusions

In conclusion, the findings from this study showed that whole bee venom and melittin were effective against all *B. burgdorferi* morphological forms in vitro, including antibiotic resistant attached biofilms. Though the findings from this in vitro study cannot be applied directly to clinical practice, it gives insight into the potential use of bee venom and its components against *B. burgdorferi*.

Supplementary Materials: The following are available online at www.mdpi.com/2079-6382/6/4/31/s1, Figure S1: The single dose effects of various antimicrobial agents on *B. burgdorferi* for as determined by SYBR Green I/PI assay (Panel A) or direct counting assay (Panel B). Figure S2: Representative Live/Dead staining images of *B. burgdorferi* log phase spirochetal cultures following single dose treatment with different antimicrobial agents. Figure S3: Representative Live/Dead staining images of *B. burgdorferi* stationary phase persister cultures following single dose treatment with different antimicrobial agents Figure S4: Representative Live/Dead staining images of *B. burgdorferi* 7-day recovery cultures following single treatment with different antimicrobial agents. Table S1: The single dose effects of various antimicrobial agents on *B. burgdorferi* as determined by SYBR Green I/PI assay (Panel A) or direct counting assay (Panel B).

Funding: This study was supported by University of New Haven and by the Lindorf Foundation, National Philanthropic Trust, Lymedisease.org and Focus on Lyme to ES. Microscopes and cameras were donated by Lymedisease.org, the Schwartz Research Foundation and Global Lyme Alliance.

Author Contributions: Designed all experiments: K.M.S., E.S. Performed all experiments: K.M.S., P.A.S.T. Analyzed the data: K.M.S., P.A.S.T., E.S. Contributed reagents/materials/analysis tools: P.A.S.T., K.G., J.P.T. wrote the manuscript: K.M.S., E.S.

References

1. Barbour, A.G.; Hayes, S.F. Biology of Borrelia species. *Microbiol. Rev.* **1986**, *50*, 381–400. [PubMed]
2. Rudenko, N.; Golovchenko, M.; Grubhoffer, L.; Oiver, J.H., Jr. Updates on *Borrelia burgdorferi* sensu lato complex with respect to public health. *Ticks Tick-borne Dis.* **2011**, *2*, 123–128. [CrossRef] [PubMed]
3. Brisson, D.; Vandermause, M.F.; Meece, J.K.; Reed, K.D.; Dykhyizen, D.E. Evolution of Northeastern and Midwestern *Borrelia burgdorferi*, United States. *Emerg. Infect. Dis.* **2010**, *16*, 911–917. [CrossRef] [PubMed]
4. Center of Disease Control and Prevention. Lyme Disease. 2016. Available online: http://www.cdc.gov/lyme/ (accessed on 13 September 2017).
5. Wormser, G.P.; Nadelman, R.B.; Dattwyler, R.J.; Dennis, D.T.; Shapiro, E.D.; Steere, A.C.; Rush, T.J.; Rahn, D.W.; Coyle, P.K.; Persing, D.H.; et al. Practice guidelines for the treatment of Lyme disease. *Clin. Infect. Dis.* **2000**, *31*, S1–S14. [CrossRef] [PubMed]
6. Sapi, E.; Kaur, N.; Anyanwu, S.; Leuke, D.F.; Data, A.; Patel, S.; Rossi, M.; Stricker, R.B. Evaluation of in vitro antibiotic susceptibility of different morphological forms of *Borrelia burgdorferi*. *Infect. Drug Resist.* **2011**, *4*, 97–113. [CrossRef] [PubMed]
7. Feng, J.; Wang, T.; Shi, W.; Zhang, S.; Sullivan, D.; Auwaerter, P.G.; Zhang, Y. Identification of novel activity against *Borrelia burgdorferi* persisters using an FDA approved drug library. *Emerg. Microbes. Infect.* **2014**, *3*. [CrossRef] [PubMed]
8. Feng, J.; Auwaerter, P.G.; Zhang, Y. Drug combinations against *Borrelia burgdorferi* persisters in vitro: Eradication achieved by using Daptomycin, Cefoperazone and Doxycycline. *PLoS ONE* **2015**, *10*, E0117207. [CrossRef] [PubMed]
9. Feng, J.; Shi, W.; Zhang, S.; Sullivan, D.; Auwaerter, P.G.; Zhang, Y. A drug combination screen identifies drugs active against amoxicillin-induced round bodies of in vitro *Borrelia burgdorferi* persisters from an FDA drug library. *Front. Microbiol.* **2016**, *7*. [CrossRef] [PubMed]
10. Feng, J.; Weitner, M.; Shi, W.; Zhang, S.; Zhang, Y. Eradication of biofilm-like microcolony structures of *Borrelia burgdorferi* by daunomycin and daptomycin but not mitomycin C in combination with doxycycline and cefuroxime. *Front. Microbiol.* **2016**, *7*. [CrossRef] [PubMed]
11. Hodzic, E.; Fen, S.; Holden, K.; Freet, K.J.; Barthold, S.W. Persistence of *Borrelia burgdorferi* following antibiotic treatment in mice. *Antimicrob. Agents Chemother.* **2008**, *52*, 1728–1736. [CrossRef] [PubMed]
12. Barthold, S.W.; Hodzic, E.; Imai, D.M.; Feng, S.; Yang, X.; Luft, B.J. Ineffectiveness of tigecycline against persistent *Borrelia burgdorferi*. *Antimicrob. Agents Chemother.* **2010**, *54*, 643–651. [CrossRef] [PubMed]
13. Embers, M.E.; Barthold, S.W.; Borda, J.T.; Bowers, L.; Doyle, L.; Hodzic, E.; Jacobs, M.B.; Hasenkampf, N.R.; Martin, D.S.; Narasimhan, S.; et al. Persistence of *Borrelia burgdorferi* in Rhesus macaques following antibiotic treatment of disseminated infection. *PLoS ONE* **2012**, *7*, E29914. [CrossRef]
14. Motaleb, M.A.; Corum, L.; Bono, J.L.; Elias, A.F.; Rosa, P.; Samuels, D.S.; Charon, N.W. *Borrelia burgdorferi* periplasmic flagella have both skeletal and motility functions. *Proc. Natl. Acad. Sci. USA* **2000**, *97*, 10899–10904. [CrossRef] [PubMed]
15. Sal, M.S.; Li, C.; Motalab, M.A.; Shibata, S.; Aizawa, S.; Charon, N.W. *Borrelia burgdorferi* uniquely regulates its motility genes and has an intricate flagellar hook-basal body structure. *J. Bacteriol.* **2008**, *190*, 1912–1921. [CrossRef] [PubMed]
16. Brorson, Ø.; Brorson, S.H. Transformation of cystic forms of *Borrelia burgdorferi* to normal, mobile spirochetes. *Infection* **1997**, *25*, 240–246. [CrossRef] [PubMed]
17. Alban, P.S.; Johnson, P.W.; Nelson, D.R. Serum-starvation-induced changes in protein synthesis and morphology of *Borrelia burgdorferi*. *Microbiology* **2000**, *146*, 119–127. [CrossRef] [PubMed]
18. Murgia, R.; Cinco, M. Induction of cystic forms by different stress conditions in *Borrelia burgdorferi*. *APMIS* **2004**, *112*, 57–62. [CrossRef] [PubMed]
19. MacDonald, A.B. Spirochetal cyst forms in neurodegenerative disorders, hiding in plain sight. *J. Med. Hypotheses* **2006**, *67*, 819–832. [CrossRef] [PubMed]

20. Miklossy, J.; Kasas, S.; Zurn, A.D.; McCall, S.; Yu, S.; McGeer, P.L. Persisting atypical and cystic forms of *Borrelia burgdorferi* and local inflammation in Lyme neuroborreliosis. *J. Neuroinflamm.* **2008**, *5*. [CrossRef] [PubMed]

21. Brorson, Ø.; Brorson, S.H.; Scythes, J.; MacAllister, J.; Wier, A.; Margulis, L. Destruction of spirochete *Borrelia burgdorferi* round-body propagules (RBs) by the antibiotic tigecycline. *Proc. Natl. Acad. Sci. USA* **2009**, *106*, 18656–18661. [CrossRef] [PubMed]

22. Sapi, E.; Bastian, S.L.; Mpoy, C.M.; Scott, S.; Rattelle, A.; Pabbati, N.; Poruri, A.; Burugu, D.; Theophilus, P.A.; Pham, T.V.; et al. Characterization of biofilm formation by *Borrelia burgdorferi* in vitro. *PLoS ONE* **2012**, *7*, 1–11. [CrossRef] [PubMed]

23. Brorson, Ø.; Brorson, S.H. In vitro conversion of *Borrelia burgdorferi* to cystic forms in spinal fluid, and transformation to mobile spirochetes by incubation in BSK-H medium. *Infection* **1998**, *26*, 144–150. [CrossRef] [PubMed]

24. Vancova, M.; Rudenko, N.; Vanecek, J.M.; Golovchenko, M.; Stand, M. Pleomorphism and viability of the Lyme disease pathogen *Borrelia burgdorferi* exposed to physiological stress conditions: A correlative cryo-fluorescence and cryo-scanning electron microscopy study. *Front. Microbiol.* **2017**, *8*, 596. [CrossRef] [PubMed]

25. Sapi, E.; Theophilus, P.A.S.; Burugu, D.; Leuke, D.F. Effect of Rpon, Rpos and Luxs pathways on the biofilm formation and antibiotic sensitivity of *Borrelia burgdorferi*. *Eur. J. Microbiol. Immunol.* **2016**, *6*, 272–286. [CrossRef] [PubMed]

26. Theophilus, P.A.; Victoria, M.J.; Socarras, K.M.; Filush, K.R.; Gupta, K.; Luecke, D.F.; Sapo, E. Effectiveness of *Stevia rebaudiana* whole leaf extract against the various morphological forms of *Borrelia burgdorferi* in vitro. *Eur. Microbiol. Immunol.* **2015**, *5*, 268–280. [CrossRef] [PubMed]

27. Raghuraman, H.; Chattopadhyay, A. Melittin: Membrane-active peptide with diverse functions. *Biosci. Rep.* **2007**, *27*, 189–223. [CrossRef] [PubMed]

28. Carter, V.; Underhill, A.; Baber, I.; Sylla, L.; Baby, M.; Larget-Thiery, I.; Zettor, A.; Bourgouin, C.; Langel, U.; Faye, I.; et al. Killer bee molecules: Antimicrobial peptides as effector molecules to target sporogonic stages of Plasmodium. *PLoS Pathog.* **2013**, *9*, E1003790. [CrossRef] [PubMed]

29. Lubke, L.L.; Garon, C.F. The antimicrobial agent melittin exhibits powerful in vitro inhibitory effects on the Lyme disease spirochete. *Clin. Infect. Dis.* **1997**, *25*, S48–S51. [CrossRef] [PubMed]

30. Alia, O.; Laila, M.; Antonious, A. Antimicrobial effect of melittin isolated from Syrian honeybee (Apis mellifera) venom and its wound healing potential. *Int. J. Pharm. Sci. Rev. Res.* **2013**, *21*, 318–324.

31. Feng, J.; Wang, T.; Zhang, S.; Shi, W.; Zhang, Y. An optimized SYBR Green I/PI assay for rapid viability assessment and antibiotic susceptibility testing for *Borrelia burgdorferi*. *PLoS ONE* **2014**, *9*, E111809. [CrossRef] [PubMed]

32. Renggli, S.; Keck, W.; Jenal, U.; Ritz, D. Role of autofluorescence in flow cytometric analyses of *Escherichia coli* treated with bactericidal antibiotics. *J. Bacteriol.* **2013**, *195*. [CrossRef] [PubMed]

33. Sapi, E.; Balasubramanian, K.; Poruri, A.; Maghsoudlou, J.S.; Socarras, K.M.; Timmaraju, A.V.; Filush, K.R.; Gupta, K.; Shaikh, S.; Theophilus, P.A.; et al. Evidence of in vivo existence of Borrelia biofilm in Borrelial lymphocytomas. *Eur. J. Microbiol. Immunol.* **2016**, *6*, 9–24. [CrossRef] [PubMed]

34. Stricker, R.B.; Johnson, L. Lyme disease: The next decade. *Infect. Drug Resist.* **2011**, *4*, 1–9. [CrossRef] [PubMed]

35. Zamai, L.; Bareggi, R.; Santavenere, E.; Vitale, M. Subtraction of autofluorescent dead cells from lymphocyte flow cytometric binding assay. *Cytometry* **1993**, *14*, 951–954. [CrossRef] [PubMed]

36. Schadow, K.H.; Simpson, W.A.; Christensen, G.D. Characteristics of adherence to plastic tissue culture plates of coagulase-negatice staphylococci exposed to subinhibitory concentrations of antimicrobial agents. *J. Infect. Dis.* **1998**, *157*, 71–77. [CrossRef]

37. Hoffman, L.R.; D'Argenio, L.A.; MacCoss, M.J.; Zhang, Z.; Jones, R.A.; Miller, S.I. Aminoglycoside antibiotics induce bacterial biofilm formation. *Nature* **2005**, *436*, 1171–1175. [CrossRef] [PubMed]

38. Kaplan, J.B. Antibiotic-induced biofilm formation. *Int. J. Artif. Organs* **2011**, *34*, 737–751. [CrossRef] [PubMed]

39. Song, N.; Duperthuy, M.; Wai, S. Sub-optimal treatment of bacterial biofilms (Review). *Antibiotics* **2016**, *5*. [CrossRef] [PubMed]

40. Kwon, Y.B.; Lee, H.J.; Han, H.J.; Mar, W.C.; Kang, S.K.; Yoon, O.B.; Beitz, A.J.; Lee, J.H. The water-soluble fraction of bee venom produces antinociceptive and anti-inflammatory effects on rheumatoid arthritis in rats. *Life Sci.* **2002**, *71*, 191–204. [CrossRef]

41. Jo, M.; Hee Park, M.H.; Kollipara, P.S.; An, B.J.; Song, H.S.; Han, S.B.; Kim, J.H.; Song, M.J.; Hong, J.T. Anti-cancer effect of bee venom toxin and melittin in ovarian cancer cells through induction of death receptors and inhibition of JAK2/STAT3 pathway. *Toxicol. Appl. Pharmacol.* **2012**, *258*, 72–81. [CrossRef] [PubMed]

42. Adade, C.M.; Olivera, I.R.S.; Pais, J.A.R.; Souto-Padrón, T. Melittin peptide kills *Trypanosoma cruzi* parasites by inducing different cell pathways. *Toxicon* **2013**, *69*, 227–239. [CrossRef] [PubMed]

43. Hood, J.L.; Jallouck, A.P.; Campbell, N.; Ratner, L.; Wickline, S.A. Cytolytic nanoparticles attenuate HIV-1 infectivity. *Antivir. Ther.* **2013**, *9*, 95–103. [CrossRef] [PubMed]

44. Nitecka-Buchta, A.; Buchta, P.; Tabeńska-Bosakowska, E.; Walcyńska-Dragoń, K.; Baron, S. Myorelaxant Effect of bee venom topical skin application in patients with RDC/TMD Ia and RDC/TMD Ib: A randomized, double blinded study. *BioMed Res. Intern.* **2014**, *2014*, 296053. [CrossRef] [PubMed]

45. Hancock, R.E.; Sahl, H.G. Antimicrobial and host-defense peptides as new anti-infective therapeutic strategies. *Nat. Biotechnol.* **2006**, *24*, 1551–1557. [CrossRef] [PubMed]

46. Mataraci, E.; Dosler, S. In vitro activities of antibiotics and antimicrobial cationic peptides alone and in combination against Methicillin-Resistant *Staphylococcus aureus* biofilms. *Antimicrob. Agents Chemother.* **2012**, *56*, 6366–6371. [CrossRef] [PubMed]

47. Dobson, A.J.; Purves, J.; Kamysz, W.; Rolff, J. Comparing selection on *S. aureus* between antimicrobial peptides and common antibiotics. *PLoS Pathog.* **2013**, *8*, E76512. [CrossRef] [PubMed]

48. Jamasbi, E.; Mularski, A.; Separovic, F. Model membrane and cell studies of antimicrobial activity of Melittin analogues. *Curr. Top. Med. Chem.* **2016**, *16*, 40–45. [CrossRef] [PubMed]

49. Wu, X.; Singh, A.K.; Wu, X.; Lyu, Y.; Bhunia, A.K.; Narsimhan, G. Characterization of antimicrobial activity against Listeria and cytotoxicity of native melittin and its mutant variants. *Colloids Surf. B Biointerfaces* **2016**, *143*, 194–205. [CrossRef] [PubMed]

50. Xu, W.; Zhu, X.; Tan, T.; Weizhong, L.; Shan, A. Design of embedded-hybrid antimicrobial peptides with enhanced cell selectivity and anti-biofilm activity. *PLoS ONE* **2014**, *9*, E98935. [CrossRef] [PubMed]

51. Hancock, R.E.W. Alteration in outer membrane permeability. *Ann. Rev. Microbiol.* **1984**, *38*, 237–264. [CrossRef] [PubMed]

52. Anderson, M.; Ulmschneider, J.P.; Ulmschneider, M.B.; White, S.H. Conformational states of melittin at a bilayer interface. *Biophys. J.* **2013**, *104*, L12–L14. [CrossRef] [PubMed]

53. Takahashi, T.; Nomura, F.; Yokoyama, Y.; Tanaka-Takiguchi, Y.; Homma, M.; Takiguchi, K. Multiple membrane interactions and versatile vesicle deformations elicited by Melittin. *Toxins* **2013**, *5*, 637–664. [CrossRef] [PubMed]

54. Mohamed, F.M.; Hammac, G.K.; Guptill, L.; Seleem, M.N. Antibacterial activity of novel cationic peptides against clinical isolates of multi-drug resistant *Staphylococcus pseudintermedius* from infected dogs. *PLoS ONE* **2014**. [CrossRef] [PubMed]

55. Brogen, K.A. Antimicrobial peptides: Pore formers or metabolic inhibitors in bacteria? *Nat. Rev. Microbiol.* **2005**, *3*, 238–250. [CrossRef] [PubMed]

56. Batoni, G.; Maisetta, G.; Brancatisano, F.L.; Esin, S.; Campa, M. Use of antimicrobial peptides against microbial biofilms: Advantages and limits. *Curr. Med. Chem.* **2011**, *18*, 256–279. [CrossRef] [PubMed]

57. Leandro, L.F.; Mendes, C.A.; Casemiro, L.A.; Vinholis, A.H.; Cunha, W.R.; de Almeida, R.; Martins, C.H. Antimicrobial activity of apitoxin, melittin and phospholipase A$_2$ of honey bee (Apis mellifera) venom against oral pathogens. *An. Acad. Bras. Cienc.* **2015**, *87*, 147–155. [CrossRef] [PubMed]

58. Strempel, N.; Strehmel, J.; Overhage, J. Potential application of antimicrobial peptides in the treatment of bacterial biofilm infections. *Curr. Pharm. Des.* **2015**, *21*, 67–84. [CrossRef] [PubMed]

59. Lewis, K. Riddle of biofilm resistance. *Antimicrob. Agents Chemother.* **2001**, *45*, 999–1007. [CrossRef] [PubMed]

60. Le, C.F.; Fang, C.M.; Sekaran, S.D. Intracellular targeting mechanisms by antimicrobial peptides. *Antimicrob. Agents Chemother.* **2017**, *61*, 12. [CrossRef] [PubMed]

61. Liu, L.; Ling, C.; Huang, X. Study on purification of melittin and its effect on anti-tumor in vitro. *Chin. J. Biochem. Pharm.* **2003**, *24*, 163–166.

62. Liu, M.; Wang, H.; Liu, L.; Wang, B.; Sun, G. Melittin-MIL-2 fusion protein as a candidate for cancer immunotherapy. *J. Transl. Med.* **2016**, *14*. [CrossRef] [PubMed]

63. Maher, S.; Mcclean, S. Melittin exhibits necrotic cytotoxicity in gastrointestinal cells which is attenuated by cholesterol. *Biochem. Pharmacol.* **2008**, *75*, 1104–1114. [CrossRef] [PubMed]

64. Jallouk, A.P.; Moley, K.H.; Omurtag, K.; Hu, G.; Lanza, G.M.; Wickline, S.A.; Hood, J.L. Nanoparticle incorporation of Melittin reduces sperm and vaginal epithelium cytotoxicity. *PLoS ONE* **2014**, *9*, E95411. [CrossRef] [PubMed]

65. Uddin, M.B.; Lee, B.H.; Nikapitiya, C.; Kim, J.H.; Kim, T.H.; Lee, H.C.; Kim, C.G.; Lee, J.S.; Kim, C.J. Inhibitory effects of bee venom and its components against viruses in vitro and in vivo. *J. Microbiol.* **2016**, *54*, 853–866. [CrossRef] [PubMed]

66. Shin, J.M.; Jeong, Y.-J.; Cho, H.J.; Park, K.K.; Chung, I.K.; Lee, I.K.; Kwak, J.Y.; Chang, H.W.; Kim, C.H.; Moon, S.K.; et al. Melittin suppresses HIF-1α/VEGF expression through inhibition of ERK and mTOR/p70S6K pathway in human cervical carcinoma cells. *PLoS ONE* **2013**, *8*, E69380. [CrossRef] [PubMed]

67. Necas, D.; Klapetek, P. Gwyddion: An open-source software for SPM data analysis. *Cent. Europ. J. Phys.* **2012**. [CrossRef]

14

Activity of Sulfa Drugs and Their Combinations against Stationary Phase *B. burgdorferi* In Vitro

Jie Feng, Shuo Zhang, Wanliang Shi and Ying Zhang *

Department of Molecular Microbiology and Immunology, Bloomberg School of Public Health,
Johns Hopkins University, Baltimore, MD 21205, USA; jfeng16@jhu.edu (J.F.);
szhang30@jhu.edu (S.Z.); wshi3@jhu.edu (W.S.)
* Correspondence: yzhang@jhsph.edu

Academic Editor: Christopher C. Butler

Abstract: Lyme disease is a most common vector-borne disease in the US. Although the majority of Lyme patients can be cured with the standard two- to four-week antibiotic treatment, at least 10%–20% of patients continue to suffer from prolonged post-treatment Lyme disease syndrome (PTLDS). While the cause for this is unclear, one possibility is that persisting organisms are not killed by current Lyme antibiotics. In our previous studies, we screened an FDA drug library and an NCI compound library on *B. burgdorferi* and found some drug hits including sulfa drugs as having good activity against *B. burgdorferi* stationary phase cells. In this study, we evaluated the relative activity of three commonly used sulfa drugs, sulfamethoxazole (Smx), dapsone (Dps), sulfachlorpyridazine (Scp), and also trimethoprim (Tmp), and assessed their combinations with the commonly prescribed Lyme antibiotics for activities against *B. burgdorferi* stationary phase cells. Using the same molarity concentration, dapsone, sulfachlorpyridazine and trimethoprim showed very similar activity against stationary phase *B. burgdorferi* enriched in persisters; however, sulfamethoxazole was the least active drug among the three sulfa drugs tested. Interestingly, contrary to other bacterial systems, Tmp did not show synergy in drug combinations with the three sulfa drugs at their clinically relevant serum concentrations against *B. burgdorferi*. We found that sulfa drugs combined with other antibiotics were more active than their respective single drugs and that four-drug combinations were more active than three-drug combinations. Four-drug combinations dapsone + minocycline + cefuroxime + azithromycin and dapsone + minocycline + cefuroxime + rifampin showed the best activity against stationary phase *B. burgdorferi* in these sulfa drug combinations. However, these four-sulfa-drug–containing combinations still had considerably less activity against *B. burgdorferi* stationary phase cells than the Daptomycin + cefuroxime + doxycycline used as a positive control which completely eradicated *B. burgdorferi* stationary phase cells. Future studies are needed to evaluate and optimize the sulfa drug combinations in vitro and also in animal models.

Keywords: *Borrelia burgdorferi*; stationary phase cells; persisters; sulfa drugs; drug combination

1. Introduction

Lyme disease, which is caused by *Borrelia burgdorferi* sensu lato complex species, is the most common vector-borne disease in the United States with an estimated 300,000 cases a year [1]. The infection is transmitted to humans by tick vectors that feed upon rodents, reptiles, birds, deer, etc. [2]. In the early stage of Lyme disease, patients often have a localized erythema migrans rash that expands as the bacteria disseminate from the cutaneous infection site via the blood stream to other parts of the body. Late-stage Lyme disease is a multi-system disorder which can cause arthritis and neurologic manifestations [1]. While the majority of Lyme disease patients can be cured if treated promptly with the standard two- four-week doxycycline, amoxicillin, or cefuroxime therapy [3], at least 10%–20%

of Lyme patients have lingering symptoms such as fatigue, muscular and joint pain, and neurologic impairment even six months after the antibiotic treatment—a set of symptoms called post-treatment Lyme disease syndrome (PTLDS) [4]. While the cause of PTLDS is unknown, several possibilities are likely to be involved, including autoimmune response [5], immune response to continued presence of antigenic debris [6], tissue damage as a result of Borrelia infection and inflammation, co-infections [7], as well as persistent infection due to *B. burgdorferi* persisters that are not killed by the current antibiotics used to treat Lyme disease [8–10]. Various studies have found evidence of *B. burgdorferi* persistence in dogs [11], mice [8,9], monkeys [10], as well as humans [12] after antibiotic treatment; however, viable organisms are very difficult to culture from the host after antibiotic treatment.

B. burgdorferi develops various forms of dormant persisters in stationary phase cultures which are tolerant to the antibiotics used to treat Lyme disease [13–16]. These persister bacteria have an altered gene expression profile, which may underlie their drug-tolerant phenotype [17]. In log phase cultures (three to five days old), *B. burgdorferi* is primarily in motile spirochetal form which is highly susceptible to current Lyme antibiotics doxycycline and amoxicillin; however, in stationary phase cultures (seven to 15 days old), increased numbers of atypical forms such as round bodies and aggregated biofilm-like microcolonies develop [13,14]. These atypical forms have been shown to have increased tolerance to doxycycline and amoxicillin when compared to the growing spirochetal forms [13–16]. In addition, that the active hits from the round body persister screens [18] overlap with those from the screens on stationary phase cells [13] indicates the stationary phase culture or cells can be used as a relevant persister model. Therefore, stationary phase cultures (seven to 15 days old) enriched in persisters have been used as a model for high-throughput drug screens against persisters [13,14,19].

We have recently identified a range of drugs with high activity against stationary phase cells enriched in persisters through screens of the FDA-approved drug library and NCI compound libraries [13,19]. Besides daptomycin, clofazimine and cephalosporin antibiotics, we also found sulfa drugs as having good activity against *B. burgdorferi* stationary phase cells as well as round body forms [19]. In addition, a recent study found that the sulfa drug dapsone had clinical benefit in the treatment of Lyme disease patients with persistent symptoms [20]. However, the relative activity of different sulfa drugs against *B. burgdorferi* stationary phase cells has not been evaluated in the same study under the same conditions. In this study, we compared the relative activity of three commonly used sulfa drugs, sulfamethoxazole (Smx), dapsone (Dps), sulfachlorpyridazine (Scp), and trimethoprim (Tmp) (a drug that also inhibits the folate pathway but is not considered a sulfa drug), and assessed their combinations with the commonly prescribed Lyme antibiotics and other antibiotics with activities against *B. burgdorferi* stationary phase cells as a persister model.

2. Results and Discussion

2.1. Comparison of the Relative Anti-Persister Activity of Commonly Used Sulfa Drugs Sulfamethoxazole, Dapsone, Sulfachlorpyridazine, and Trimethoprim for Their Activity against Stationary Phase B. burgdorferi Culture

To compare the activity of sulfamethoxazole, dapsone, sulfachlorpyridazine, and trimethoprim against *B. burgdorferi* stationary phase cells, we tested them on the same seven-day-old *B. burgdorferi* stationary phase culture with the same molarity concentrations (10, 20, and 40 µM), using doxycycline and persister drug daptomycin as controls. Compared to the drug-free control (residual viability 91%), the three sulfa drugs and trimethoprim (residual viability 88%–92%, Figure 1) showed little or no activity against stationary phase *B. burgdorferi* cultures at the low concentration (10 µM). Meanwhile, the doxycycline control also showed no activity (residual viability 91%, Figure 1) against the stationary phase *B. burgdorferi*. At the 10 µM concentration, we only found persister drug daptomycin showed good activity (residual viability 48%, Figure 1) against the stationary phase *B. burgdorferi* culture. To confirm results of the plate reader SYBR Green I/PI assay, we performed a microscope counting SYBR Green I/PI assay on the antibiotic-treated samples. The microscope counting results were in agreement with the plate reader results (Figure 1).

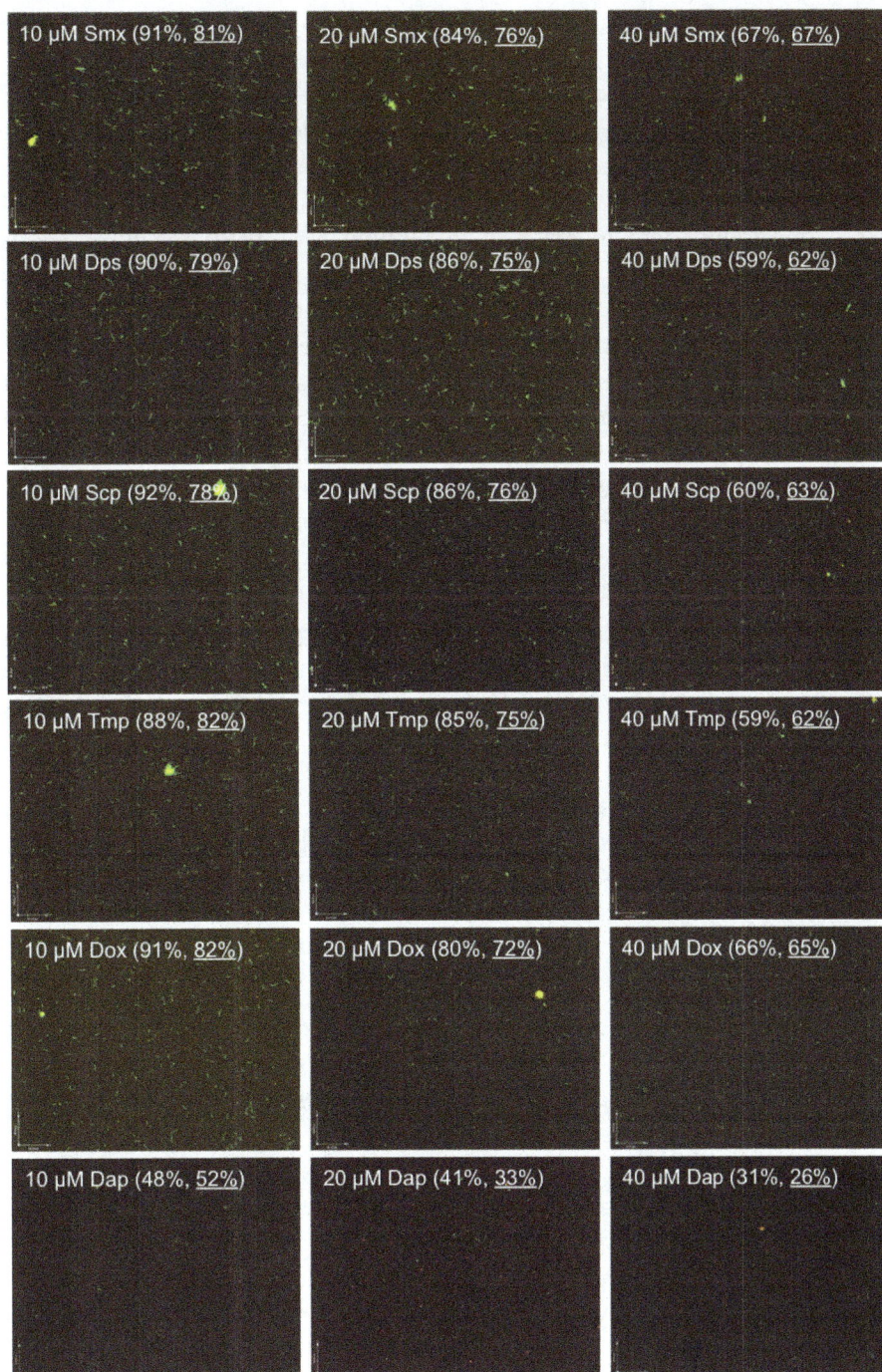

Figure 1. Comparison of anti-persister activity of sulfamethoxazole, dapsone, sulfachlorpyridazine and trimethoprim with doxycycline and daptomycin as controls. A seven-day-old *B. burgdorferi* stationary phase culture containing aggregated microcolonies was incubated for seven days with sulfamethoxazole (Smx), dapsone (Dps), sulfachlorpyridazine (Scp), trimethoprim (Tmp), doxycycline (Dox) and daptomycin (Dap) at the same drug concentrations of 10, 20 or 40 μM, respectively, followed by viability assessment using the SYBR Green I/PI assay. Representative images were taken using epifluorescence microscopy at 100× magnification. The calculated percentage and direct counting percentage (underlined) of residual viable cells are shown in brackets. The green cells stained by SYBR Green I dye indicate live cells while the red cells stained by PI dye indicate dead cells.

At the higher concentration (20 µM), the three sulfa drugs and trimethoprim had some activity (residual viability 86%–84%, Figure 1) against the *B. burgdorferi* stationary phase culture. We did not observe a statistically significant difference in the activity of these four drugs. The three sulfa drugs and trimethoprim (residual viability 86%–84%) showed slightly less activity than doxycycline (residual viability 80%) but considerably less activity than daptomycin (residual viability 41%) at the 20 µM concentration (Figure 1).

We found a dose-dependent increase in the killing activity of the three sulfa drugs and trimethoprim against the stationary phase *B. burgdorferi*, resulting in 59%–67% residual viability (Figure 1) at the highest concentration (40 µM). Dapsone, sulfachlorpyridazine and trimethoprim showed very similar activity against stationary phase *B. burgdorferi* with the 59%, 60% and 59% residual viability, respectively, at 40 µM; however, sulfamethoxazole was the less active drug among the three sulfa drug and trimethoprim as shown by 67% residual viability after the drug treatment for seven days (Figure 1). Meanwhile, we observed that dapsone, sulfachlorpyridazine and trimethoprim showed better activity than the doxycycline control (residual viability 66%) at the high concentration (40 µM). However, the three sulfa drugs and trimethoprim still could not eradicate stationary phase *B. burgdorferi* even at 40 µM. After the seven-day drug treatment of sulfamethoxazole, dapsone, sulfachlorpyridazine and trimethoprim, we could still find many green (live) *B. burgdorferi* cells in aggregated microcolony form, round body form and spirochetal form under the microscope revealed by the SYBR Green I/PI viability assay (Figure 1). As shown in our previous studies [13,14,18], daptomycin showed impressive activity (residual viability 31%) against stationary phase *B. burgdorferi* at 40 µM, as shown by mostly red (dead) cells and red microcolonies (Figure 1). Although dapsone, sulfachlorpyridazine, and trimethoprim showed better activity than doxycycline at 40 µM, their activity is relatively weak compared to daptomycin. We also noticed that sulfamethoxazole showed the weakest activity (residual viability 67%) among the sulfa drugs evaluated and is close to the activity of doxycycline (residual viability 66%) at the high concentration (40 µM).

2.2. Comparison of the Relative Anti-Persister Activity of Sulfamethoxazole, Dapsone, Sulfachlorpyridazine, and Trimethoprim in Drug Combinations at Respective Serum Drug Concentrations

Comparison with the same molar concentration of sulfamethoxazole, dapsone, sulfachlorpyridazine, and trimethoprim could reflect the relative activity of these drugs, while testing the activity of these drugs and their drug combination at their respective serum concentration would provide clinically relevant information. To evaluate effective drug combinations that kill *B. burgdorferi* stationary phase culture at their serum concentrations, we tested sulfamethoxazole (15 µg/mL), dapsone (3 µg/mL), sulfachlorpyridazine (3 µg/mL), and trimethoprim (3 µg/mL) alone and their combinations with doxycycline (4 µg/mL), cefuroxime (5 µg/mL) and ciprofloxacin (3 µg/mL) on a seven-day-old *B. burgdorferi* stationary phase culture. Using these clinically relevant concentrations, except sulfamethoxazole (residual viability 84%), sulfachlorpyridazine (residual viability 84%) and sulfamethoxazole + trimethoprim (residual viability 86%), all the other drugs or drug combinations showed some killing activity compared to the drug-free control (residual viability 95%) (p < 0.01, Table 1). Sulfamethoxazole (residual viability 84%), dapsone (residual viability 83%), sulfachlorpyridazine (residual viability 84%), and trimethoprim (residual viability 84%) showed some killing activity compared to the drug-free control (residual viability 95%) (Table 1), but the differences between their activities were statistically insignificant (p > 0.05).

Interestingly, trimethoprim (residual viability 84%) did not show synergy in the drug combinations with sulfamethoxazole (combination residual viability 86%), dapsone (combination residual viability 85%) and sulfachlorpyridazine (combination residual viability 86%). The results showed that the three sulfa drugs and trimethoprim combined with doxycycline (residual viability 85%), cefuroxime (residual viability 83%) and ciprofloxacin (residual viability 82%) were indeed more active (combination residual viability 74%–78%) than the single drugs (Table 1). However, we did not find significant differences in the activity among these drug combinations. As shown in our previous studies [14,18], cefuroxime combined with doxycycline showed better activity (residual viability 78%) than either one alone (Table 1). However, cefuroxime/doxycycline and cefuroxime/ciprofloxacin combined with sulfamethoxazole, dapsone, sulfachlorpyridazine or trimethoprim did not show higher activity (residual viability 74%–77%).

Our genomic analysis did not identify dihydropteroate synthase and dihydrofolate reductase in B. burgdorferi B31, which respectively are the known targets of sulfa drugs and trimethoprim in other bacteria. Therefore, sulfa drugs and trimethoprim may work on B. burgdorferi B31 through some different and unknown pathways. This may explain why the sulfa drugs and trimethoprim combination did not show a synergistic effect against B. burgdorferi as would be expected with other bacteria, but instead showed more activity when combined with doxycycline, cefuroxime and ciprofloxacin (Table 1).

Table 1. Relative activity of drugs at blood drug combinations on a seven-day-old B. burgdorferi stationary phase culture [a].

Drugs	Ctrl	Smx	Smx + Tmp	Dps	Dps + Tmp	Scp	Scp + Tmp	Tmp
Ctrl	95%	84% [b]	86%	83%	85%	84% [b]	86% [b]	84%
Dox	85%	76%	76%	77%	76%	76%	78%	76%
CefU	83%	77%	76%	77%	76%	74%	76%	75%
Cip	82%	78%	77%	77%	77%	76%	77%	77%
CefU + Dox	78%	76%	77%	77%	77%	76%	77%	77%
CefU + Cip	78%	76%	76%	75%	76%	77%	76%	74%

[a] A seven-day-old stationary phase culture of B. burgdorferi was treated with the indicated drugs at their respective serum concentration (Smx 15 μg/mL, Dps 3 μg/mL, Scp 3 μg/mL, Tmp 3 μg/mL, Dox 4 μg/mL, CefU 5 μg/mL and Cip 3 μg/mL) for seven days. Residual viability of B. burgdorferi after the antibiotic treatment was calculated according to the regression equation and ratio of Green I/PI assay [13]. Viabilities are the average of three replicates.
[b] P-values of the standard t-test for all treated groups versus the drug-free control were less than 0.01 except the data marked with "b".

2.3. Effect of Dapsone Drug Combinations with Clinically Used Drugs on Stationary Phase B. burgdorferi Culture

Dapsone improved chronic Lyme disease/PTLDS patients' clinical symptoms in a recent study [20]. To identify more effective dapsone drug combinations that kill B. burgdorferi stationary phase cells, we tested some dapsone drug combinations with clinically used antibiotics (cefuroxime, azithromycin, rifampin and minocycline). The plate reader results were also confirmed with the microscope counting after SYBR Green I/PI viability staining (Figure 2). The results showed that some drug combinations (Figure 2h–n) were indeed much more effective than single drugs (Figure 2c–g). Dapsone (residual viability 84%, Figure 2d) showed slightly better activity against the seven-day-old stationary phase culture (residual viability 93%, Figure 2a) than the other three clinically used antibiotics azithromycin (residual viability 88%, Figure 2e), rifampin (residual viability 87%, Figure 2f) and minocycline (residual viability 86%, Figure 2g). Both two-drug combinations dapsone/minocycline and dapsone/rifampin showed better activity, with 78% and 81% residual viable (green) cells (Figure 2h,k) remaining, respectively, in comparison to the single drugs (residual viability 84%–87%, Figure 2d,f,g). Interestingly, when cefuroxime was added to the drug combination dapsone/rifampin, the anti-persister activity of these compounds was markedly increased as shown by the 65% residual viable cells remaining (Figure 2l), compared to the dapsone/rifampin combination (residual viability 81%, Figure 2k). We also noted that rifampin/dapsone/minocycline showed better cooperative activity (residual viability 66%, Figure 2m) than the azithromycin/dapsone/minocycline combination (residual viability 72%, Figure 2i), indicating rifampin is more important than azithromycin in combination with dapsone and minocycline. Not surprisingly, the four-drug combinations were more active (residual viability 58% and 60%, Figure 2j,n) than the three-drug combinations (residual viability 65%–72%, Figure 2i,l,m). However, in contrast to the three-drug combination, azithromycin combined with dapsone/minocycline/cefuroxime was slightly more active (residual viability 58%, Figure 2j) than the rifampin four-drug combination (rifampin/dapsone/minocycline/cefuroxime, residual viability 60%, Figure 2n).

Sulfa drugs have recently been shown to have activity against *B. burgdorferi* persisters [13,14], and more recently, dapsone has been shown to improve the symptoms of patients with persistent Lyme disease [20]. Nevertheless, the relative activity of commonly used sulfa drugs such as sulfamethoxazole, dapsone and drug trimethoprim has not been compared under the same conditions. In this study, we found that the different sulfa drugs dapsone, sulfachlorpyridazine, sulfamethoxazole and trimethoprim, when used alone at their respective blood concentrations, had similar but limited activity against *B. burgdorferi* stationary phase cells. However, at the same molar concentrations, trimethoprim had comparable activity to dapsone, both of which seem to be slightly more active than sulfachlorpyridazine and sulfamethoxazole (Figure 1).

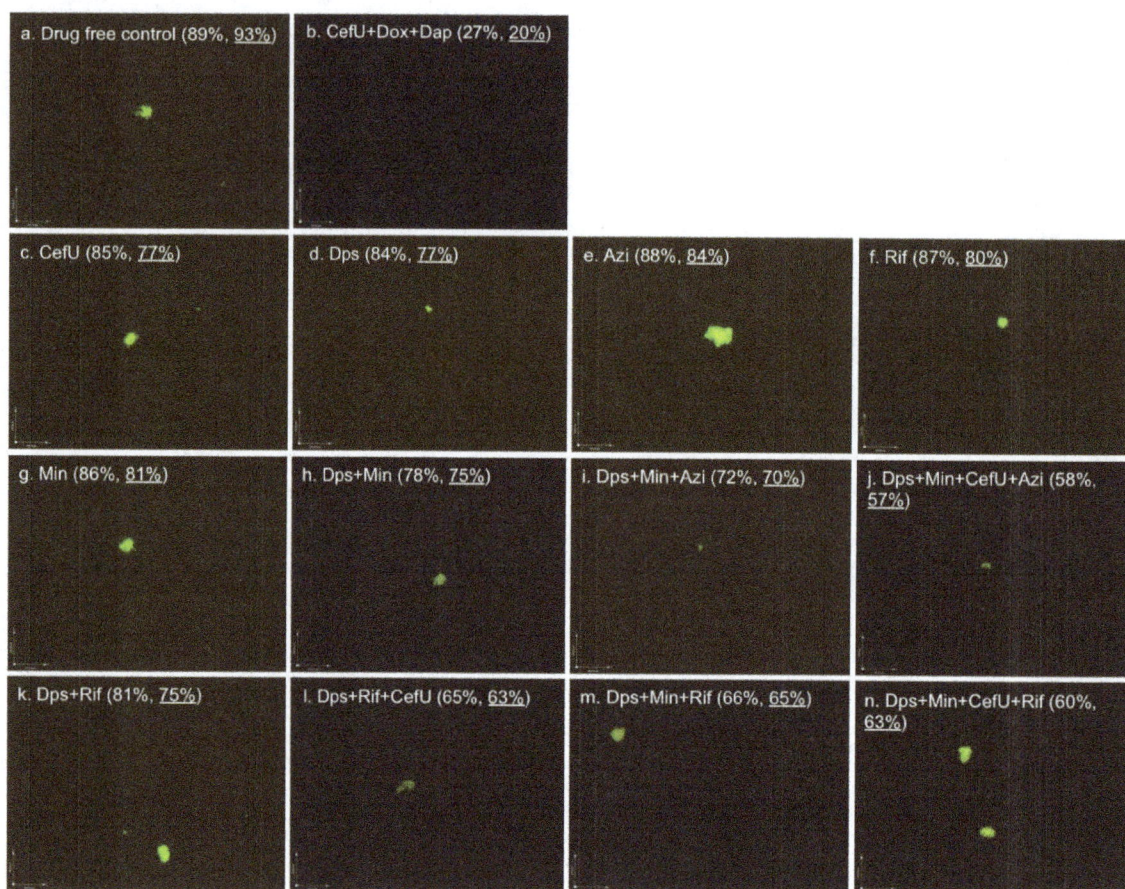

Figure 2. Effect of antibiotics alone or in combinations on stationary phase *B. burgdorferi* culture. A seven-day-old *B. burgdorferi* stationary phase culture was incubated with the indicated drugs or drug combinations at a final concentration of 5 μg/mL for each antibiotic for seven days, followed by SYBR Green I/PI staining and epifluorescence microscopy (100× magnification). The calculated percentage and direct counting percentage (underlined) of residual viable cells are shown in brackets. Abbreviations: CefU, cefuroxime; Dps, dapsone; Azi, azithromycin; Rif, rifampin; Min, minocycline; Dox, doxycycline; Dap: daptomycin.

Although the sulfa drugs had some activity against *B. burgdorferi* stationary phase cells, their activities were enhanced when the sulfa drugs were combined with doxycycline, cefuroxime, ciprofloxacin, rifampin, or azithromycin, and the combination effects were more active than those of the respective single drugs. Among them, the oral four-drug combinations dapsone + minocycline + cefuroxime + azithromycin and dapsone + minocycline + cefuroxime + rifampin showed the best activity (residual viable cells at 58% and 60%, respectively, Figure 2j,n) against stationary phase *B. burgdorferi*. However, the sulfa drug combinations containing even up to four drugs still had considerably less activity against *B. burgdorferi* stationary phase cells than the best drug combination of daptomycin + cefuroxime + doxycycline (residual viable cells at 27%), used as a positive control (Figure 2b). As in our previous study [21], the daptomycin + cefuroxime + doxycycline drug combination could eradicate all *B. burgdorferi* cells as shown by all red (dead) cells or lack of aggregated biofilm-like microcolony structures under the microscope (Figure 2b).

In our previous studies [14,18,21], we used subculture to compare the samples with less than 30% viability after drug treatment to confirm whether the drugs eradicated the bacteria completely. However, in this study, most borrelia were still viable after sulfa drug or drug combination treatment with viable cells above 60%. In this case, the recovery subculture would not find any difference between these samples, and therefore we did not perform subculture tests in this study.

It is worth noting the present study was conducted in vitro and as such the findings may have limitations. The levels of antibiotics in in vitro systems and the degree of protein binding in BSK medium are quite different from human serum, and it remains to be seen if the differences in the relative activity of sulfa drugs and their combinations in vitro can be validated in vivo in animal models or in patients.

2.4. Effect of Sulfamethoxazole, Dapsone, Sulfachlorpyridazine, and Trimethoprim on Growing B. burgdorferi

We also determined the minimum inhibitory concentration (MIC) of sulfamethoxazole, dapsone, sulfachlorpyridazine and trimethoprim on growing *B. burgdorferi* using the standard microdilution method. Our results showed that the three sulfa drugs and trimethoprim could only partly inhibit the growth of *B. burgdorferi*, but failed to completely inhibit the growth, even at 200 μg/mL (Figure 3c–l). Sulfamethoxazole and trimethoprim showed an obvious inhibition effect at the lowest concentration (Figure 3c,g), and their combination nearly completely inhibited the growth of *B. burgdorferi* at 200 μg/mL (Figure 3l). However, even the 200 μg/mL of these drugs still could not completely inhibit the growth of *B. burgdorferi* compared to the start culture (Figure 3d,f,h,l). This result is in disagreement with our previous test in which sulfamethoxazole showed a low MIC (less than 0.25 μg/mL) [13]. There are several possible reasons for the discrepant results. First, in this study we used an animal-passaged *B. burgdorferi* strain instead of the previous unpassaged ATCC strain. Second, we could only selectively check some wells in the 96-well plate by counting chamber in the previous study, but in this study we checked every well directly in the 96-well plate with the BZ-X710 fluorescence microscopy. This greatly improved the experimental accuracy. In this study, we also found an obvious growth-inhibiting effect of sulfamethoxazole even at very low concentrations (0.4 μg/mL) (Figure 3c) compared to the drug-free control (Figure 3a). This inhibiting effect led to incorrect MIC determination because of the lack of a day 0 start culture control in the previous study. Besides the comparison to the drug-free control (Figure 3b), the sulfamethoxazole-treated *B. burgdorferi* culture grew mainly in microcolony form instead of spirochetal form (Figure 3c,d), which could also have led to difficulties and inaccuracy of the counting chamber method used in the previous study. Meanwhile, consistent with our previous experiment [13], doxycycline and amoxicillin, included as controls, did not show growth of *B. burgdorferi*, even at the lowest concentration of 0.2 μg/mL (Figure 3m–p).

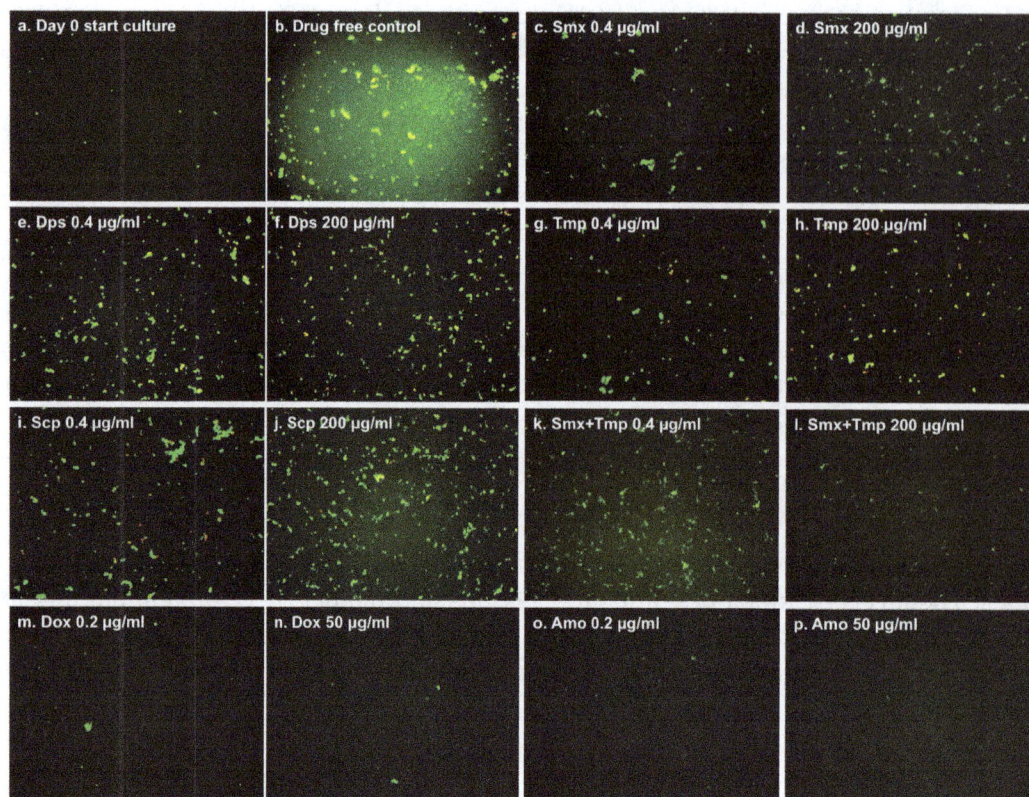

Figure 3. Effect of antibiotics on growing *B. burgdorferi* culture (five days old). The 10^4 spirochetes in 90 μL fresh BSK-H medium as start culture (**a**) were incubated in 96-well microplate at 33 °C and 5% CO_2. The 10 μL two-fold diluted antibiotics (200 μg/mL to 0.4 μg/mL) (**c–l**) and 10 μl DMSO as the drug-free control (**b**) were added to the start culture. After a five-day incubation, the cell proliferation of every well was assessed using the SYBR Green I/PI assay and BZ-X710 All-in-One fluorescence microscope (KEYENCE, Inc., Itasca, IL, USA).

3. Experimental Section

3.1. Strain, Media and Culture Techniques

Low passaged *Borrelia burgdorferi* strain B31 5A19 was kindly provided by Monica Embers [16,22]. The *B. burgdorferi* B31 strain was grown in BSK-H medium (HiMedia Laboratories Pvt. Ltd., Mumbai, India) and supplemented with 6% rabbit serum (Sigma-Aldrich, St. Louis, MO, USA). All culture medium was filter-sterilized by 0.2 μm filter. Cultures were incubated in sterile 15 mL conical tubes (BD Biosciences, CA, USA) in microaerophilic incubator (33 °C, 5% CO_2) without antibiotics. After incubation for seven to 10 days, stationary-phase *B. burgdorferi* culture (about 10^7 spirochetes/mL) was transferred into a 96-well plate for evaluation with the drugs or their combinations.

3.2. Drugs

The following drugs were obtained from Sigma-Aldrich, St. Louis, MO, USA and dissolved in suitable solvents as suggested by the Clinical and Laboratory Standards Institute to make a 5 mg/mL stock solution: doxycycline (Dox), cefuroxime (CefU), ciprofloxacin (Cip), sulfamethoxazole (Smx), dapsone (Dps), sulfachlorpyridazine (Scp), trimethoprim (Tmp), azithromycin (Azi), rifampin (Rif), minocycline (Min) and daptomycin (Dap). The drug stock solutions were filter-sterilized using a 0.2 μm filter and stored at −20 °C.

3.3. Microscopy

The *B. burgdorferi* cultures were examined using a Zeiss AxioImager M2 microscope with epifluorescence illumination. Pictures were taken using a SPOT slider camera. The SYBR Green I/PI viability assay was performed to assess cell viability using the ratio of green/red fluorescence to determine the live:dead cell ratio, respectively, as described previously [14]. This residual cell viability reading was confirmed by analyzing three representative images of the bacterial culture using epifluorescence microscopy. Image Pro-Plus software was used to quantitatively determine the fluorescence intensity.

3.4. Evaluation of Drugs and Drug Combinations for Their Activities against B. burgdorferi Stationary Phase Cultures

For assessing the activity of drugs and drug combinations against stationary phase *B. burgdorferi*, 5 μL aliquots of the drugs were added to 96-well plate containing 100 μL of the seven-day-old stationary phase *B. burgdorferi* culture to obtain the desired drug concentration. Different drugs and drug combinations were evaluated at concentrations close to their Cmax values (maximum serum concentration). The plate was then sealed and was incubated at 33 °C and 5% CO_2 without shaking for seven days when the residual viable cells remaining were calculated according to the regression equation and ratios of Green/Red fluorescence obtained by the SYBR Green I/PI viability assay, and then confirmed using epifluorescence microscopy as described [23]. Untreated groups were used as controls.

3.5. Minimum Inhibitory Concentration (MIC) Determination

The standard microdilution method was used to determine the MIC based on inhibition of visible growth of *B. burgdorferi* by microscopy. *B. burgdorferi* cells (1×10^4) were inoculated into each well of a 96-well microplate containing 90 mL fresh BSK-H medium per well. Antibiotics were two-fold diluted from 200 μg/mL to 0.4 μg/mL. Each diluted compound (10 μL) was added to the culture. All experiments were run in triplicate. The 96-well plate was sealed and placed in an incubator at 33 °C for five days. Cell proliferation was assessed using the SYBR Green I/PI assay and BZ-X710 All-in-One fluorescence microscope (KEYENCE, Inc.) after the incubation.

3.6. Statistical Analysis

All experiments were run in triplicate. Statistical analyses were performed using Student's *t*-test.

4. Conclusions

In summary, dapsone, sulfachlorpyridazine and trimethoprim showed very similar activity against stationary phase *B. burgdorferi* at the same molarity concentration, and sulfamethoxazole was the least active drug among them. However, at blood concentrations, all four drugs had similar activity. It is worth noting that trimethoprim did not show synergy in the drug combinations with the three sulfa drugs at their serum concentrations. However, sulfa drugs and trimethoprim, when combined with other antibiotics such as doxycycline, ciprofloxacin and cefuroxime, were more active than the respective single drugs. However, none of the sulfa drug combinations were as effective as the daptomycin drug combination control since they were unable to completely eradicate *B. burgdorferi* stationary phase cells. Future studies are needed to optimize the drug combinations in vitro and to evaluate the sulfa drugs and their drug combinations in vivo.

Acknowledgments: We acknowledge the support of our work by the Steven & Alexandra Cohen Foundation, the Global Lyme Alliance, the Lyme Disease Association, and NatCapLyme. We thank Richard Horowitz for suggesting some drug combinations tested in this study. Ying Zhang was supported in part by NIH grants AI099512 and AI108535.

Author Contributions: Ying Zhang conceived the experiments; Jie Feng, Wanliang Shi, Shuo Zhang, performed the experiments; Jie Feng and Ying Zhang analyzed the data; Jie Feng and Ying Zhang wrote the paper.

References

1. CDC. Lyme Disease. Available online: http://www.cdc.gov/lyme/ (accessed on 13 September 2015).
2. Radolf, J.D.; Caimano, M.J.; Stevenson, B.; Hu, L.T. Of ticks, mice and men: Understanding the dual-host lifestyle of lyme disease spirochaetes. *Nat. Rev. Microbiol.* **2012**, *10*, 87–99. [CrossRef] [PubMed]
3. Wormser, G.P.; Dattwyler, R.J.; Shapiro, E.D.; Halperin, J.J.; Steere, A.C.; Klempner, M.S.; Krause, P.J.; Bakken, J.S.; Strle, F.; Stanek, G.; et al. The clinical assessment, treatment, and prevention of lyme disease, human granulocytic anaplasmosis, and babesiosis: Clinical practice guidelines by the infectious diseases society of america. *Clin. Infect. Dis.* **2006**, *43*, 1089–1134. [CrossRef] [PubMed]
4. CDC. Post-Treatment Lyme Disease Syndrome. Available online: http://www.cdc.gov/lyme/postLDS/index.html (accessed on 18 September 2016).
5. Steere, A.C.; Gross, D.; Meyer, A.L.; Huber, B.T. Autoimmune mechanisms in antibiotic treatment-resistant lyme arthritis. *J. Autoimmun.* **2001**, *16*, 263–268. [CrossRef] [PubMed]
6. Bockenstedt, L.K.; Gonzalez, D.G.; Haberman, A.M.; Belperron, A.A. Spirochete antigens persist near cartilage after murine lyme borreliosis therapy. *J. Clin. Investig.* **2012**, *122*, 2652–2660. [CrossRef] [PubMed]
7. Swanson, S.J.; Neitzel, D.; Reed, K.D.; Belongia, E.A. Coinfections acquired from ixodes ticks. *Clin. Microbiol. Rev.* **2006**, *19*, 708–727. [CrossRef] [PubMed]
8. Hodzic, E.; Feng, S.; Holden, K.; Freet, K.J.; Barthold, S.W. Persistence of *Borrelia burgdorferi* following antibiotic treatment in mice. *Antimicrob. Agents Chemother.* **2008**, *52*, 1728–1736. [CrossRef] [PubMed]
9. Hodzic, E.; Imai, D.; Feng, S.; Barthold, S.W. Resurgence of persisting non-cultivable *Borrelia burgdorferi* following antibiotic treatment in mice. *PLoS ONE* **2014**, *9*, e86907. [CrossRef] [PubMed]
10. Embers, M.E.; Barthold, S.W.; Borda, J.T.; Bowers, L.; Doyle, L.; Hodzic, E.; Jacobs, M.B.; Hasenkampf, N.R.; Martin, D.S.; Narasimhan, S.; et al. Persistence of *Borrelia burgdorferi* in rhesus macaques following antibiotic treatment of disseminated infection. *PLoS ONE* **2012**, *7*, e29914. [CrossRef]
11. Straubinger, R.K.; Summers, B.A.; Chang, Y.F.; Appel, M.J. Persistence of *Borrelia burgdorferi* in experimentally infected dogs after antibiotic treatment. *J. Clin. Microbiol.* **1997**, *35*, 111–116. [PubMed]
12. Marques, A.; Telford, S.R., 3rd; Turk, S.P.; Chung, E.; Williams, C.; Dardick, K.; Krause, P.J.; Brandeburg, C.; Crowder, C.D.; Carolan, H.E.; et al. Xenodiagnosis to detect *Borrelia burgdorferi* infection: A first-in-human study. *Clin. Infect. Dis.* **2014**, *58*, 937–945. [CrossRef] [PubMed]
13. Feng, J.; Wang, T.; Shi, W.; Zhang, S.; Sullivan, D.; Auwaerter, P.G.; Zhang, Y. Identification of novel activity against *Borrelia burgdorferi* persisters using an FDA approved drug library. *Emerg. Microb. Infect.* **2014**. [CrossRef] [PubMed]
14. Feng, J.; Auwaerter, P.G.; Zhang, Y. Drug combinations against *Borrelia burgdorferi* persisters in vitro: Eradication achieved by using daptomycin, cefoperazone and doxycycline. *PLoS ONE* **2015**, *10*, e0117207. [CrossRef] [PubMed]
15. Sharma, B.; Brown, A.V.; Matluck, N.E.; Hu, L.T.; Lewis, K. *Borrelia burgdorferi*, the causative agent of lyme disease, forms drug-tolerant persister cells. *Antimicrob. Agents Chemother.* **2015**, *59*, 4616–4624. [CrossRef] [PubMed]
16. Caskey, J.R.; Embers, M.E. Persister development by *Borrelia burgdorferi* populations in vitro. *Antimicrob. Agents Chemother.* **2015**, *59*, 6288–6295. [CrossRef] [PubMed]
17. Feng, J.; Shi, W.; Zhang, S.; Zhang, Y. Persister mechanisms in borrelia burgdorferi: Implications for improved intervention. *Emerg. Microbes Infect.* **2015**. [CrossRef] [PubMed]
18. Feng, J.; Shi, W.; Zhang, S.; Sullivan, D.; Auwaerter, P.G.; Zhang, Y. A drug combination screen identifies drugs active against amoxicillin-induced round bodies of in vitro *Borrelia burgdorferi* persisters from an FDA drug library. *Front. Microbiol.* **2016**. [CrossRef] [PubMed]
19. Feng, J.; Weitner, M.; Shi, W.; Zhang, S.; Sullivan, D.; Zhang, Y. Identification of additional anti-persister activity against *Borrelia burgdorferi* from an FDA drug library. *Antibiotics* **2015**. [CrossRef] [PubMed]
20. Horowitz, R.; Freeman, P. The use of dapsone as a novel "persister" drug in the treatment of chronic lyme disease/post treatment lyme disease syndrome. *J. Clin. Exp. Dermatol. Res.* **2016**. [CrossRef]

21. Feng, J.; Weitner, M.; Shi, W.; Zhang, S.; Zhang, Y. Eradication of biofilm-like microcolony structures of *Borrelia burgdorferi* by daunomycin and daptomycin but not mitomycin C in combination with doxycycline and cefuroxime. *Front. Microbiol.* **2016**. [CrossRef] [PubMed]

22. Purser, J.E.; Norris, S.J. Correlation between plasmid content and infectivity in *Borrelia burgdorferi*. *Proc. Natl. Acad. Sci. USA* **2000**, *97*, 13865–13870. [CrossRef] [PubMed]

23. Feng, J.; Wang, T.; Zhang, S.; Shi, W.; Zhang, Y. An optimized SYBR Green I/PI assay for rapid viability assessment and antibiotic susceptibility testing for *Borrelia burgdorferi*. *PLoS ONE* **2014**, *9*, e111809. [CrossRef] [PubMed]

15

Veterinary Students' Knowledge and Perceptions About Antimicrobial Stewardship and Biosecurity

Laura Hardefeldt [1,2,*] ⓘ, Torben Nielsen [3], Helen Crabb [1,2], James Gilkerson [1], Richard Squires [4], Jane Heller [5], Claire Sharp [6], Rowland Cobbold [7], Jacqueline Norris [8] ⓘ and Glenn Browning [1,2]

[1] Asia-Pacific Centre for Animal Health, Department of Veterinary Biosciences, Faculty of Veterinary and Agricultural Sciences, Melbourne Veterinary School, University of Melbourne, Parkville, VIC 3050, Australia; helen.crabb@unimelb.edu.au (H.C.); jrgilk@unimelb.edu.au (J.G.); glenfb@unimelb.edu.au (G.B.)

[2] National Centre for Antimicrobial Stewardship, Peter Doherty Institute, Grattan St, Carlton, VIC 3050, Australia

[3] School of Animal and Veterinary Sciences, University of Adelaide, Roseworthy, SA 5371, Australia; torben.nielsen@adelaide.edu.au

[4] College of Public Health, Medical and Veterinary Sciences, James Cook University, Townsville, QLD 4810, Australia; richard.squires@jcu.edu.au

[5] School of Animal and Veterinary Sciences, Charles Sturt University, Wagga Wagga, NSW 2650, Australia; jheller@csu.edu.au

[6] School of Veterinary and Life Sciences, Murdoch University, Perth, WA 6150, Australia; c.sharp@murdoch.edu.au

[7] School of Veterinary Science, University of Queensland, Gatton, QLD 4343, Australia; r.cobbold@uq.edu.au

[8] Sydney School of Veterinary Science, University of Sydney, Sydney, NSW 2006, Australia; jacqui.norris@sydney.edu.au

* Correspondence: laura.hardefeldt@unimelb.edu.au

Abstract: A better understanding of veterinary students' perceptions, attitudes, and knowledge about antimicrobial stewardship and biosecurity could facilitate more effective education of future veterinarians about these important issues. A multicenter cross-sectional study was performed by administering a questionnaire to veterinary students expected to graduate in 2017 or 2018 in all Australian veterinary schools. Four hundred and seventy-six of 1246 students (38%) completed the survey. Many students were unaware of the high importance of some veterinary drugs to human medicine, specifically enrofloxacin and cefovecin (59% and 47% of responses, respectively). Fewer than 10% of students would use appropriate personal protective equipment in scenarios suggestive of Q fever or psittacosis. Students expected to graduate in 2018 were more likely to select culture and susceptibility testing in companion animal cases (OR 1.89, 95% CI 1.33–2.69, $p < 0.001$), and were more likely to appropriately avoid antimicrobials in large animal cases (OR 1.75, 95% CI 1.26–2.44, $p = 0.001$) than those expected to graduate in 2017. However, 2018 graduates were less likely to correctly identify the importance rating of veterinary antimicrobials for human health (OR 0.48, 95% CI 0.34–0.67, $p < 0.001$) than 2017 graduates. Students reported having a good knowledge of antimicrobial resistance, and combating resistance, but only 34% thought pharmacology teaching was adequate and only 20% said that teaching in lectures matched clinical teaching. Efforts need to be made to harmonize preclinical and clinical teaching, and greater emphasis is needed on appropriate biosecurity and antimicrobial stewardship.

Keywords: education; antimicrobial resistance; personal protective equipment; antimicrobial stewardship; antibiotic

1. Introduction

The association between antimicrobial use and increasing antimicrobial resistance (AMR) in animals has long been established [1–10]. Direct [11–20] or indirect [13,17,21,22] contact with animals can result in human–animal exchange of multidrug-resistant pathogens. Despite this established relationship, there is still widespread inappropriate prescribing of antimicrobials in all sectors of veterinary practice in Australia [23–26], indicating a need for antimicrobial stewardship (AMS) programs. Antimicrobial stewardship was conceptualized in the 1970s within the human health sector and has recently been defined as "a coherent set of actions which promote using antimicrobials responsibly" [27]. According to the World Health Organisation, "education of healthcare workers and medical students on rational antimicrobial prescribing or AMS is an integral part of all AMR containment activities" [28]. We would argue that education of veterinarians is equally important.

Biosecurity also plays an important role in controlling antimicrobial resistance. In veterinary medicine, biosecurity is the set of preventative measures designed to reduce the risk of transmission of infectious diseases. The biosecurity habits of veterinarians have been investigated and 45% report contracting a zoonosis during their career and the reported use of personal protective equipment (PPE) was poor [29]. Equine veterinarians in Australia are reported as having up to 23-times-higher odds of carrying methicillin-resistant *Staphylococcus aureus* (MRSA) than controls [30], a trend that persists globally. Equine veterinarians who report use of PPE have 65% lower odds of carriage of MRSA compared with those not reporting PPE utilization [31]. There has been no investigation into veterinary students' knowledge of and behavior regarding biosecurity or use of personal protective equipment.

Understanding the perceptions of veterinary students in different phases of their education is critical in guiding future education about AMS and resistance, in understanding the reasons for inappropriate antimicrobial use by recent graduates, and in guiding education about biosecurity measures. There is considerable literature on the knowledge and perceptions of medical students regarding AMS [32–38], but no studies to date on veterinary students. One United Kingdom study took a 'One Health' approach to this topic; however, the numbers of students from each sector responding to the survey were small and comparisons could not be made. Findings were largely consistent with previous research. Students recognized the global challenge of AMR but failed to recognize their personal prescribing practices as significantly contributing to the problem and mostly felt underprepared to prescribe antimicrobials appropriately [39]. To address the gap in understanding veterinary student knowledge and attitudes, we conducted a comprehensive survey of students in the last two years of their training across all Australian veterinary schools to assess the adequacy of current educational efforts and the factors influencing student attitudes and perceptions about AMS and biosecurity.

2. Results

Of the 1246 Australian veterinary students graduating in 2017 or 2018, 476 (38%) completed the survey, with a further 30 responses incomplete and subsequently discarded. Students from all universities were represented and a significant sample was obtained from 6 of the 7 Australian veterinary schools (Table 1). Responses were obtained from 2017 graduates (227/476, 48%) and 2018 graduates (249/476, 52%). Students with varied interest areas completed the survey (Table 1). Overall, 88% of respondents thought veterinary use of antimicrobials had a moderate or strong contribution to overall AMR (Figure 1). Content analysis revealed the reasons for the contribution of veterinary antimicrobial use to overall AMR included overuse of antimicrobials (27% of respondents), overuse of antimicrobials in food animals (18% of respondents), and low use of culture and susceptibility (C & S) testing (7% of respondents). The residual variation due to university effects (variation partition coefficient) was 10–13% for outcomes of treatment and biosecurity, with most variance attributable to within-university and between-students.

Table 1. Demographics of 2017 and 2018 graduating Australian veterinary students ($n = 476$) responding to antimicrobial stewardship questionnaire.

Exposures	Number of responses (%)	University response rate, %
University		
Charles Sturt University (2018 graduates only)	7 (1.5)	11
James Cook University	55 (12)	37
Murdoch University	65 (14)	26
University of Adelaide	81 (17)	72
University of Melbourne	170 (36)	71
University of Queensland	53 (11)	22
University of Sydney	44 (9)	23
Year of graduation		
2017	227 (47)	
2018	249 (52)	
Area of interest		
Small animal	201 (42)	
Mixed practice	182 (38)	
Public health, government, industry, research	25 (5)	
Equine	23 (5)	
Bovine	18 (4)	
Undecided	27 (6)	

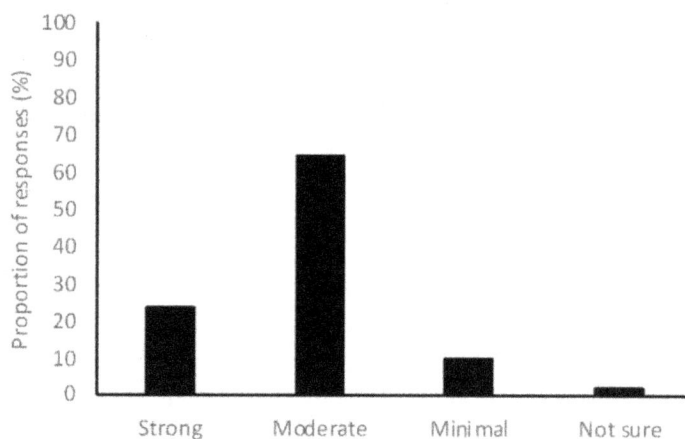

Figure 1. Proportion of 2017 and 2018 graduating Australian veterinary students ($n = 476$) responding to a survey indicating how much they think antimicrobial use by veterinarians contributes to the overall burden of antimicrobial resistance.

Over 80% of students correctly identified amoxycillin and penicillin as first-line therapies (86% and 84%, respectively) (Figure 2). All other antimicrobials were correctly categorized by fewer than 75% of respondents. Amoxycillin/clavulanate (second line) and enrofloxacin (third line) were incorrectly categorized into lower levels by 59% of respondents (for both drugs). Similarly, cefovecin (third line) was also commonly categorized into a lesser category (47% of respondents). Chloramphenicol (first line) was the only antimicrobial to be frequently categorized into a higher level (63% of respondents) (Figure 2). In the mixed effects model, 2018 graduates were significantly less likely to correctly identify the importance rating of antimicrobials than 2017 graduates, after adjusting for their area of interest and the random effect of place of study (OR 0.48, 95% CI 0.34–0.67, $p < 0.001$).

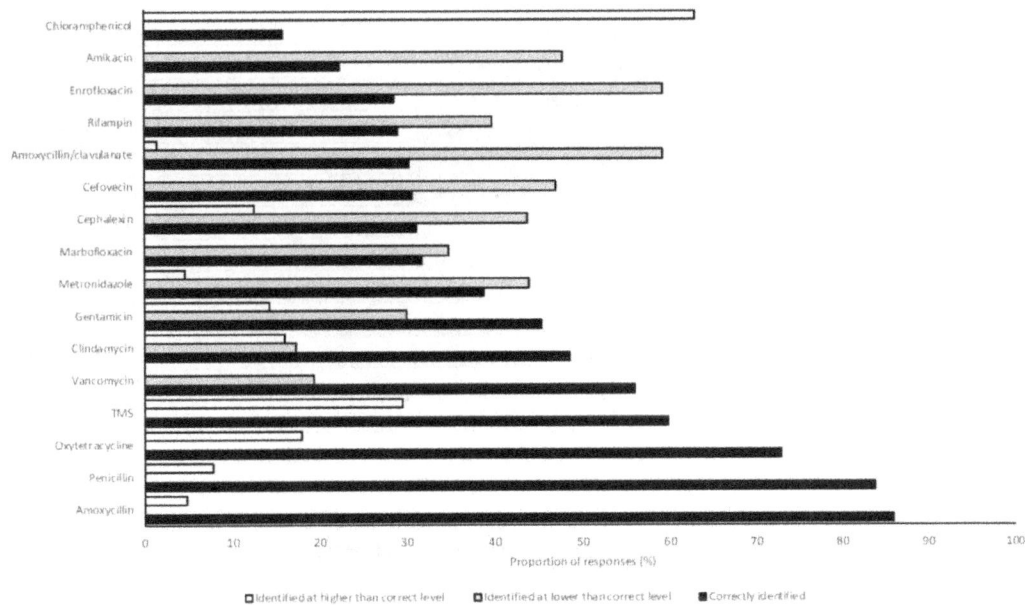

Figure 2. Proportions of 2017 and 2018 graduating Australian veterinary students (*n* = 476) responding to a survey correctly identifying the level of importance of antimicrobials in human medicine and identifying a level lower than or higher than that assigned by the Australian Strategic Technical Advisory Panel on Antimicrobial Resistance [40]. TMS, trimethoprim sulphonamide.

Veterinary students were asked to indicate whether they would always, frequently, rarely, or never use systemic antimicrobials for a range of clinical scenarios. All scenarios were designed in such a way that systemic antimicrobials were rarely or never indicated. Always and frequently were combined, as were rarely or never, for ease of evaluation. Dog spey was the only scenario in which the vast majority of respondents indicated that antimicrobials were rarely or never indicated (91%) (Figure 3). After adjusting for their area of interest and the random effect of place of study, the 2018 graduates were significantly more likely to propose appropriate prescribing in large animal scenarios than 2017 graduates (OR 1.75, 95% CI 1.26–2.44, *p* = 0.001). In small animal scenarios, there was no difference in the appropriateness of prescribing by 2017 and 2018 graduates (OR 0.96, 95% CI 0.68–1.36, *p* = 0.83). There was no difference between students with small animal, mixed practice, or large animal practice interests in either small or large animal scenarios.

Veterinary students were asked to indicate whether they would always, frequently, rarely, or never utilize C & S testing for a range of clinical scenarios. At least 24% of students reported that they would perform C & S testing in each scenario, and at least 50% of students reported that they would always or frequently perform C & S in each of 13 of the 17 scenarios (Figure 4). Severe and recurrent infections were the scenarios most frequently associated with high rates of C & S testing. The most important factors that influenced students' decisions to perform C & S testing were persistent infections (84%), recurring infections (71%), severe infections (38%), and client finances (32%). In small animal scenarios, 2018 graduates were significantly more likely to always or frequently perform C & S testing than 2017 graduates (OR 1.89, 95% CI 1.33–2.69, *p* < 0.001). There was no difference between year levels in large animal scenarios (OR 0.90, 95% CI 0.64–1.26, *p* = 0.537).

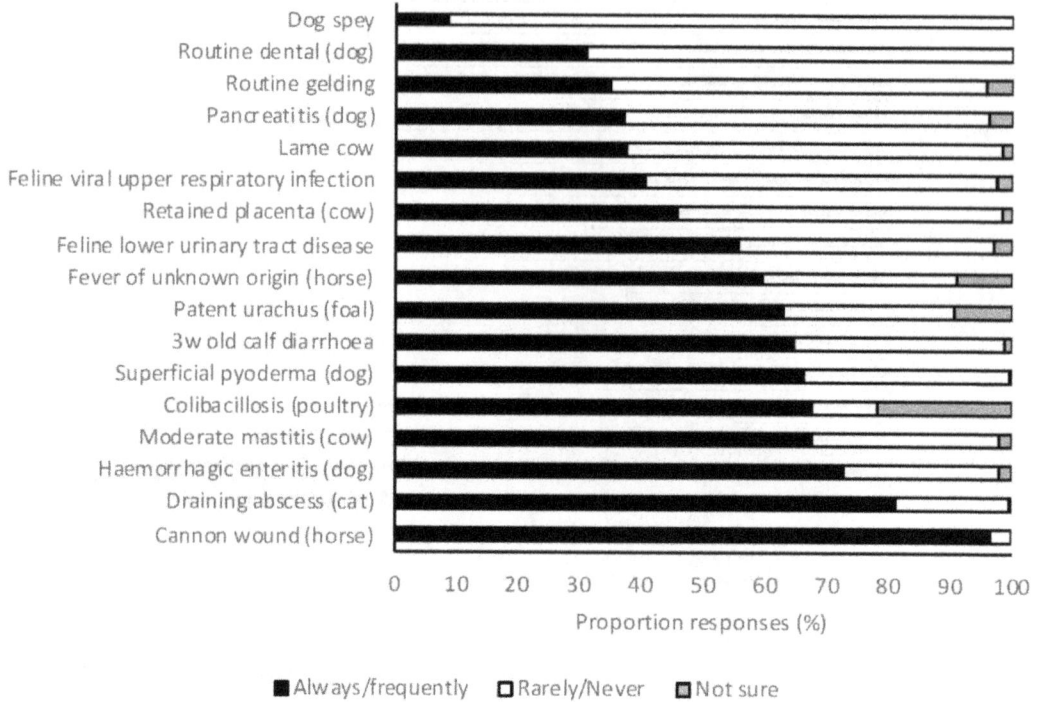

Figure 3. The frequency with which 2017 and 2018 graduating Australian veterinary students (*n* = 476) responding to a survey would treat a range of clinical scenarios with systemic antimicrobials.

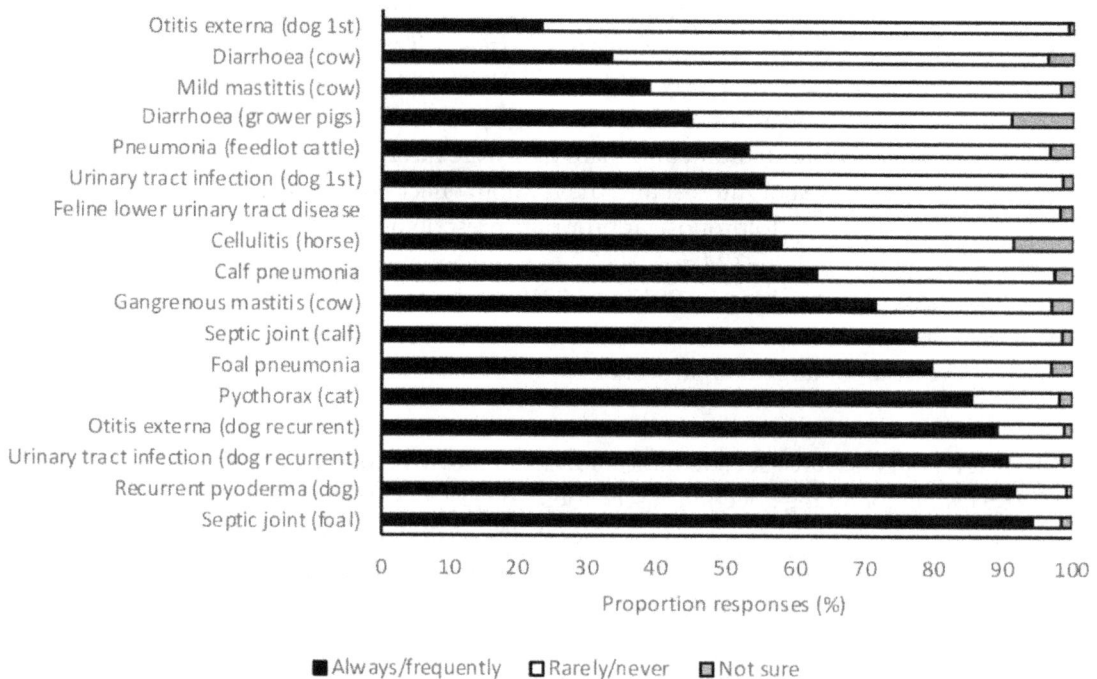

Figure 4. The frequency with which 2017 and 2018 graduating Australian veterinary students (*n* = 476) responding to a survey would perform culture and susceptibility for a range of clinical scenarios.

Appropriate use of PPE procedures and biosecurity were reported by the majority of students for routine examination of dogs and cats, cattle, and horses (97%, 98%, and 86%, respectively) (Figure 5). However, there were four scenarios in which the proposed use of PPE was insufficient for more than 90% of respondents: respiratory disease in a galah (*Elophus roseicapilla*), aborted fetal material from a horse, poor conception rates in goats, and dystocia in a mare (7%, 7%, 4%, and 4% of responses were appropriate, respectively). Students graduating in 2018 were significantly more likely to propose use of appropriate PPE in large animal scenarios than 2017 graduates (OR 1.15, 95% CI 1.02–1.29, $p = 0.021$). There was no difference in the appropriateness of use of PPE between year levels for small animal (OR 1.10, 95% CI 0.77–1.57, $p = 0.606$) or large animal scenarios (OR 1.39, 95% CI 0.97–1.99, $p = 0.07$). Students from the University of Sydney were significantly more likely to use appropriate PPE for large animal scenarios than students from all other universities (OR 1.23–1.55, $p < 0.05$ for all). This was largely due to an increased awareness of psittacosis, for which University of Sydney students were more likely to use appropriate PPE than students from other universities (OR 2.2–4.8, $p < 0.05$ for all). There were no differences between students based on area of interest.

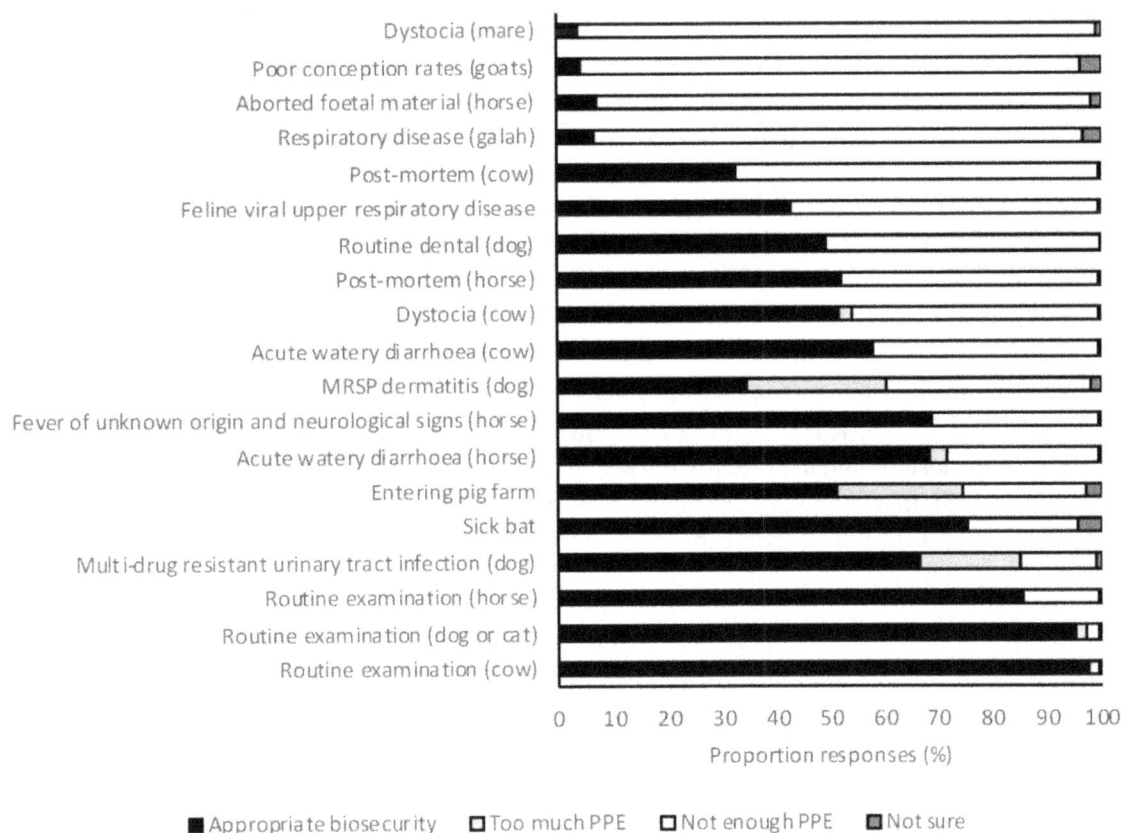

Figure 5. The frequency with which 2017 and 2018 graduating Australian veterinary students ($n = 476$) responding to survey applied appropriate biosecurity for a range of clinical scenarios. PPE, personal protective equipment; MRSP, multi-drug resistant *Staphylococcus pseudintermedius*

Students reported having a good understanding of the mechanisms of AMR and AMS (Figure 6). However, most respondents suggested that prudent antimicrobial use and pharmacology were taught less than was perceived necessary. Students also indicated that what they were taught in clinical practice about antimicrobial use was often different to what they were taught in preclinical learning activities (Figure 6). Students were largely aware of at least one of the antimicrobial prescribing guidelines currently available (83%), but rarely reported referring to these frequently (12%). Students had similar awareness of biosecurity guidelines, with 79% having at least heard of one of the biosecurity guidelines available for veterinarians in Australia. Biosecurity guidelines were also rarely referred to by students (3.5%).

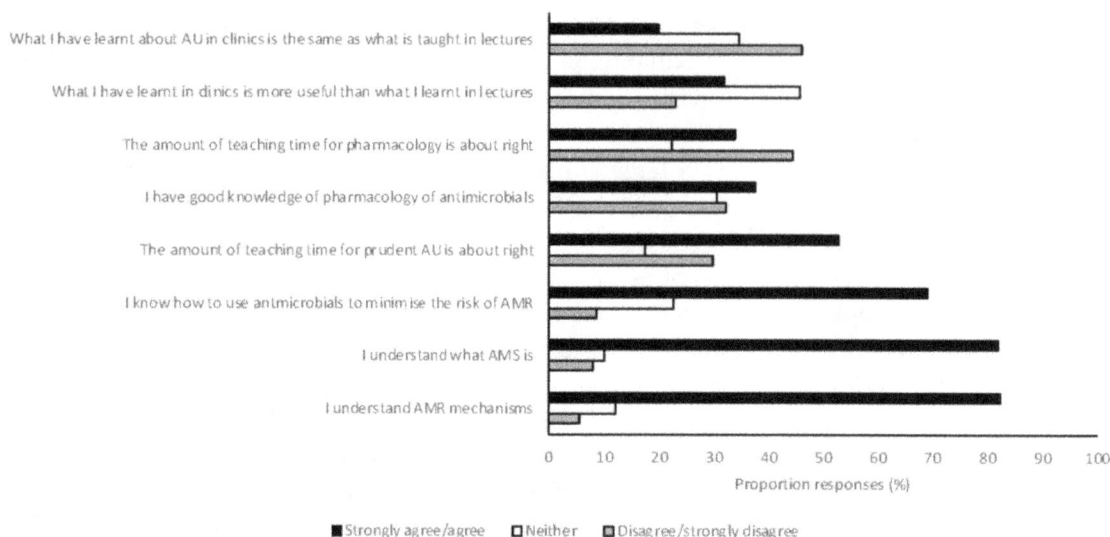

Figure 6. The opinion of Australian veterinary students, graduating in 2017 and 2018 and responding to a survey (n = 476), about the teaching of antimicrobial resistance and antimicrobial stewardship. AMR, antimicrobial resistance; AMS, antimicrobial stewardship; AU, antimicrobial use.

3. Discussion

To our knowledge, this is the first multicenter study investigating veterinary students' knowledge and attitudes about AMS. This survey is also unique in its comparison of 2 years of veterinary students, gaining valuable insight into the progressive acquisition of AMS principles. Most students completing this survey thought that veterinary use of antimicrobials contributed moderately to the overall issue of AMR. This is consistent with a recent study of veterinarians in Australia [41]. There is little consensus between prescribing professions in Australia as to the proportional role of each in the evolution of AMR [42]. Students identified overuse of antimicrobials, especially in food animals, and low use of C & S, leading to inappropriate use of antimicrobials, as the main reasons underlying this contribution. In Australia, use of antimicrobials in food animals is modest in most industries, with most reports of multi-resistant organisms coming from companion animal species [20,43–46]. With evidence that both direct [11–19] and indirect [13,17,21,22] contact with animals can result in human acquisition of multidrug-resistant pathogens of animal origin, and high rates of pet ownership [47] in Australia, AMR in companion animal species is likely to pose the biggest risk to the community in Australia. Low use of C & S, due to the high cost of this testing, has been identified as a barrier to AMS in Australia [41]. As there is no obvious solution to this issue, rates of C & S testing are unlikely to increase.

Ratings of the importance of antimicrobials in human health in Australia are assigned by the Australian Strategic Technical Advisory Group on AMR (ASTAG) [40]. Amoxycillin-clavulanate, enrofloxacin, and cefovecin were rated lower than by ASTAG by many students who responded to this survey (59%, 59%, and 47%, respectively). A recent survey of Australian veterinarians found that amoxycillin-clavulanate and cefovecin were frequently used in veterinary practice [48]. Antimicrobial use guidelines largely recommend amoxycillin alone as a first-line therapy and cefovecin is registered for use in Australia only after C & S testing [49]. Chloramphenicol was rated higher than by ASTAG by 63% of students in this survey. The adverse effects of chloramphenicol on people, and low use of this drug in clinical veterinary practice in Australia, may contribute to students erroneously believing that chloramphenicol has a higher importance rating. Students expected to graduate in 2018 were less likely to correctly identify the importance rating of antimicrobials than 2017 graduates (OR 0.48, 95% CI 0.34–0.67, p < 0.001), suggesting that greater exposure to use of antimicrobials during clinical teaching in the final year of veterinary school may lead to a greater awareness of antimicrobial importance ratings.

In a recent survey, a high proportion of equine veterinarians [24] indicated that they would always or frequently use antimicrobials for an uncomplicated wound, and the survey described here also found that a very high proportion of students (97%) would always or frequently use antimicrobials for an uncomplicated wound over the cannon in a horse. Best-practice clinical guidelines do not recommend antimicrobials for uncomplicated wounds in horses [50,51]. Many students also indicated that they would always or frequently use antimicrobials for an uncomplicated draining abscess in a cat and hemorrhagic diarrhea in a dog (81% and 73%, respectively) even though guidelines recommend against such use [50,52]. However, some small animal textbooks [53,54] still recommend antimicrobials for hemorrhagic diarrhea, highlighting the need for harmonization of recommendations. Use of guidelines in preference to textbooks will also assist, as these should be more dynamic in their recommendations as an evolving evidence base arises. The rate of use of antimicrobials for abscesses in cats was assessed in a survey in 2011 and 52% (468/893) of respondents indicated that antimicrobials were not routinely prescribed (authors' unpublished data). Students' perceptions that use in these scenarios is warranted is concerning and efforts should be made to improve education in these areas. Students expected to graduate in 2018 were more likely to use antimicrobials appropriately in large animal scenarios than those expected to graduate in 2017 (OR 1.75, 95% CI 1.26–2.44, $p = 0.001$), suggesting that exposure to large animal clinical practice may be teaching students inappropriate antimicrobial use. In contrast, clinical experience did appear to improve student knowledge of the rating on antimicrobial importance, as described above. Contemporary research on the prescribing practices of Australian veterinarians showed that recent veterinary graduates were less likely to use antimicrobials appropriately than older graduates [23]. It was speculated that this may be due to inadequacies in preclinical and/or clinical university teaching, clinical teaching in the final year, or other challenges faced by recent graduates (greater fear of adverse events, workplace culture, or peer pressure). The hierarchical structure of veterinary practice has recently been identified as a barrier to effective AMS in veterinary practices [41]. This study suggests that universities should endeavor to promote AMS in both university teaching hospitals and associated extramural veterinary practices.

Many students indicated they would always or frequently perform C & S testing in a range of scenarios in both large and small animal practice. Clearly there is a shift in behavior following the transition to clinical practice, as such high rates of C & S testing are not seen in clinical veterinary practice in Australia [26]. In small animal scenarios, 2018 graduates were more likely to perform C & S than 2017 graduates (OR 1.89, 95% CI 1.33–2.69, $p < 0.001$). Exposure to the low use of C & S in clinical practice may influence student decision-making in their final year of study. As seen in surveys of veterinarians in practice [41], severe and recurrent infections were most frequently recognized as always or frequently necessitating C & S testing. Restricted client finances were identified by 34% of practicing veterinarians as a barrier to C & S testing [41], and this was also recognized by students, with 32% indicating that this was an important factor in deciding whether or not to perform C & S.

There were four scenarios in which the vast majority of students indicated that they would use insufficient PPE. Two of these scenarios suggested commonly known zoonoses in Australian veterinarians. The first was avian psittacosis (respiratory disease in a galah), for which only 7% of respondents would use appropriate PPE, while the second was Q fever (poor conception rates in goats), for which only 4% of respondents would use appropriate PPE. The other two scenarios in which students indicated that they would use insufficient PPE described the recently identified risk of psittacosis after contact with fetal membranes in horses [55]. Personal protective equipment for Hendra virus infection in a horse was also concerningly inadequate given the wide publicity and educational effort given to this zoonosis in Australia (inadequate PPE selected by 31% of respondents). Students attending the University of Sydney were more likely to use appropriate PPE for the scenario suggestive of chlamydial abortion in horses. No differences were found between students attending different universities in their responses to the scenario suggestive of infection with Hendra virus. Hendra virus has caused fatal disease in veterinarians in Australia and this zoonosis has received much attention across the profession. Students should be aware of the measures needed to protect themselves, and others, from such zoonoses. Further studies are needed to clarify the methods used to convey this message to students and may be useful in providing effective means for conveying other key messages.

Students in this survey frequently thought that more time should be spent on teaching pharmacology. Veterinary pharmacology is taught as a stand-alone subject in 5 of the 7 veterinary schools in Australia [56–58] and is integrated in the other courses. Similarly, surveys of medical students in the United Kingdom, France, and the United States of America have demonstrated that students also desire more education in this area [35–38]. Many students (45%) indicated that clinical teaching of antimicrobial use was not consistent with preclinical teaching, and many students (32%) felt that clinical teaching was more useful. However, students graduating in 2017, with higher levels of exposure to clinical teaching, had lower levels of compliance with guidelines compared with students graduating in 2018 before entering the clinical environment. This suggests that preclinical teaching is superior in the teaching of appropriate antimicrobial use. Efforts should be made to ensure consistency of teaching between preclinical and clinical teachers, and to ensure that appropriate AMS measures are in place in the clinical environment. Awareness of the existence of guidelines for antimicrobial use was high amongst this cohort of students, but utilization of these guidelines was low. Poor guideline utilization has been identified as an issue in medical hospitals [59], but the reasons are likely to be different for veterinary students. Understanding how guidelines are utilized in veterinary practice will allow for methods to be developed to optimize uptake. Malalignment of textbooks and current guidelines may contribute to differences in clinical behavior and further investigation is warranted.

Enrolment bias may occur with surveys such as this as respondents are self-selected. This factor may bias the results towards respondents that are more interested in AMS and therefore have more awareness of appropriate antimicrobial use. This survey had a good response rate, however, and high numbers of responses from 6 of the 7 universities. The results are unlikely affected by enrolment bias. Poor participation from one university was likely due to the differing graduation pattern at this school, with students graduating in August. For this reason, there were no 2017 graduate responses. While students in this survey reported having a good understanding of the mechanisms of AMR, the present study did not assess the understanding of AMR mechanisms. Further study is needed to confirm the perceptions of students.

4. Materials and Methods

We conducted a cross-sectional multicenter study of the knowledge and attitudes of Australian veterinary students regarding AMS and biosecurity during October and November 2017. The source population comprised the national veterinary students expected to graduate in 2017 or 2018. All 2018 graduates had completed, or were near completion of, preclinical training but were yet to start the immersive clinical phase of training. All 2017 graduates had completed, or were near completion of, the clinical phase of training and were scheduled to graduate within 2 months of completion of the survey. Participation was voluntary and responses were anonymous. Students were recruited via email, social media, and by a researcher in class in some instances. Sample size calculations were performed to determine the number of respondents required to make appropriate inferences from the survey. To be 95% certain that our estimate of the population prevalence of veterinary students selecting a given treatment was within 5% of the true population prevalence, a total of 308 completed surveys were required. To detect a 15% difference between 2017 and 2018 graduates in the proportion answering correctly in any one part of the questionnaire, 388 completed surveys were required. To allow for comparisons between universities, 44–54 students from each university were required to complete the survey, which took into account the number of students in university year levels [60].

A questionnaire was developed using REDCap electronic data capture tools (Vanderbilt University, Nashville, TN, USA) [61] that consisted of 6 sections and 88 questions (available as Supplementary Materials). The initial section asked for demographic details about the respondents and their opinion of the degree to which veterinary antimicrobial use contributes to community AMR.

Questionnaire Section 2 required respondents to indicate whether 16 named antimicrobials were first-, second-, or third-line therapies (as defined by the ASTAG) [40] with low importance rating agents classified first-line therapies, medium importance rating agents classified as second line, and high importance rating agents classified as third-line therapies). Section 3 required respondents to indicate the frequency (always, frequently, sometimes, rarely, never, or not sure) with which they would use antimicrobials for 17 specific scenarios (both medical and surgical). Section 4 required respondents to indicate the frequency (always, frequently, sometimes, rarely, never, or not sure) with which they would submit samples for culture and susceptibility (C & S) testing for 17 specific scenarios. Section 5 required respondents to indicate the level of biosecurity they would undertake for 19 specific scenarios. The final section required respondents to indicate their knowledge of common guidelines and their opinion about the quantity and quality of teaching on AMS within their program. All questions were closed except for one requesting the respondent's opinion about the community impact of veterinary antimicrobial use. The survey was pretested with 2 recently graduated veterinarians and no changes were made.

The entire section of each part of the survey had to be completed by the respondent to be included in the analysis. Descriptive statistics were computed, with percentages reported for the proportion of the total number of respondents answering a particular question. Answers to questions that used a 5-point Likert scale were condensed into 3 categories (agree/strongly agree, neutral, disagree/strongly disagree). Differences in proportions were tested using χ^2 test. An overall knowledge score was assessed for each section using antimicrobial use and biosecurity guidelines and by calculating the total proportion of correct answers.

A multilevel logistic regression model was used to identify individual student-level characteristics that were associated with correct identification of the importance rating of antimicrobials, appropriate antimicrobial usage, appropriate use of C & S testing, and correct use of PPE and biosecurity. Where students indicated they did not know the answer, these questions were discarded from the proportion of correct answers for this student. Results from the university with low numbers of responses were excluded from investigations of the effect of place of study. We started all analysis with a null model that included our binomial dependent variable and added the predictor variable of place of study to see whether the model was improved. Unconditional associations between each of the hypothesized explanatory variables (year level, veterinary school attended, species of interest) and the outcome of interest were examined using odds ratios. For the multivariable model, the outcome of interest was parameterized as a function of the explanatory variables. The random effect of university was tested in the model using a likelihood ratio test. Plausible two-way interactions were tested at an alpha level of 0.05. Where interactions were present, odds ratios are presented for each group. Analysis was performed using Stata, version 14.2 (StataCorp LLC, College Station, TX, USA).

Questions with open responses were openly coded and analyzed by one researcher (LYH) using content analysis and qualitative data analysis principles [62–65]. The code structure was developed using an inductive approach.

This research was approved by the University of Melbourne Faculty of Veterinary and Agricultural Sciences Human Ethics Advisory Group under Approval No. 1750016.1.

5. Conclusions

In conclusion, this research has identified some gaps in the AMS education of veterinary students in Australia. Specifically, that the antimicrobials with a high importance rating that are in common use in veterinary practice should be identifiable by students. In addition, the lack of knowledge about appropriate use of PPE was concerning. Student perceptions and approaches indicate that preclinical AMS teaching is superior to clinical teaching and harmonization is recommended. Efforts are needed to improve guideline utilization by veterinarians, as this has been associated with more appropriate use of antimicrobials in human medicine [66,67] and in a veterinary teaching hospital [68]. Further research is needed into the barriers to usage and implementation of guidelines in the veterinary profession.

Acknowledgments: This research was funded by the National Health and Medical Research Council through the Centres of Research Excellence Programme, Grant no. 1079625.

Author Contributions: L.H. contributed to conceiving and designing the questionnaire, contributed to data collection, analyzed the data, and wrote the paper. T.N. contributed to data collection and assisted with data analysis and manuscript editing. H.C. assisted with data analysis and manuscript editing. J.G. contributed to questionnaire design and manuscript editing. R.S., J.H., C.S., R.C., and J.N. contributed to data collection and manuscript editing. G.B. contributed to conceiving and designing the questionnaire, data analysis, and manuscript editing.

References

1. Lowrance, T.C.; Loneragan, G.H.; Kunze, D.J.; Platt, T.M.; Ives, S.E.; Scott, H.M.; Norby, B.; Echeverry, A.; Brashears, M.M. Changes in antimicrobial susceptibility in a population of *Escherichia coli* isolated from feedlot cattle administered ceftiofur crystalline-free acid. *Am. J. Vet. Res.* **2007**, *68*, 501–507. [CrossRef] [PubMed]

2. Schmidt, J.W.; Griffin, D.; Kuehn, L.A.; Brichta-Harhay, D.M. Influence of therapeutic ceftiofur treatments of feedlot cattle on fecal and hide prevalences of commensal *Escherichia coli* resistant to expanded-spectrum cephalosporins, and molecular characterization of resistant isolates. *Appl. Environ. Microbiol.* **2013**, *79*, 2273–2283. [CrossRef] [PubMed]

3. Alali, W.Q.; Scott, H.M.; Norby, B.; Gebreyes, W.; Loneragan, G.H. Quantification of the bla(cmy-2) in feces from beef feedlot cattle administered three different doses of ceftiofur in a longitudinal controlled field trial. *Foodborne Pathog. Dis.* **2009**, *6*, 917–924. [CrossRef] [PubMed]

4. Jiang, X.; Yang, H.; Dettman, B.; Doyle, M.P. Analysis of fecal microbial flora for antibiotic resistance in ceftiofur-treated calves. *Foodborne Pathog. Dis.* **2006**, *3*, 355–365. [CrossRef] [PubMed]

5. Leite-Martins, L.R.; Mahu, M.I.; Costa, A.L.; Mendes, A.; Lopes, E.; Mendonca, D.M.; Niza-Ribeiro, J.J.; de Matos, A.J.; da Costa, P.M. Prevalence of antimicrobial resistance in enteric *Escherichia coli* from domestic pets and assessment of associated risk markers using a generalized linear mixed model. *Prev. Vet. Med.* **2014**, *117*, 28–39. [CrossRef] [PubMed]

6. Rentala, M.; Lahti, E.; Kuhalampi, J.; Pesonen, S.; Jarvinen, A.K.; Saijonmaa-Koulumies, L.; Honkanen-Buzalski, T. Antimicrobial resistance in *Staphlococcus* spp., *Escherichia coli* and *Enterococcus* spp. in dogs given antibiotics for chronic dermatological disorders compared with non-treated control dogs. *Acta Vet. Scand.* **2004**, *45*, 37–45. [CrossRef]

7. Kanwar, N.; Scott, H.M.; Norby, B.; Loneragan, G.H.; Vinasco, J.; McGowan, M.; Cottell, J.L.; Chengappa, M.M.; Bai, J.; Boerlin, P. Effects of ceftiofur and chlortetracycline treatment strategies on antimicrobial susceptibility and on tet(a), tet(b), and bla cmy-2 resistance genes among *E. coli* isolated from the feces of feedlot cattle. *PLoS ONE* **2013**, *8*, e80575. [CrossRef] [PubMed]

8. Ahmed, M.O.; Clegg, P.D.; Williams, N.J.; Baptiste, K.E.; Bennett, M. Antimicrobial resistance in equine faecal *Escherichia coli* isolates from north west England. *Ann. Clin. Microbiol. Antimicrob* **2010**, *9*, 12. [CrossRef] [PubMed]

9. Berge, A.C.; Epperson, W.B.; Pritchard, R.H. Assessing the effect of a single dose florfenicol treatment in feedlot cattle on the antimicrobial resistance patterns in faecal *Escherichia coli*. *Vet. Res.* **2005**, *36*, 723–734. [CrossRef] [PubMed]

10. Chambers, L.; Yang, Y.; Littier, H.; Ray, P.; Zhang, T.; Pruden, A.; Strickland, M.; Knowlton, K. Metagenomic analysis of antibiotic resistance genes in dairy cow feces following therapeutic administration of third generation cephalosporin. *PLoS ONE* **2015**, *10*, e0133764. [CrossRef] [PubMed]

11. Weese, J.S.; Dick, H.; Willey, B.M.; McGeer, A.; Kreiswirth, B.N.; Innis, B.; Low, D.E. Suspected transmission of methicillin-resistant *Staphylococcus aureus* between domestic pets and humans in veterinary clinics and in the household. *Vet. Microbiol.* **2006**, *115*, 148–155. [CrossRef] [PubMed]

12. Platell, J.L.; Cobbold, R.N.; Johnson, J.R.; Heisig, A.; Heisig, P.; Clabots, C.; Kuskowski, M.A.; Trott, D.J. Commonality among fluoroquinolone-resistant sequence type st131 extraintestinal *Escherichia coli* isolates from humans and companion animals in Australia. *Antimicrob. Agents Chemother.* **2011**, *55*, 3782–3787. [CrossRef] [PubMed]

13. Liu, W.; Liu, Z.; Yao, Z.; Fan, Y.; Ye, X.; Chen, S. The prevalence and influencing factors of methicillin-resistant *Staphylococcus aureus* carriage in people in contact with livestock: A systematic review. *Am. J. Infect. Control* **2015**, *43*, 469–475. [CrossRef] [PubMed]

14. Oppliger, A.; Moreillon, P.; Charriere, N.; Giddey, M.; Morisset, D.; Sakwinska, O. Antimicrobial resistance of *Staphylococcus aureus* strains acquired by pig farmers from pigs. *Appl. Environ. Microbiol.* **2012**, *78*, 8010–8014. [CrossRef] [PubMed]

15. Dohmen, W.; Bonten, M.J.; Bos, M.E.; van Marm, S.; Scharringa, J.; Wagenaar, J.A.; Heederik, D.J. Carriage of extended-spectrum beta-lactamases in pig farmers is associated with occurrence in pigs. *Clin. Microbiol. Infect.* **2015**, *21*, 917–923. [CrossRef] [PubMed]

16. Schwaber, M.J.; Navon-Venezia, S.; Masarwa, S.; Tirosh-Levy, S.; Adler, A.; Chmelnitsky, I.; Carmeli, Y.; Klement, E.; Steinman, A. Clonal transmission of a rare methicillin-resistant *Staphylococcus aureus* genotype between horses and staff at a veterinary teaching hospital. *Vet. Microbiol.* **2013**, *162*, 907–911. [CrossRef] [PubMed]

17. Ishihara, K.; Saito, M.; Shimokubo, N.; Muramatsu, Y.; Maetani, S.; Tamura, Y. Methicillin-resistant *Staphylococcus aureus* carriage among veterinary staff and dogs in private veterinary clinics in Hokkaido, Japan. *Microbiol. Immunol.* **2014**, *58*, 149–154. [CrossRef] [PubMed]

18. Paterson, G.K.; Harrison, E.M.; Craven, E.F.; Petersen, A.; Larsen, A.R.; Ellington, M.J.; Torok, M.E.; Peacock, S.J.; Parkhill, J.; Zadoks, R.N.; et al. Incidence and characterisation of methicillin-resistant *Staphylococcus aureus* (MRSA) from nasal colonisation in participants attending a cattle veterinary conference in the UK. *PLoS ONE* **2013**, *8*, e68463. [CrossRef] [PubMed]

19. Paul, N.C.; Moodley, A.; Ghibaudo, G.; Guardabassi, L. Carriage of methicillin-resistant *Staphylococcus pseudintermedius* in small animal veterinarians: Indirect evidence of zoonotic transmission. *Zoonoses Public Health* **2011**, *58*, 533–539. [CrossRef] [PubMed]

20. Worthing, K.A.; Abraham, S.; Pang, S.; Coombs, G.W.; Saputra, S.; Jordan, D.; Wong, H.S.; Abraham, R.J.; Trott, D.J.; Norris, J.M. Molecular characterization of methicillin-resistant *Staphylococcus aureus* isolated from Australian animals and veterinarians. *Microb. Drug Resist.* **2018**, *24*, 203–212. [CrossRef] [PubMed]

21. Grinberg, A.; Kingsbury, D.D.; Gibson, I.R.; Kirby, B.M.; Mack, H.J.; Morrison, D. Clinically overt infections with methicillin-resistant *Staphylococcus aureus* in animals in New Zealand: A pilot study. *N. Z. Vet. J.* **2008**, *56*, 237–242. [PubMed]

22. Boost, M.; Ho, J.; Guardabassi, L.; O'Donoghue, M. Colonization of butchers with livestock-associated methicillin-resistant *Staphylococcus aureus*. *Zoonoses Public Health* **2013**, *60*, 572–576. [CrossRef] [PubMed]

23. Hardefeldt, L.Y.; Browning, G.F.; Thursky, K.; Gilkerson, J.R.; Billman-Jacobe, H.; Stevenson, M.A.; Bailey, K.E. Antimicrobials used for surgical prophylaxis by companion animal veterinarians in Australia. *Vet. Microbiol.* **2017**, *203*, 301–307. [CrossRef] [PubMed]

24. Hardefeldt, L.Y.; Browning, G.F.; Thursky, K.; Gilkerson, J.R.; Billman-Jacobe, H.; Stevenson, M.A.; Bailey, K.E. Antimicrobials used for surgical prophylaxis by equine veterinary practitioners in Australia. *Equine Vet. J.* **2017**, *50*, 65–72. [CrossRef] [PubMed]

25. Hardefeldt, L.Y.; Browning, G.F.; Thursky, K.; Gilkerson, J.R.; Billman-Jacobe, H.; Stevenson, M.A.; Bailey, K.E. Antimicrobials used for surgical prophylaxis by bovine veterinary practitioners in Australia. *Vet. Rec.* **2017**, *50*, 65–72. [CrossRef]

26. Hardefeldt, L.Y.; Holloway, S.; Trott, D.J.; Shipstone, M.; Barrs, V.R.; Malik, R.; Burrows, M.; Armstrong, S.; Browning, G.F.; Stevenson, M. Antimicrobial prescribing in dogs and cats in Australia: Results of the Australasian Infectious Disease Advisory Panel survey. *J. Vet. Intern. Med.* **2017**, *31*, 1100–1107. [CrossRef] [PubMed]

27. Dyar, O.J.; Huttner, B.; Schouten, J.; Pulcini, C.; Esgap. What is antimicrobial stewardship? *Clin. Microbiol. Infect.* **2017**, *23*, 793–798. [PubMed]

28. World Health Organisation. Who Evolving Treat of AMR, Options for Action. Available online: http://apps.who.int/iris/bitstream/10665/44812/1/9789241503181_eng.pdf (accessed on 30 January 2018).

29. Dowd, K.; Taylor, M.; Toribio, J.A.; Hooker, C.; Dhand, N.K. Zoonotic disease risk perceptions and infection control practices of Australian veterinarians: Call for change in work culture. *Prev. Vet. Med.* **2013**, *111*, 17–24. [CrossRef] [PubMed]

30. Jordan, D.; Simon, J.; Fury, S.; Moss, S.; Giffard, P.; Maiwald, M.; Southwell, P.; Barton, M.D.; Axon, J.E.; Morris, S.G.; et al. Carriage of methicillin-resistant *Staphylococcus aureus* by veterinarians in australia. *Aust. Vet. J.* **2011**, *89*, 152–159. [CrossRef] [PubMed]

31. Anderson, M.E.; Lefebvre, S.L.; Weese, J.S. Evaluation of prevalence and risk factors for methicillin-resistant *Staphylococcus aureus* colonization in veterinary personnel attending an international equine veterinary conference. *Vet. Microbiol.* **2008**, *129*, 410–417. [CrossRef] [PubMed]

32. Khan, A.K.A.; Banu, G.; K, K.R. Antibiotic resistance and usage-a survey on the knowledge, attitude, perceptions and practices among the medical students of a southern Indian teaching hospital. *J. Clin. Diagn. Res.* **2013**, *7*, 1613–1616.

33. Huang, Y.; Gu, J.; Zhang, M.; Ren, Z.; Yang, W.; Chen, Y.; Fu, Y.; Chen, X.; Cals, J.W.; Zhang, F. Knowledge, attitude and practice of antibiotics: A questionnaire study among 2500 Chinese students. *BMC Med. Educ.* **2013**, *13*, 163. [CrossRef] [PubMed]

34. Scaioli, G.; Gualano, M.R.; Gili, R.; Masucci, S.; Bert, F.; Siliquini, R. Antibiotic use: A cross-sectional survey assessing the knowledge, attitudes and practices amongst students of a school of medicine in Italy. *PLoS ONE* **2015**, *10*, e0122476. [CrossRef] [PubMed]

35. Minen, M.T.; Duquaine, D.; Marx, M.A.; Weiss, D. A survey of knowledge, attitudes, and beliefs of medical students concerning antimicrobial use and resistance. *Microb. Drug Resist.* **2010**, *16*, 285–289. [CrossRef] [PubMed]

36. Dyar, O.J.; Howard, P.; Nathwani, D.; Pulcini, C.; ESGAP. Knowledge, attitudes, and beliefs of French medical students about antibiotic prescribing and resistance. *Med. Mal. Infect.* **2013**, *43*, 423–430. [CrossRef] [PubMed]

37. Dyar, O.J.; Pulcini, C.; Howard, P.; Nathwani, D.; ESGAP. European medical students: A first multicentre study of knowledge, attitudes and perceptions of antibiotic prescribing and antibiotic resistance. *J. Antimicrob. Chemother.* **2014**, *69*, 842–846. [CrossRef] [PubMed]

38. Abbo, L.M.; Cosgrove, S.E.; Pottinger, P.S.; Pereyra, M.; Sinkowitz-Cochran, R.; Srinivasan, A.; Webb, D.J.; Hooton, T.M. Medical students' perceptions and knowledge about antimicrobial stewardship: How are we educating our future prescribers? *Clin. Infect. Dis.* **2013**, *57*, 631–638. [CrossRef] [PubMed]

39. Dyar, O.J.; Hills, H.; Seitz, L.T.; Perry, A.; Ashiru-Oredope, D. Assessing the knowledge, attitudes and behaviors of human and animal health students towards antibiotic use and resistance: A pilot cross-sectional study in the UK. *Antibiotics* **2018**, *7*, 10. [CrossRef] [PubMed]

40. Australian Strategic and Technical Advisory Group on Antimicrobial Resistance. Importance Rating and Summary of Antibacterials Used in Human Health in Australia. Available online: http://www.health.gov.au/internet/main/publishing.nsf/content/1803C433C71415CACA257C8400121B1F/$File/ratings-summary-Antibacterial-uses-humans.pdf (accessed on 5 February 2018).

41. Hardefeldt, L.Y.; Gilkerson, J.R.; Billman-Jacobe, H.; Stevenson, M.A.; Thursky, K.; Bailey, K.E.; Browning, G.F. Barriers to and enablers of implementing antimicrobial stewardship programs in veterinary practices. *J. Vet. Intern. Med.* **2018**. [CrossRef] [PubMed]

42. Zhuo, A.; Labbate, M.; Norris, J.M.; Gilbert, G.L.; Ward, M.; Bajorek, B.; Degeling, C.; Rowbotham, S.; Dawson, A.; Nguyen, K.A.; et al. What are the opportunities and challenges to improving antibiotic prescribing practices through a one health approach: Results of a comparative survey of doctors, dentists, and veterinarians in Australia. *BMJ Open* **2018**, *8*, e020439. [CrossRef] [PubMed]

43. Abraham, S.; O'Dea, M.; Trott, D.J.; Abraham, R.J.; Hughes, D.; Pang, S.; McKew, G.; Cheong, E.Y.; Merlino, J.; Saputra, S.; et al. Isolation and plasmid characterization of carbapenemase (imp-4) producing *Salmonella enterica* typhimurium from cats. *Sci. Rep.* **2016**, *6*, 35527. [CrossRef] [PubMed]

44. Saputra, S.; Jordan, D.; Worthing, K.A.; Norris, J.M.; Wong, H.S.; Abraham, R.; Trott, D.J.; Abraham, S. Antimicrobial resistance in coagulase-positive *Staphylococci* isolated from companion animals in Australia: A one year study. *PLoS ONE* **2017**, *12*, e0176379. [CrossRef] [PubMed]

45. Saputra, S.; Jordan, D.; Mitchell, T.; Wong, H.S.; Abraham, R.J.; Kidsley, A.; Turnidge, J.; Trott, D.J.; Abraham, S. Antimicrobial resistance in clinical *Escherichia coli* isolated from companion animals in Australia. *Vet. Microbiol.* **2017**, *211*, 43–50. [CrossRef] [PubMed]

46. Worthing, K.A.; Abraham, S.; Coombs, G.W.; Pang, S.; Saputra, S.; Jordan, D.; Trott, D.J.; Norris, J.M. Clonal diversity and geographic distribution of methicillin-resistant *Staphylococcus pseudintermedius* from Australian animals: Discovery of novel sequence types. *Vet. Microbiol.* **2018**, *213*, 58–65. [CrossRef] [PubMed]

47. Animal Medicines Australia. Pet Ownership in Australia. Available online: http://animalmedicinesaustralia. org.au/wp-content/uploads/2016/11/AMA_Pet-Ownership-in-Australia-2016-Report_sml.pdf (accessed on 3 February 2018).

48. Hardefeldt, L.Y.; Selinger, J.; Stevenson, M.A.; Gilkerson, J.R.; Crabb, H.; Billman-Jacobe, H.; Thursky, K.; Bailey, K.E.; Awad, M.; Browning, G.F. Population wide assessment of antimicrobial use in companion animals using a novel data source—A cohort study using pet insurance data. *J. Antimicrob. Chemother.* **2018**, in review.

49. Zoetis Australia Pty Ltd. Convenia. Available online: http://websvr.infopest.com.au/LabelRouter? LabelType=L&Mode=1&ProductCode=60461 (accessed on 2 October 2017).

50. Asia Pacific Centre for Animal Health; National Centre for Antimicrobial Stewardship. Australian Veterinary Prescribing Guidelines. Available online: www.fvas.unimelb.edu.au/vetantibiotics (accessed on 13 September 17).

51. British Equine Veterinary Association. Protect Me. Available online: http://www.beva.org.uk/useful-info/ Vets/Guidance/AMR (accessed on 13 September 17).

52. Spohr, A.; Schjoth, B.; Wiinberg, B.; Houser, G.; Willesen, J.; Jesson, L.R.; Guardabassi, L.; Schjaerff, M.; Eriksen, T.; Jensen, V.F. Antibiotic Use Guidelines for Companion Animal Practice. Danish Small Animal Veterinary Association. Available online: https://www.ddd.dk/sektioner/familiedyr/ antibiotikavejledning/Documents/AntibioticGuidelines%20-%20v1.4_jun15.pdf (accessed on 18 April 2018).

53. Plunkett, S.J. Gastrointestinal emergencies. In *Emergency Procedures for the Small Animal Veterinarian3: Emergency*, 3rd ed.; Plunkett, S.J., Ed.; Saunders Elsevier: London, UK, 2013; p. 288.

54. Shaw, D.H.; Ihle, S.L. Gastrointestinal diseases. In *Small Animal Internal Medicine*; Shaw, D.H., Ihle, S.L., Eds.; Blackwell Publishing: Ames, IA, USA, 2008.

55. Chan, J.; Doyle, B.; Branley, J.; Sheppeard, V.; Gabor, M.; Viney, K.; Quinn, H.; Janover, O.; McCready, M.; Heller, J. An outbreak of psittacosis at a veterinary school demonstrating a novel source of infection. *One Health* **2017**, *3*, 29–33. [CrossRef] [PubMed]

56. University of Queensland. Bachelor of Veterinary Science Study Planner. Available online: https://planner. science.uq.edu.au/content/bvsc-hons (accessed on 22 September 2017).

57. University of Adelaide. Doctor of Veterinary Medicine. Available online: http://www.adelaide.edu.au/ degree-finder/dvetm_drvetmedi.html (accessed on 22 September 2017).

58. Secombe, C.; (Murdoch University, Perth, WA, Australia); Wereszka, M.; (University of Sydney, Camden, NSW, Australia); Raidal, S.; (Charles Sturt, Perth, WA, Australia); Squires, R.; (James Cook University, Townsville, QLD, Australia). Personal communication, 2017.

59. Cortoos, P.J.; De Witte, K.; Peetermans, W.E.; Simoens, S.; Laekeman, G. Opposing expectations and suboptimal use of a local antibiotic hospital guideline: A qualitative study. *J. Antimicrob. Chemother.* **2008**, *62*, 189–195. [CrossRef] [PubMed]

60. Cochran, W.G. *Sampling Techniques, 3d ed.*; Wiley: New York, NY, USA, 1977; 428p.

61. Harris, P.A.; Taylor, R.; Thielke, R.; Payne, J.; Gonzalez, N.; Conde, J.G. Research electronic data capture (REDCap)—A metadata-driven methodology and workflow process for providing translational research informatics support. *J. Biomed. Inform.* **2009**, *42*, 377–381. [CrossRef] [PubMed]

62. Pope, C.; Ziebland, S.; Mays, N. Qualitative research in health care. Analysing qualitative data. *BMJ* **2000**, *320*, 114–116. [CrossRef] [PubMed]

63. Liamputtong, P. Making sense of qualitative data: The analysis process. In *Qualitative Research Methods*, 3rd ed.; Oxford University Press: Melbourne, Australia, 2009; pp. 277–296.

64. Morse, J. 'Emerging from the data': The cognitive process of analysis in qualitative inquiry. In *Issues in Qualitative Research Methods*; Sage: Thousand Oaks, CA, USA, 1994; pp. 23–43.

65. Bradley, E.H.; Curry, L.A.; Devers, K.J. Qualitative data analysis for health services research: Developing taxonomy, themes, and theory. *Health Serv. Res.* **2007**, *42*, 1758–1772. [CrossRef] [PubMed]

66. Talpaert, M.J.; Gopal Rao, G.; Cooper, B.S.; Wade, P. Impact of guidelines and enhanced antibiotic stewardship on reducing broad-spectrum antibiotic usage and its effect on incidence of *Clostridium difficile* infection. *J. Antimicrob. Chemother.* **2011**, *66*, 2168–2174. [CrossRef] [PubMed]

67. Ozgun, H.; Ertugrul, B.M.; Soyder, A.; Ozturk, B.; Aydemir, M. Peri-operative antibiotic prophylaxis: Adherence to guidelines and effects of educational intervention. *Int. J. Surg.* **2010**, *8*, 159–163. [CrossRef] [PubMed]

68. Weese, J.S. Investigation of antimicrobial use and the impact of antimicrobial use guidelines in a small animal veterinary teaching hospital: 1995–2004. *J. Am. Vet. Med. A* **2006**, *228*, 553–558. [CrossRef] [PubMed]

16

Point Prevalence Surveys of Antimicrobial Use among Hospitalized Children

Sumanth Gandra [1,*], Sanjeev K. Singh [2], Dasaratha R. Jinka [3], Ravishankar Kanithi [4], Ashok K. Chikkappa [5], Anita Sharma [6], Dhanya Dharmapalan [7], Anil Kumar Vasudevan [2], Onkaraiah Tunga [5], Akhila Akula [4], Garima Garg [6], Yingfen Hsia [8] [iD], Srinivas Murki [9], Gerardo Alvarez-Uria [3] [iD], Mike Sharland [8] and Ramanan Laxminarayan [1,10]

[1]   Center for Disease Dynamics, Economics & Policy, New Delhi 110020, India; ramanan@cddep.org
[2]   Department of Infection Control & Microbiology, Amrita Institute of Medical Sciences, Amrita University, Ponekkara, Kochi 682041, India; sanjeevksingh@aims.amrita.edu (S.K.S.); vanilkumar@aims.amrita.edu (A.K.V.)
[3]   Department of Infectious Diseases & Department of Paediatrics, Rural Development Trust Hospital, Bathalapalli 515661, India; jdashrath86@gmail.com (D.R.J.); gerardouria@gmail.com (G.A.-U.)
[4]   Department of Paediatrics, Sowmya Children's Hospital, Hyderabad 500038, India; ravineonatologist@gmail.com (R.K.); akhi0602@gmail.com (A.A.)
[5]   Department of Paediatrics, Rural Development Trust Hospital, Kalyanadurgam 515761, India; ashokkld1971@yahoo.com (A.K.C.); onkaraiahtunga@gmail.com (O.T.)
[6]   Department of Microbiology & Department of Paediatric Intensive Care Unit, Fortis Hospital, Mohali 160062, India; anita.sharma@fortishealthcare.com (A.S.); Garima.garg@fortishealthcare.com (G.G.)
[7]   Department of Paediatrics, Dr Yewale's Multispeciality Hospital for Children, Navi Mumbai 400703, India; drdhanyaroshan@gmail.com
[8]   Paediatric Infectious Diseases Research Group, Institute of Infection and Immunity, St. Georges University, London SW17 0RE, UK; yhsia@sgul.ac.uk (Y.H.); Mike.Sharland@stgeorges.nhs.uk (M.S.)
[9]   Department of Neonatology, Fernandez Hospital, Hyderabad 500029, India; srinivasmurki2001@gmail.com
[10]   Princeton Environmental Institute, Princeton University, Princeton, NJ 08544, USA
*   Correspondence: gandra@cddep.org

Academic Editor: Christopher C. Butler

Abstract: The prevalence of antimicrobial resistance in India is among the highest in the world. Antimicrobial use in inpatient settings is an important driver of resistance, but is poorly characterized, particularly in hospitalized children. In this study, conducted as part of the Global Antimicrobial Resistance, Prescribing, and Efficacy in Neonates and Children (GARPEC) project, we examined the prevalence of and indications of antimicrobial use, as well as antimicrobial agents used among hospitalized children by conducting four point prevalence surveys in six hospitals between February 2016 and February 2017. A total of 681 children were hospitalized in six hospitals across all survey days, and 419 (61.5%) were prescribed one or more antimicrobials (antibacterials, antivirals, antifungals). Antibacterial agents accounted for 90.8% (547/602) of the total antimicrobial prescriptions, of which third-generation cephalosporins (3GCs) accounted for 38.9% (213/547) and penicillin plus enzyme inhibitor combinations accounted for 14.4% (79/547). Lower respiratory tract infection (LRTI) was the most common indication for prescribing antimicrobials (149 prescriptions; 24.8%). Although national guidelines recommend the use of penicillin and combinations as first-line agents for LRTI, 3GCs were the most commonly prescribed antibacterial agents (55/149 LRTI prescriptions; 36.9%). In conclusion, 61.5% of hospitalized children were on at least one antimicrobial agent, with excessive use of 3GCs. Hence there is an opportunity to limit their inappropriate use.

Keywords: point prevalence survey; antimicrobial use; children; hospital; India

1. Introduction

Antimicrobial resistance is rising across the globe, with prevalence in India reported as being among the highest [1,2]. A recent study reported that resistance to last-resort antimicrobials increased between 2008 and 2014 [3]. In 2014, 57% of *Klebsiella pneumoniae* and 10% of *Escherichia coli* blood culture isolates were observed to be carbapenem resistant. The high proportion of bacterial infections due to extended spectrum beta-lactamase (ESBL)-producing organisms is one reason for the high consumption of carbapenems in India. Among 51 countries for which antimicrobial resistance surveillance data were available in 2014, India had the highest proportion of third-generation cephalosporin-resistant *E. coli* (83%), an indirect marker for ESBL production [4].

Antimicrobial selection pressure is a primary driver of resistance development [5], and there is an urgent need to reduce antimicrobial overuse and misuse. Surveillance of antimicrobial use in hospitals can provide an insight into patterns of antimicrobial use, help highlight differences in prescribing practices among hospitals, and identify opportunities for improvement. Information on antimicrobial use from point prevalence surveys (PPSs) could be used to design, implement, and assess the effects of antimicrobial policies [6]. To date, only one multicenter (>2 hospitals) study describing antimicrobial use among hospitalized children has been published in India [7]. However, this study did not collect information on the total number of children admitted to various wards and thus could not estimate the rate of antimicrobial use per patient. In this study, we examined the prevalence of and indications of antimicrobial use, as well as the antimicrobial agents used among hospitalized children, by conducting four PPSs in six hospitals in India.

2. Methods

As part of the Global Antimicrobial Resistance, Prescribing, and Efficacy in Neonates and Children (GARPEC) study, the participating hospitals were asked to conduct a one-day cross-sectional hospital based PPSs in all pediatric and neonatal wards four times between 1 February 2016 and 28 February 2017. The Antibiotic Resistance and Prescribing in European Children (ARPEC) project PPS methodology was utilized for this study [8]. Four single-day PPSs on antimicrobial use were conducted between 1 February 2016 and 28 February 2017. The first PPS was conducted between 1 February and 31 March 2016; the second between 1 May and 30 June 2016; the third between 1 September and 31 October 2016; and the fourth between 1 December 2016 and 28 February 2017. Four PPSs were conducted to increase the precision of measurement of antimicrobial use and to examine the variation of antimicrobial use at different time points.

Each hospital needed to register providing the name, geographic location and type of hospital (primary, secondary and tertiary level and teaching vs. nonteaching hospital). Hospitals were asked to conduct the survey only on a weekday during the designated months of each round of PPS. All neonates and pediatric hospitalized patients younger than 18 years of age, present in the ward at 8:00 a.m., were included in the survey. Detailed data were recorded only for patients with an active antimicrobial prescription at 8 am on the day of survey.

At the time of initiation of the study on 1 February 2016, five hospitals were enrolled into the study. Three additional hospitals were enrolled by 1 May 2016 and did not participate in the first round of PPS. Among the eight hospitals, two were rural general trust hospitals, three were stand-alone private children's hospitals, two were private tertiary care hospitals and one was a private mother and child care center with inborn neonatal services. One tertiary care hospital had teaching services in pediatrics and neonatal departments. Two stand-alone pediatric hospitals and the mother and child care center had teaching services in neonatal departments. PPSs were conducted in the neonatal intensive care units and neonatal wards of all eight hospitals and the pediatric units (including pediatric intensive care units) of only six hospitals (one hospital had only neonatal services and the other hospital restricted the study to neonatal units). In this study, we examined the antimicrobial use patterns among the pediatric units of six hospitals. Antimicrobial use in neonatal intensive care units and general neonatal wards were not examined in this study.

Hospital, department, and de-identified patient data were collected using a standardized web-based electronic data entry form on the Research Electronic Data Capture (REDCap)® developed for the GARPEC project. For children receiving antimicrobials (antibiotics, antifungal and antivirals, antiparasital agents), data were collected on patient sex, age, weight, ventilation status, comorbid conditions, number of antimicrobials, antimicrobial name, dose per administration, dose units, number of doses each day, route of administration, reason for treatment, treatment indication (community versus healthcare associated) or prophylaxis, and whether treatment was empirical or targeted. We included all diagnoses for which antimicrobials were prescribed even if there was more than one diagnosis. Ethics approval was received for all participating hospitals from their respective institutional human research ethics committees.

Categorical variables were expressed as percentages, and the chi-squared test or Fisher's exact test was used, as appropriate, for comparisons. Statistical significance was defined as $p < 0.05$. The statistical analyses were performed using STATA 12.1 (StataCorp, College Station, TX, USA).

3. Results

At the six participating hospitals, the total number of beds for all four survey days ranged from 24 to 517, and the bed occupancy ranged from 15.1% to 79.8% (Table 1).

Table 1. Characteristics, bed occupancy, and antimicrobial prescription in six hospitals in India in 2016.

Hospital ID	Hospital Characteristics	Total Beds	Total Patients (N)	Bed Occupancy (%)	Intensive Care Beds (Yes/No)	Patients on Antimicrobials (N)	Patients on Antimicrobials (%)
A *	Rural general hospital	149	92	61.7	Y	51	55.4
B	Stand-alone pediatric	112	79	70.5	Y	57	72.2
C *	Rural general hospital	119	95	79.8	N	76	80.0
D #	Tertiary care hospital	517	385	74.5	Y	212	55.1
E *	Tertiary care hospital	24	14	58.3	Y	13	92.9
F **	Stand-alone pediatric	106	16	15.1	Y	10	62.5
All		1027	681	66.3		419	61.5

Note: Hospitals A, B, and F have only medical intensive care units; Hospitals D and E have surgical intensive care beds available in addition to medical. * Did not participate in the first point prevalence survey; ** Did not participate in the second point prevalence survey; # Has teaching services in pediatric departments.

A total of 681 children were hospitalized in six hospitals across all survey days, and 419 (61.5%) were prescribed one or more antimicrobials. The percentage of children on antimicrobials in the six hospitals ranged from 55.1% to 92.9% (Table 1). One antimicrobial was prescribed to 291 patients, two antimicrobials were prescribed to 85 patients, and three or more were prescribed to 43 patients. The percentages of patients on antimicrobials for the four PPSs were 61.3% (73/119), 59.4% (104/175), 63.6% (133/209), and 61.2% (109/178), respectively.

Of the 419 children receiving antimicrobials, 147 (35.1%) were less than one year old, and 248 (59.2%) were male (Table 2).

Only one hospital (Hospital D) had two dedicated surgical wards. The remaining five hospitals had general pediatric wards, where both medical and surgical patients were admitted. Pediatric intensive care units were present in five hospitals, of which two had dedicated surgical intensive care units. General pediatric wards accounted for 78.5% (329) of children on antimicrobials, and intensive care units accounted for the remaining 21.5% (90) (Table 2). The percentage of patients on antimicrobials was significantly higher in intensive care units than in general pediatric wards (73.4% vs. 59.0%; $p = 0.003$). The average number of antimicrobials per patient was higher in intensive care units (mean 1.5; range 1–4) than in general pediatric wards (mean 1.4; range 1–5). In 419 patients with an antimicrobial prescription, 343 (81.8%) were prescribed for treatment of active infection and 76 (18.2%) for prophylaxis. Lower respiratory tract infections (LRTIs) (117, 27.9%), sepsis (66, 15.7%), and prophylaxis for surgical disease (49, 11.7%) were the three most common reasons for prescribing antimicrobials (Table 2).

Table 2. Percentages of hospitalized children on antimicrobials in six hospitals in India in 2016.

Characteristic	Number of Children (N = 419)	Percentage of Children	Number of Prescriptions (N = 602)	Percentage of Prescriptions
Underlying comorbid conditions	256	61.1	359	59.6
No underlying disease	163	38.9	243	40.4
Age category				
Age < 1	147	35.1	197	32.7
Age 1–6	173	41.2	255	43.2
Age 7–12	79	18.8	118	19.6
Age > 12	20	4.8	32	5.5
Gender				
Male	248	59.2	354	58.6
Ward activity				
Intensive care units	90	21.5	138	22.9
General wards	329	78.5	464	77.1
Diagnosis *				
Lower respiratory tract infection (LRTI)	117	27.9	149	24.8
Sepsis	67	15.9	90	15.0
Prophylaxis for surgical disease	50	11.9	77	12.8
Treatment for surgical disease	34	8.1	64	10.6
Prophylaxis for medical problems	29	6.9	41	6.6
Other	80	19.0	116	19.3
Upper respiratory infections (URTI)	17	4.1	23	3.8
Urinary tract infections (UTI)	18	4.3	22	3.7
GI tract infections	19	4.5	21	3.5
Indication *				
Community-acquired infection (CAI)	233	55.6	313	52.0
Healthcare-associated infection (HAI)	40	9.5	55	9.1
Unknown	79	18.9	116	19.3
Prophylaxis (medical and surgical)	79	18.9	118	19.6

* Total can be more than 100% as one patient can have more than one diagnosis.

Of the 602 total antimicrobial prescriptions, 313 (52%) were for community-acquired infections (CAIs), 55 (9.1%) were for healthcare associated infections (HAI), and 116 (19.3%) were for unknown indications (CAI or HAI) (Table 2). Of the 602 prescriptions, 118 (19.6%) were for medical and surgical prophylaxis. Among the 313 prescriptions for CAIs, 283 (90.4%) were empiric, whereas 35 (63.6%) of 55 prescriptions for HAIs were empiric. Of the 313 antimicrobial prescriptions for CAIs, the majority were prescribed for LRTI (133 prescriptions; 42.5%) and sepsis (54 prescriptions; 17.3%).

Antibacterial agents accounted for 90.8% (547 of 602) of total antimicrobial prescriptions. Of the 547 antibacterial prescriptions, the three most common classes of antibiotics prescribed were third-generation cephalosporins (213 of 547 prescriptions; 38.9%), penicillin plus enzyme inhibitor combinations (78 of 547 prescriptions; 14.3%), and aminoglycosides (57 of 547 prescriptions; 10.4%) (Table 3).

The top three classes of antibacterial agents and their order were similar in each of the four PPSs. Carbapenems and fluoroquinolones accounted for less than 5% each of total antibacterial prescriptions, respectively (Table 3).

Of the prescriptions for carbapenems, 55.5% (15/27) were prescribed in intensive care units. The top three reasons for prescribing carbapenems were sepsis (4 HAI and 1 CAI), LRTI (3 CAI and 1 HAI), and central nervous system infections (2 CAI and 1 unknown). Overall, the three most commonly prescribed antimicrobials were ceftriaxone (111 of 602 prescriptions; 18.4%), amoxicillin-clavulanic acid (69 of 602 prescriptions; 11.5%), and cefotaxime (58 of 602 prescriptions; 9.6%) (Figure 1).

Table 3. Antimicrobial prescriptions for all indications among hospitalized children in six hospitals in India in 2016.

	All	Hospital A	Hospital B	Hospital C	Hospital D	Hospital E	Hospital F
Children on ≥1 antimicrobials	432	93	108	95	388	14	14
Total number of prescriptions	**602**	**77**	**90**	**91**	**306**	**26**	**12**
Third-generation cephalosporins	213	25	44	16	108	12	8
Penicillin + enzyme inhibitors	78	13	3	44	16	1	1
Others *	73	13	16	19	22	3	0
Aminoglycosides	57	11	4	1	31	10	0
Penicillins	35	4	1	0	29	0	1
Metronidazole	33	0	2	2	29	0	0
Carbapenems	27	2	3	1	21	0	0
Fluoroquinolones	20	1	6	0	13	0	0
First/second-generation cephalosporins	18	0	0	0	18	0	0
Macrolides	16	1	6	2	6	0	1
Glycopeptides	14	3	3	0	8	0	0
Trimethoprim/sulfa	12	3	1	4	4	0	0
Tetracycline	6	1	1	2	1	0	1

* Others included chloramphenicol, clindamycin, linezolid, doxycycline, tigecycline, colistin, and antituberculosis, antifungal, antiviral, and antimalarial agents.

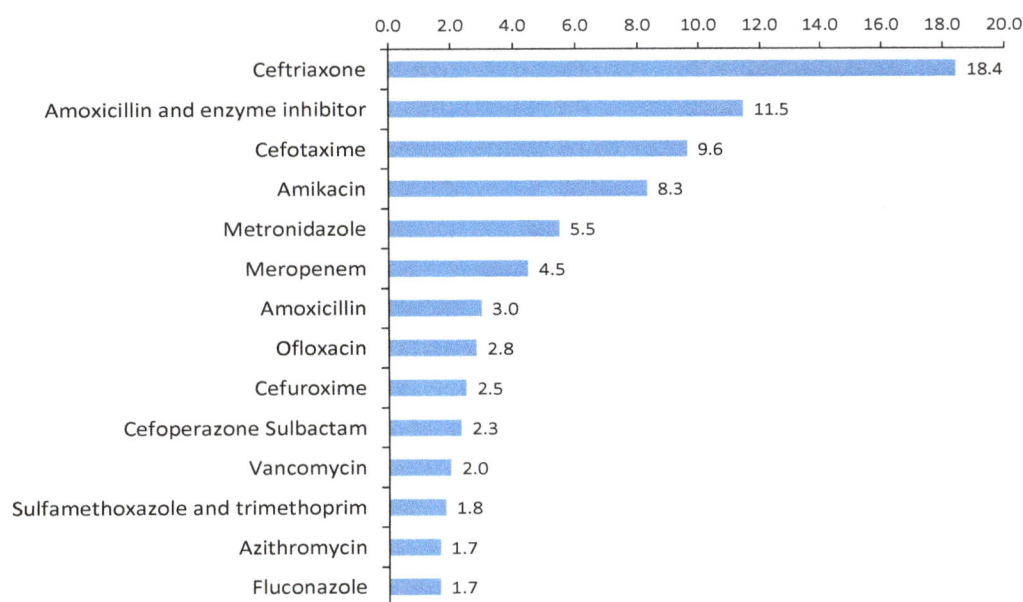

Figure 1. Prescribed antimicrobials among hospitalized children, ranked by overall drug utilization 75% (DU75%).

The five diagnoses associated with the highest rates of antimicrobial prescribing were LRTI (149 of 602 prescriptions; 24.8%), sepsis (90 of 602 prescriptions; 15%), prophylaxis for surgical disease (77 of 602 prescriptions; 12.8%), treatment of surgical disease (64 of 602 prescriptions; 10.6%), and prophylaxis for medical problems (41 of 602 prescriptions; 6.8%) (Table 2). The two most commonly prescribed antibacterial classes for LRTI were third-generation cephalosporins (55 of 149 prescriptions; 36.9%) and penicillin plus enzyme inhibitor combinations (46 of 149 prescriptions; 30.9%). For LRTI, third-generation cephalosporins were mainly used as monotherapy (38/55) and in combination in 17 other cases, mostly with macrolides (5/17). The two most common antibacterial agents prescribed for sepsis were the third-generation cephalosporins (40 of 90 prescriptions; 44.4%) and amikacin (11 of 90 prescriptions; 12.2%). For sepsis cases, third-generation cephalosporins were mainly used as monotherapy (26/40) and in combination in 14 other cases, mostly with amikacin (8/14).

In cases of prophylaxis for surgical disease, the two most commonly prescribed antibacterial classes were third-generation cephalosporins (29 of 64 prescriptions; 37.7%) and aminoglycosides (16 of 64 prescriptions; 25%). Third-generation cephalosporins were used as monotherapy in 9 cases and in combination in 20 other cases, mostly with aminoglycosides (8/20) and with both aminoglycosides and metronidazole (4/20). Third-generation cephalosporins were the most commonly used antibacterial agents (14/41) used for medical prophylaxis. They were used as monotherapy in six patients in combination mainly with aminoglycosides in eight patients (4/8).

4. Discussion

To the best of our knowledge, this is the first published multicenter study to estimate the prevalence of antimicrobial use among hospitalized children in India. The percentage of hospitalized children who received at least one antimicrobial agent was 61.5% in this study. In the global Antibiotic Resistance and Prescribing in European Children (ARPEC) PPS study conducted in 2012, involving 226 hospitals from 41 countries, the overall percentage of hospitalized children on antimicrobials was 42.5%, which was much lower than the 61.5% in our study [8]. The percentage of patients on antimicrobials in our study was higher than reported in Turkey (54.6%) [9], Italy (47%) [10], Australia (46%) [11], the United Kingdom (40.9%) [12], Latvia (39%) [13], and the United States (33%) [14]. However, it was lower than in Iran (66.6%) [15] and China (78.2%) [16]. Consistent with previous studies, we observed that the majority of the antimicrobial usage was for therapeutic purposes rather than prophylaxis [8,10–12,15].

LRTI was the most common indication for prescribing antimicrobials, a finding consistent with PPSs among hospitalized children in several other countries [10–13]. Third-generation cephalosporins were the most commonly prescribed antibiotics for LRTI in this study. Similar findings were reported by another Indian study, which reviewed antibiotic prescription practices among hospitalized children in two private hospitals in central India [17]. However, the Indian National Center for Disease Control and Prevention (NCDC) guidelines [18] and the INDIACLEN task force guidelines for pneumonia [19] recommend ampicillin or ampicillin plus gentamicin or amoxicillin-clavulanic acid as first-line therapy for LRTI among hospitalized children older than two months. Third-generation cephalosporins are recommended in hospitalized children only when they deteriorate on first-line agents.

Consistent with our findings, third-generation cephalosporins were the most commonly prescribed antimicrobials in Eastern Europe (35.7%) and Asia (28.6%) in the global ARPEC study [8], as well as in Turkey (18.4%) [9], Italy (20%) [10], Latvia (28%) [13], and Iran (43.5%) [15]. However, in Australia and the United Kingdom, penicillin plus enzyme inhibitor combinations were the most commonly prescribed antimicrobials [11,12]. Carbapenem prescription in this study was lower than in Turkey (12.7%) [9], Italy (6%) [10], and Iran (5.2%) [15], but higher than in Australia (3.2%) [11] and Latvia (0.5%) [13]. However, it is possible that carbapenem consumption has been underestimated because of the lack of representation of tertiary care centers with large numbers of intensive care unit beds in this study.

The study has several strengths. First, the repeated PPSs in the six hospitals increased the robustness of our estimates of antimicrobial prescription among hospitalized children. Second, the six participating hospitals represented diverse settings that are commonly seen in India. Two hospitals were small stand-alone children hospitals in urban areas, two were part of a rural general hospital, and two were part of large tertiary care referral centers. Thus we were able to capture antimicrobial prescribing practices in different hospital settings. Third, we examined for the variation of antimicrobial use at different times of the year. Interestingly, the percentages of children on antimicrobials and the antimicrobial prescription patterns in each of the four PPSs were similar when compared with combined data from all four PPSs. We did not observe any temporal variation in antimicrobial prescribing.

The study also has several limitations, however. First, we did not collect data on the duration of therapy, nor the microbiology and antimicrobial susceptibility results, which could help indicate the appropriateness of antimicrobial prescribing; Second, although we included hospitals with different characteristics, we did not include large academic centers and hospitals from all regions of India. This would require a much larger study. Thus, our results may not be generalizable to all healthcare settings and geographic regions of the country. Similarly, as all hospitals included in the study were from the private sector, the results may not be generalizable to public sector hospitals. The choice of antibiotics may differ in public hospitals as the national and state drug policies often define the types of antibiotics procured and prescribed in the public sector hospitals. The public sector hospitals are also obliged to follow national prescribing guidelines; Third, five out of six hospitals did not have dedicated surgical wards or other specialized units such as hematology-oncology or cardiology, which limited our ability to study variation of antimicrobial use across different hospital units; Fourth, with Hospital D having most number of beds and patients in the study, the results could have been biased affecting the representativeness of the data; Fifth, the date of the survey was chosen as per the convenience of the site principal investigator within the specified months. However, we have not taken additional steps to minimize the Hawthorne effect. As the physicians knew that their antimicrobial prescriptions were being studied, the results might have been affected. Sixth, 79 (19%) of the prescriptions had unknown indications (where it was not known whether the infection was community acquired or healthcare associated), however, we have not taken additional efforts to identify the indications.

Our study identified an opportunity to improve antimicrobial use for LRTI among hospitalized children. The current guidelines recommend the use of third-generation cephalosporins only when there is deterioration in the effectiveness of first-line agents. However, in our study, the majority of hospitalized children with LRTI were on third-generation cephalosporins. A recent study assessing the antibiotic susceptibility of the major bacterial pathogens isolated from community-acquired pneumonia among both adults and children in India indicated high susceptibility to first-line agents (ampicillin and amoxicillin-clavulanic acid) [20]. In this study, 91.8% of *Streptococcus pneumoniae* isolates were susceptible to amoxicillin. Similarly, 91.1% of *Haemophilus influenzae* isolates were susceptible to ampicillin, and 97% of the *H. influenzae* isolates were susceptible to amoxicillin-clavulanic acid [20]. This study reinforces that third-generation cephalosporins can be avoided as first-line therapy for LRTI. We also observed that third-generation cephalosporins were the most commonly used antibiotics for surgical prophylaxis. However, the published international guidelines recommend use of first- and second-generation cephalosporins for surgical prophylaxis instead of third-generation cephalosporins [21].

Reviewing national antimicrobial resistance surveillance data obtained both from adults and children, in 2014, 83% of the *E. coli* isolates were resistant to third-generation cephalosporins in India, which was much higher than in Australia (9%), the United Kingdom (11%), Argentina (14%), the United States (16%), South Africa (19%), and China (62%) [22,23]. Use of third-generation cephalosporins is associated with increased the risk of colonization with ESBL-producing bacteria [24]. Third-generation cephalosporin exposure in children could lead to colonization at a very young age, which could facilitate the spread of ESBL-producing bacteria to other family members, leading to a further increase in ESBL Enterobacteriaceae infections and subsequently the consumption of carbapenems in India. Our findings indicate the need for increased compliance with NCDC and INDIACLEN treatment guidelines for the management of LRTI in children.

In conclusion, 61.5% of the hospitalized children were on at least one antimicrobial agent. We observed an excessive use of third-generation cephalosporins for LRTI. There is an opportunity to limit the use of third-generation cephalosporins by following the recommended national treatment guidelines for management of LRTI.

Acknowledgments: S.G. and R.L. are supported by Global Antibiotic Resistance Partnership (GARP), funded by the Bill & Melinda Gates Foundation.

Author Contributions: M.S., S.G., and R.L. conceptualized and designed the study. S.G. and Y.H. performed the analysis and created figures and tables. S.G. drafted the manuscript. All authors interpreted the analysis. All authors reviewed, revised, and approved the final manuscript.

References

1. Laxminarayan, R.; Matsoso, P.; Pant, S.; Brower, C.; Rottingen, J.A.; Klugman, K.; Davies, S. Access to effective antimicrobials: A worldwide challenge. *Lancet* **2016**, *387*, 168–175. [CrossRef]

2. Laxminarayan, R.; Duse, A.; Wattal, C.; Zaidi, A.K.; Wertheim, H.F.; Sumpradit, N.; Vlieghe, E.; Hara, G.L.; Gould, I.M.; Goossens, H.; et al. Antibiotic resistance: The need for global solutions. *Lancet Infect. Dis.* **2013**, *13*, 1057–1098. [CrossRef]

3. Gandra, S.; Mojica, N.; Klein, E.Y.; Ashok, A.; Nerurkar, V.; Kumari, M.; Ramesh, U.; Dey, S.; Vadwai, V.; Das, B.R.; et al. Trends in antibiotic resistance among major bacterial pathogens isolated from blood cultures tested at a large private laboratory network in India, 2008–2014. *Int. J. Infect. Dis.* **2016**, *50*, 75–82. [CrossRef] [PubMed]

4. Gelband, H.; Miller-Petrie, M.; Pant, S.; Gandra, S.; Levinson, J.; Barter, D.; White, A.; Laxminarayan, R. *The State of the World's Antibiotics, 2015*; Center for Disease Dynamics, Economics & Policy: New Delhi, India, 2015.

5. World Health Organisation (WHO). WHO's First Global Report on Antibiotic Resistance Reveals Serious, Worldwide Threat to Public Health. Available online: http://www.who.int/mediacentre/news/releases/2014/amr-report/en/ (accessed on 18 March 2017).

6. Skoog, G.; Struwe, J.; Cars, O.; Hanberger, H.; Odenholt, I.; Prag, M.; Skarlund, K.; Ulleryd, P.; Erntell, M. Repeated nationwide point-prevalence surveys of antimicrobial use in Swedish hospitals: Data for actions 2003–2010. *Euro. Surveill.* **2016**, *21*. [CrossRef] [PubMed]

7. Sanjeev Singh, T.J.; Versporten, A.; Sengupta, S.; Fini, P.; Sharland, M.; Kumar, K.R.; Goossens, H. A point prevalence surveillance study from pediatric and neonatal specialty hospitals in India. *J. Pediatr. Infect. Dis.* **2014**, *9*, 151–155.

8. Versporten, A.; Bielicki, J.; Drapier, N.; Sharland, M.; Goossens, H. The worldwide Antibiotic Resistance and Prescribing in European Children (ARPEC) point prevalence survey: Developing hospital-quality indicators of antibiotic prescribing for children. *J. Antimicrob. Chemother.* **2016**, *71*, 1106–1117. [CrossRef] [PubMed]

9. Ceyhan, M.; Yildirim, I.; Ecevit, C.; Aydogan, A.; Ornek, A.; Salman, N.; Somer, A.; Hatipoglu, N.; Camcioglu, Y.; Alhan, E.; et al. Inappropriate antimicrobial use in Turkish pediatric hospitals: A multicenter point prevalence survey. *Int. J. Infect. Dis.* **2010**, *14*, e55–e61. [CrossRef] [PubMed]

10. De Luca, M.; Dona, D.; Montagnani, C.; Lo Vecchio, A.; Romanengo, M.; Tagliabue, C.; Centenari, C.; D'Argenio, P.; Lundin, R.; Giaquinto, C.; et al. Antibiotic prescriptions and prophylaxis in Italian children: Is it time to change? Data from the ARPEC project. *PLoS ONE* **2016**, *11*, e0154662. [CrossRef] [PubMed]

11. Osowicki, J.; Gwee, A.; Noronha, J.; Palasanthiran, P.; McMullan, B.; Britton, P.N.; Isaacs, D.; Lai, T.; Nourse, C.; Avent, M.; et al. Australia-wide point prevalence survey of the use and appropriateness of antimicrobial prescribing for children in hospital. *Med. J. Aust.* **2014**, *201*, 657–662. [CrossRef] [PubMed]

12. Gharbi, M.; Doerholt, K.; Vergnano, S.; Bielicki, J.A.; Paulus, S.; Menson, E.; Riordan, A.; Lyall, H.; Patel, S.V.; Bernatoniene, J.; et al. Using a simple point-prevalence survey to define appropriate antibiotic prescribing in hospitalised children across the UK. *BMJ Open* **2016**, *6*, e012675. [CrossRef] [PubMed]

13. Sviestina, I.; Mozgis, D. Antimicrobial usage among hospitalized children in Latvia: A neonatal and pediatric antimicrobial point prevalence survey. *Medicina* **2014**, *50*, 175–181. [CrossRef] [PubMed]

14. Pakyz, A.L.; Gurgle, H.E.; Ibrahim, O.M.; Oinonen, M.J.; Polk, R.E. Trends in antibacterial use in hospitalized pediatric patients in United States academic health centers. *Infect. Control Hosp. Epidemiol.* **2009**, *30*, 600–603. [CrossRef] [PubMed]

15. Fahimzad, A.; Eydian, Z.; Karimi, A.; Shiva, F.; Sayyahfar, S.; Kahbazi, M.; Rahbarimanesh, A.; Sedighi, I.; Arjmand, R.; Soleimani, G.; et al. Surveillance of antibiotic consumption point prevalence survey 2014: Antimicrobial prescribing in pediatrics wards of 16 Iranian hospitals. *Arch. Iran. Med.* **2016**, *19*, 204–209. [PubMed]

16. Xie, D.S.; Xiang, L.L.; Li, R.; Hu, Q.; Luo, Q.Q.; Xiong, W. A multicenter point-prevalence survey of antibiotic use in 13 Chinese hospitals. *J. Infect. Public Health* **2015**, *8*, 55–61. [CrossRef] [PubMed]

17. Sharma, M.; Damlin, A.; Pathak, A.; Stalsby Lundborg, C. Antibiotic prescribing among pediatric inpatients with potential infections in two private sector hospitals in Central India. *PLoS ONE* **2015**, *10*, e0142317. [CrossRef] [PubMed]

18. National Center for Disease Control. National Treatment Guidelines for Antimicrobial Use in Infectious Diseases. 2016. Available online: http://pbhealth.gov.in/amr_guideline7001495889.Pdf (accessed on 26 January 2017).

19. Arora, N.K.; Awasthi, S.; Gupta, P.; Kabra, S.K.; Mathew, J.L.; Nedunchelian, K.; Niswade, A.K.; Patel, A.; Rewal, S.; Sethi, G.R.; et al. Rational use of antibiotics for pneumonia. *Indian Pediatr.* **2010**, *47*, 11–18. [CrossRef]

20. Torumkuney, D.; Chaiwarith, R.; Reechaipichitkul, W.; Malatham, K.; Chareonphaibul, V.; Rodrigues, C.; Chitkins, D.S.; Dias, M.; Anandan, S.; Kanakapura, S.; et al. Results from the survey of antibiotic resistance (SOAR) 2012–14 in Thailand, India, South Korea and Singapore. *J. Antimicrob. Chemother.* **2016**, *71*, 3628. [CrossRef] [PubMed]

21. Bratzler, D.W.; Dellinger, E.P.; Olsen, K.M.; Perl, T.M.; Auwaerter, P.G.; Bolon, M.K.; Fish, D.N.; Napolitano, L.M.; Sawyer, R.G.; Slain, D.; et al. Clinical practice guidelines for antimicrobial prophylaxis in surgery. *Surg. Infect.* **2013**, *14*, 73–156. [CrossRef] [PubMed]

22. Resistancemap. Center for Disease Dynamics, Economics & Policy. Available online: https://resistancemap.cddep.org/resmap/resistance/ (accessed on 24 September 2015).

23. Hu, F.P.; Guo, Y.; Zhu, D.M.; Wang, F.; Jiang, X.F.; Xu, Y.C.; Zhang, X.J.; Zhang, C.X.; Ji, P.; Xie, Y.; et al. Resistance trends among clinical isolates in China reported from CHINET surveillance of bacterial resistance, 2005–2014. *Clin. Microbiol. Infect.* **2016**, *22*, S9–S14. [CrossRef] [PubMed]

24. Paterson, D.L.; Bonomo, R.A. Extended-spectrum beta-lactamases: A clinical update. *Clin. Microbiol. Rev.* **2005**, *18*, 657–686. [CrossRef] [PubMed]

17

Lysoquinone-TH1, a New Polyphenolic Tridecaketide Produced by Expressing the Lysolipin Minimal PKS II in *Streptomyces albus*

Torben Hofeditz [1], **Claudia Eva-Maria Unsin** [2], **Jutta Wiese** [3], **Johannes F. Imhoff** [3], **Wolfgang Wohlleben** [2,4], **Stephanie Grond** [1,*] and **Tilmann Weber** [2,5,*] ⓘ

[1] Institut für Organische Chemie, Eberhard Karls Universität Tübingen, Auf der Morgenstelle 18, 72076 Tübingen, Germany; torben.hofeditz@gmx.de

[2] Interfakultäres Institut für Mikrobiologie und Infektionsmedizin, Eberhard Karls Universität Tübingen, Auf der Morgenstelle 28, 72076 Tübingen, Germany; claudia_unsin@yahoo.de (C.E.-M.U.); wolfgang.wohlleben@biotech.uni-tuebingen.de (W.W.)

[3] GEOMAR, Helmholtz-Zentrum für Ozeanforschung Kiel, Düsternbrooker Weg 20, 24105 Kiel, Germany; jwiese@geomar.de (J.W.); jimhoff@geomar.de (J.F.I.)

[4] German Center for Infection Research (DZIF), partner site Tübingen, Auf der Morgenstelle 28, 72076 Tübingen, Germany

[5] The Novo Nordisk Foundation Center for Biosustainability, Technical University of Denmark, Kemitorvet bygning 220, 2800 Kongens Lyngby, Denmark

[*] Correspondence: stephanie.grond@uni-tuebingen.de (S.G.); tiwe@biosustain.dtu.dk (T.W.)

Abstract: The structural repertoire of bioactive naphthacene quinones is expanded by engineering *Streptomyces albus* to express the lysolipin minimal polyketide synthase II (PKS II) genes from *Streptomyces tendae* Tü 4042 (*llpD-F*) with the corresponding cyclase genes *llpCI-CIII*. Fermentation of the recombinant strain revealed the two new polyaromatic tridecaketides lysoquinone-TH1 (**7**, identified) and TH2 (**8**, postulated structure) as engineered congeners of the dodecaketide lysolipin (**1**). The chemical structure of **7**, a benzo[a]naphthacene-8,13-dione, was elucidated by NMR and HR-MS and confirmed by feeding experiments with [1,2-^{13}C$_2$]-labeled acetate. Lysoquinone-TH1 (**7**) is a pentangular polyphenol and one example of such rare extended polyaromatic systems of the benz[a]napthacene quinone type produced by the expression of a minimal PKS II in combination with cyclases in an artificial system. While the natural product lysolipin (**1**) has antimicrobial activity in nM-range, lysoquinone-TH1 (**7**) showed only minor potency as inhibitor of Gram-positive microorganisms. The bioactivity profiling of lysoquinone-TH1 (**7**) revealed inhibitory activity towards phosphodiesterase 4 (PDE4), an important target for the treatment in human health like asthma or chronic obstructive pulmonary disease (COPD). These results underline the availability of pentangular polyphenolic structural skeletons from biosynthetic engineering in the search of new chemical entities in drug discovery.

Keywords: lysolipin; minimal PKS II; cyclases; benz[a]naphthacene quinone; tridecaketide; aromatic polyketide; pentacyclic angular polyphenol; extended polyketide chain

1. Introduction

Polyketides are a large family of structurally-diverse natural products, mainly produced by bacteria, fungi, and plants. Their biosynthesis is catalyzed by distinct enzymes, termed type I polyketide synthases (PKS), type II PKS, type III PKS or variants thereof [1]. They exhibit broad ranges of pharmacological properties for use in clinical applications [2].

Many bacterial aromatic polyketides, such as the clinically used tetracycline, are biosynthesized by type II polyketide synthases (PKS II). Each PKS II contains a minimal set of enzymes (minPKS) that is required to synthesize a polyketide chain of defined length usually primed by acetyl-CoA and extended with malonyl-CoA to polycyclic products [3]. A minimal PKS II consists of two β-ketoacyl synthases (KS_α and KS_β) and one acyl carrier protein (ACP). KS_α is responsible for loading malonyl-CoA extender onto the PKS II system and also for the iterative Claisen condensations to extend the polyketide chain. KS_β, also referred to as chain length factor (CLF), is contributing to control the polyketide chain length [4]. Diverse cyclization patterns convert the polyketones to an enormous variety of structural polycyclic skeletons [5].

The final bioactive polycyclic PKS II natural products are aromatic compounds and often arise from additional enzymatic conversions, among them cyclases (CYC) [6], reductases (KR) [7], oxidases [8] and decarboxylating enzymes [2,9] or amidotransferases [10] for insertion of nitrogen or glycosyl transferases [11].

Lysolipin I (1) from *Streptomyces* Tü 4042 [12] and other members of microbial aromatic polyketides, such as pradimicin A (2) [13], fredericamycin A (3) [14], benastatin A (4) [15], bequinostatin C (4a) [16] and xantholipin (5) [17], are among the largest type II PKS products that have been described. They differentiate from the important groups of the smaller angucyclinones and anthracyclines (A-type, resp. B in Figure 1). They have distinct pentangular polycyclic aromatic core structures with pyridone, piperidone or lactone rings, respectively, added to a hexacyclic core structure as in xantholipin (5), lysolipin (1) or fredericamycins (3, 3a) [18] (Figure 1). This additional ring F varies in δ-position with different substituents next to the amide. Several lysolipin derivatives have been described. While lysolipin I (1) carries a methoxy substituent at C-24, derivatives of lysolipin have been engineered which have a methyl group at this position (Patent WO2007079715 (A3), Combinature Biopharm, Berlin, Germany).

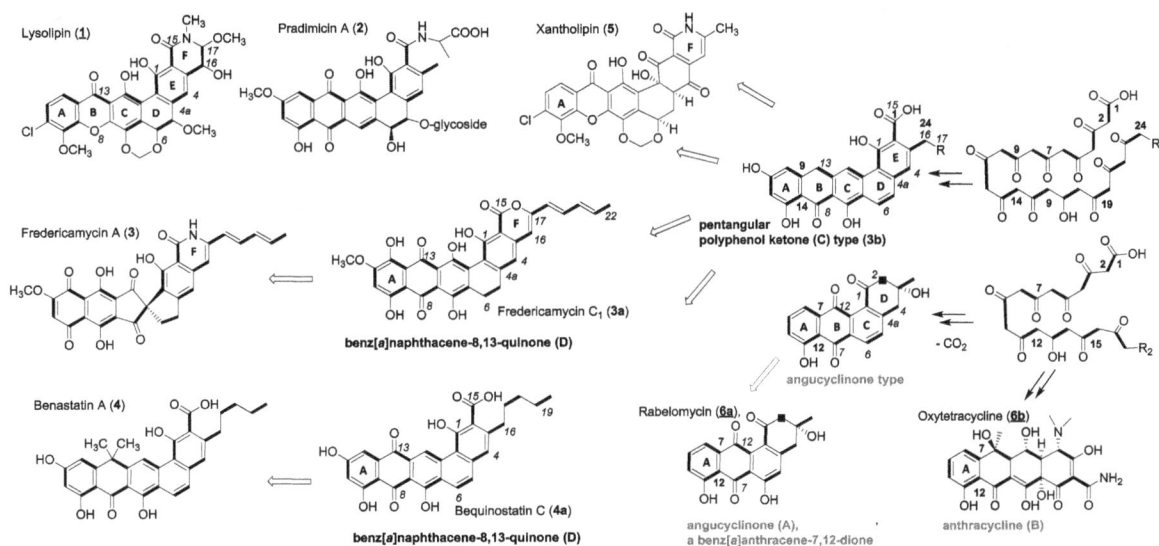

Figure 1. Chemical structures of PKS II products (1–6) and examples of biosynthetic congeners (3a, b, 4a). PKS chains (acetate units bold) of angucyclinone (A) and anthracycline (B) type structures start to cyclize with ring A at C-7/C-12. Benz[a]naphthacene (C) and benz[a]naphthacene quinone (D) type structures cyclize starting with C-9/C-14 according to polyketide chain numbering (green). Variations of δ-substituents of ring-F highlighted in red. R = H or alkyl-, allylic carbon chains (usual chemical nomenclature in blue).

Several biosynthetic gene clusters of these large PKS-II antibiotics are known and have been subject to extensive genetic and biochemical characterization [18–23]. In the biosynthetic pathways of pentangular polyaromatic polyketides, e.g., 1–5, the respective cyclized polyphenols (3b) and polyphenolic quinones (**3a**) have been demonstrated as pathway intermediates; they have also been obtained as products of genetic engineering efforts (Figure 2). Therefore, we regard the class of pentangular quinones as the metabolic hub of the important aromatic polyketide products.

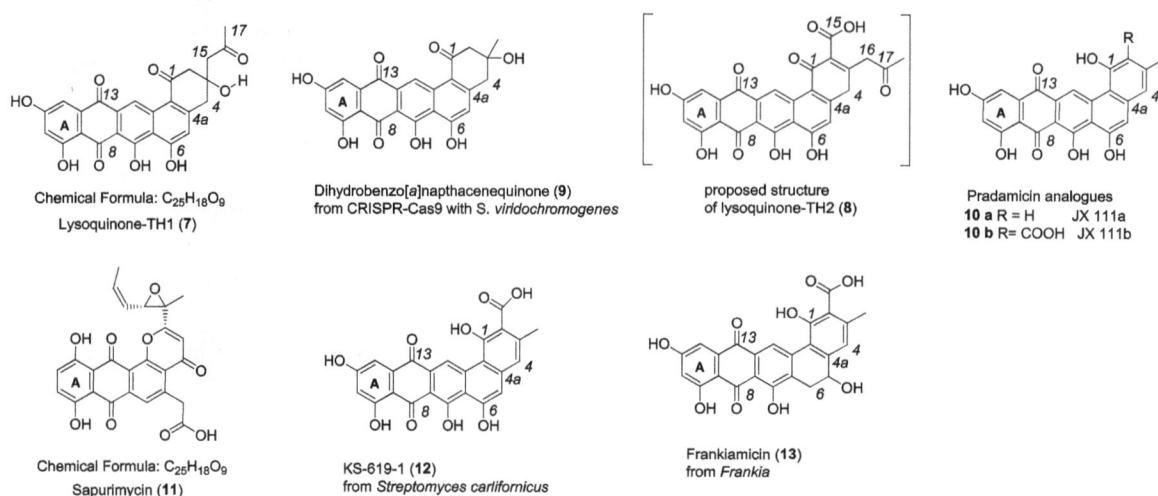

Figure 2. Chemical structure of lysoquinone-TH1 (**7**, identified), lysoquinone-TH2 (**8**, proposed), the constitutional isomer sapurimycin (**11**) and structurally related pentangular polyketides **9**–**13**.

Here, we report that the heterologous expression of the lysolipin minimal PKS II genes, which comprise *llpF*, coding for the ketosynthase α (KSα), *llpE*, coding for the ketosynthase β (KSβ), and *llpD*, coding for the ACP, in combination with genes encoding the cyclases (*llpCI-CIII*) in the host *S. albus* J1074 resulted in the production of novel metabolites (Figure 2). The structure elucidation of the novel bioactive lysoquinone-TH1 (**7**), strong evidence for its tridecaketide backbone from the doubly labeled [1,2-$^{13}C_2$]-acetate-feeding experiments, and the potent bioactivity as potent phosphodiesterase inhibitor are discussed.

2. Results and Discussion

2.1. Heterologous Production of Lysoquinone-TH 1 (7) in S. albus

The lysolipin gene cluster has been identified on a 42-kb genomic region in *Streptomyces tendae* Tü 4042 and analyzed by sequence comparison and heterologous expression in *S. albus* [21]. For this study, the genes coding for the minimal PKS II (*llpD-F*) and cyclases (*llpCI-CIII*) were amplified by PCR from the cosmid 4H04 encoding the complete lysolipin (**1**) gene cluster. The 4.1-kb PCR fragment was cloned into the vector pSET152*ermE**p [24] under control of the constitutive promoter *ermE**p yielding plasmid pCU1 (Figure S1). pCU1 was introduced into *S. albus* J1074 by intergeneric conjugation and the minimal PKS II and cyclase genes were heterologously expressed in culture. The recombinant strain expressing the minimal PKS and cyclases changed the color of the nutrient media (R5) and colonies on plates from yellowish to dark brown. In comparison, *S. albus* strain containing a pSET152*ermE**p plasmid without insert does not show the phenotype.

Thus, this strain gained the ability to produce new substances. Thin layer chromatography (TLC) analysis revealed a strong red fraction proved to be not identical to lysolipin (**1**).

2.2. Isolation and Structure Elucidation of Lysoquinone-TH1 (7)

Starting from the newly observed colored product, we developed a work-up procedure towards the isolation of the pure compound for structure elucidation and biological profiling from a four liter fermentation broth in M65 medium. Acetone and methanol extractions removed water soluble and other unwanted compounds. Filtration with RP-18 material preceded the preparative HPLC purification using a C_4 column and H_2O (Ammonium formate, TFA): acetonitrile as solvents (see Supplemental Materials). Thereby, 3.4 mg of purified red compound (lysoquinone-TH1, **7**) were obtained from a four-liter fermentation broth from medium supplemented with sterile adsorber resin XAD-16 and subsequently characterized by TLC, LC-mass spectrometry (MS) and NMR-analysis (Figures S2–S5).

HR-ESI-MS data for the red metabolite **7** revealed a m/z = 461.087756 $[M-H]^-$ ((Δppm = 0.11 ppm) and suggested the molecular formula for **7** to be $C_{25}H_{18}O_9$ (M_R = 462,4). Consistently low resolution ESI-MS monitoring of the crude extracts exhibited m/z = 461.1 $[M-H]^-$ and 463.2 $[M+H]^+$) ions with stronger ionization in the negative mode. Thus, the sum formula for compound **7** proposed 17 degrees of unsaturation and implied a large aromatic ring system.

The LC-MS/MS fragmentation analysis of lysoquinone-TH1 (**7**) gave evidence for a mass difference of m/z 58 with m/z = 403.1 $[M-C_3H_6O-H]^-$ as the only fragmentation product, which was assigned to a McLafferty rearrangement and a neutral loss of acetone (Figure S2). These results indicated a stable substance in MS-fragmentation.

One- and two-dimensional NMR-data (^{1}H-NMR, ^{13}C-NMR, HMBC, HSQC, COSY) yielded ten proton signals; one aliphatic methyl-, one methylene group, four protons with methylene character and four aromatic protons (Figures S3–S5). The carbon to proton correlation (HSQC experiments) pointed to two isolated methylene groups with diasterotopic protons. These doublet protons (δ_H = 2.67, 2.91 and δ_H = 3.01, 3.25 ppm) underlined that they only couple within the methylene group, each (J = 15.9 Hz), and suggest a ring structure. Furthermore, a methyl group singlet (δ_H = 2.18 ppm) next to an aliphatic carbonyl group (δ_C = 207.8) implied no other direct substituents. However, this carbonyl group is adjacent to a methylene group (δ_H = 2.70, δ_C = 53.3 ppm), attached to a quaternary carbon (δ_C = 71.0 ppm) as part of the aliphatic ring system (C-1-C-4, C-4a, C-14b). The proton at δ_H = 9.48 indicated an aromatic proton with exceptional low field shift from two carbonyl groups (C-1, C-13) in spatial proximity. In consistence with the recorded ^{13}C-NMR- and ^{1}H-NMR-data, the HMBC-experiment unambiguously delivered assigned key correlations due to well separated signals which established the connectivity to the whole scaffold of lysoquinone-TH1 (**7**) and a full structural assignment (Table S1) to a pentangular polyphenolic core (Figure S4). Lysoquinone-TH1 (**7**) is a 3-(2-oxo-propyl)-decorated dihydrobenz[a]napthacene-8,13-quinone, a novel compound to the best of our knowledge.

Additionally, the purification protocol revealed another violet fraction with obviously a second compound (proposed as lysoquinone-TH2, **8**) not identical to lysolipin (**1**). However, only minute amounts were observed in production cultures, and presumably a distinct instability did not allow for purification and full structure elucidation. HR-ESI-MS data from extract fractions of the violet metabolite **8** revealed a m/z = 487.0670 $[M-H]^-$ (Δppm = 0.1 ppm) and suggested the molecular formula for **8** to be $C_{26}H_{16}O_{10}$ (M_R = 488.4). In comparison to **7**, 19 instead of 17 degrees of unsaturation were calculated. A large aromatic ring system is also concluded. The isolation of **8** was not achieved to allow for NMR studies. Thus, the analytical MS/MS and the UV-data of lysoquinone-TH1 (**7**) in addition to the knowledge of the mentioned McLafferty rearrangement are pointing to structure **8**. This proposed compound was named lysoquinone-TH2 (**8**) and resembles the C-2 carboxyl analogue of **7** as a yet unknown structure.

In comparison to **7**, the only known constitutional isomer sapurimycin (**11**, $C_{25}H_{18}O_9$) [25] is an annealed tetracyclic ring system. The rare moiety of a reduced ring E of angular naphthacene quinone of **7** is only known from metabolite **9**, generated via CRISPR-Cas9 technology with *S. viridochromogenes* [26]. JX111a (**10a**), JX111b (**10b**), and further precursors of pradimicin A (**2**) [27], KS-619-1 (**12**) [28], and frankiamicin (**13**) from *Frankia* [29] display a similar structural skeleton to lysoquinone-TH1 (**7**) and to the proposed structure lysoquinone-TH2 (**8**) (Figure 2). It could be anticipated that the benz[a]napthacene carbon skeleton originates from a native tridecaketide polyketide chain for the lysoquinones **7** and **8** from the min PKS while the parent natural product of strain *S*. Tü4042 lysolipin I (**1**) has a dodecaketide backbone.

2.3. Feeding Experiment with [1,2-$^{13}C_2$]-Labeled Acetate

For validating the biogenesis of lysoquinone-TH1 (7) a feeding experiment with the doubly ^{13}C-labeled [1,2-$^{13}C_2$] acetate was carried out, and lysoquinone-TH1 (7) was purified from the culture and subjected to NMR spectroscopy. All carbon atoms turned out to be enriched [30] with highly specific incorporation rates between 2.0 and 7.3 (Figure 3, Figure S4 and S6, Table S1). The specific coupling constants from NMR analysis again confirmed the structure of lysoquinone-TH1 (7) and suggest a polyketide origin assembled from 13 acetate extender units (tridecaketide, Figure 2). It is therefore among the largest polyketides formed by a minimal PKS II (LlpD, E, F) with cyclases (LlpCI–CIII) via heterologous expression. It could be anticipated that the proposed structure of lysoquinone-TH2 (8) further corroborates the native tridecaketide precursor and carries the additional carboxyl group (C-15) of the final extender acetate unit. The continuous labeled-acetate chain of 7 corresponds with the pattern of the further post-PKS-processed antibiotic lysolipin I (1) [31].

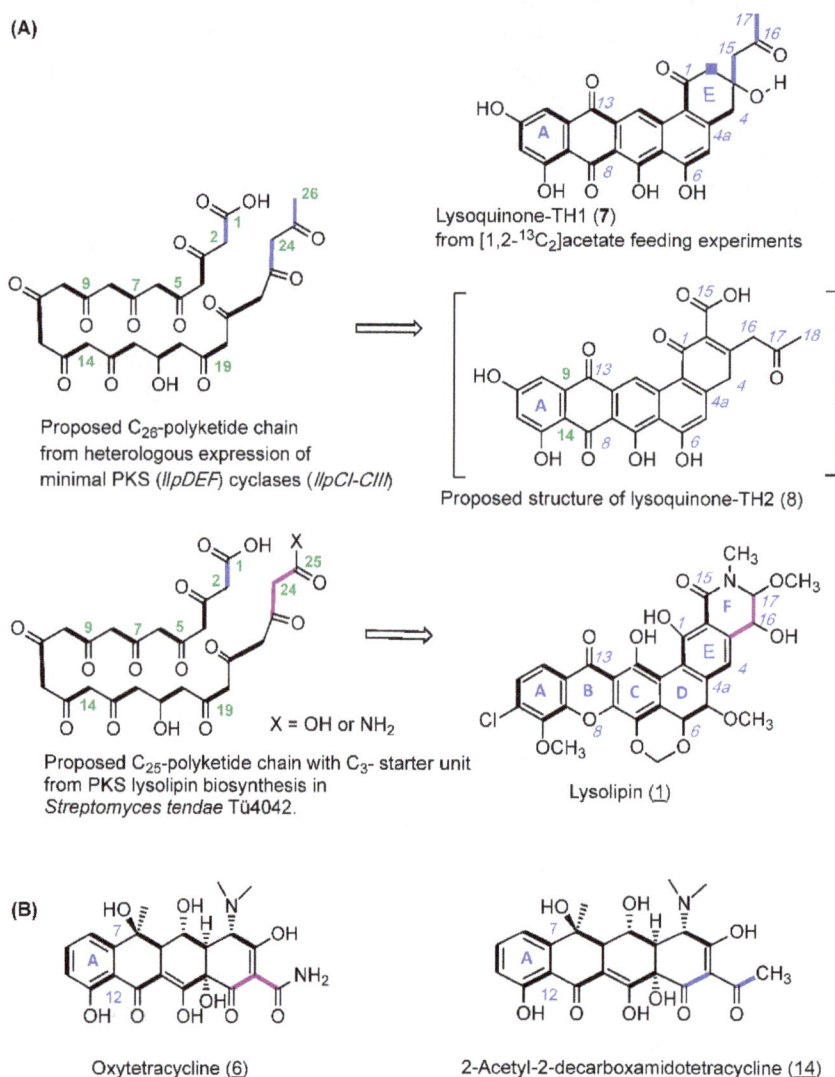

Figure 3. (**A**) Biosynthetic origin of lysoquinone-TH1 (7) and the proposed structure of lysoquinone-TH2 (8): Biosynthesis hypothesis from feeding experiments with doubly labeled [1,2-$^{13}C_2$] acetate with the S. albus host strain and heterologous expression of the lysolipin minimal PKS genes (*llpD-F*) and cyclase genes (*llpCI-CIII*). (**B**) Oxytetracycline (6) from a biosynthesis primed with malonamide in the wild-type producer, and with two acetate units in the mutant producer.

A specific feature of the lysolipin polyketide biosynthesis is the priming by a malonate-derived starter unit [31]. However, in the identified lysoquinone-TH1 (**7**) as well as in the proposed structure of lysoquinone-TH2 (**8**), two acetate units replace the original C_3-malonyl/malonamide starter unit. Respective observations were also made for oxytetracycline (**6b**) with a malonamide starter unit since heterologous expression of the oxytetracycline minimal PKS of *Streptomyces rimosus* in *S. coelicolor* yielded tetracycline analogue **14** with two acetate units priming the polyketide backbone instead [32] (Figure 3). Co-expressing the *oxyD* gene with the oxytetracyline minimal PKS in heterologous expression experiments has shown that it is presumably responsible for generating the characteristic malonamate starter unit. OxyD codes for an amidotransferase and is homologous to the putative amidotransferase LlpA of lysolipin biosynthesis. Therefore, priming of the PKS biosynthesis with malonamate and and formation of a N-heterocyclic product does not require additional enzymes [10].

Studies on hybrid PKS pathways with benastatin A (**4**) revealed isolated hybrid PKS-II products with the number of extender units increased if shorter starter units were used. In analogy, based on the observations on the identified lysoquinone-TH 1 (**7**) and the proposed structure of lysoquinone-TH2 (**8**) it can be anticipated that the number of elongation steps is dependent on the length of the polyketide chain [33] fitting into the substrate pocket of the $KS\alpha/KS\beta$-complex.

2.4. Biological Activity of Lysoquinone-TH1 (7)

Lysolipin (**1**) is highly active against various Gram-positive bacteria and shows antifungal activity. While the molecular target of lysolipin (**1**) still remains elusive, there is strong indication that this xanthone antibiotic targets the bacterial cell envelope [12,34].

Because of the high antibiotic activity of lysolipin (**1**) in nM-range, biological assays with lysoquinone-TH1 (**7**) were performed. Only weak antibiotic activities at 100 μM concentration of lysoquinone-TH1 (**7**) were observed against the Gram-positive strains *Staphylococcus lentus*, *Staphylococcus epidermidis* and *Propionibacterium acnes* with inhibition of 39%, 66% and 74%, respectively, in comparison to the positive control chloramphenicol [35]. Therefore, no IC_{50} values were determined.

KS-619-1 (**12**) and K-259-2 are representing inhibitors of the cyclic nucleotide phosphodiesterase (PDE4) [28,36–38]. The enzyme PDE4 is a very attractive target for the treatment of asthma, chronic obstructive pulmonary disease (COPD), psoriasis, schizophrenia, diet induced obesity, glucose intolerance and multiple sclerosis [39–44]. PDE4 addresses cyclic nucleotides like cAMP and cGMP and degrades these cellular messengers. However, these messengers possess regulatory functions in almost all cells so it is regarded an important target [45], therefore, detailed studies with different inhibitors are needed to evaluate an ideally selective bioactivity.

For profiling lysoquinone-TH1 (**7**), an enzyme assay using PDE-4B2 was carried out according to Schulz et al. [39]. A clearly defined IC_{50} value could not be determined in this assay due to an additional luminescence signal derived from the chromophore of lysoquinone-TH1 (**7**), an extensive polyaromatic skeleton. However, an IC_{50} range of 10–20 μM could be inferred from the assays against the PDE-4B2 enzyme. The MIC (minimal inhibition concentration) of lysoquinone-TH1 (**7**) was determined to a value of 2.33 μM (±0.04) corresponding to 3.368 log(nM) (±0.007) (Figure S7). The standard used in these assays was rolipram ($IC_{50} = 0.8$ μM (±0.1)) [39], an optimized and approved drug. Lysoquinone-TH1 (**7**), a completely new substance, is only 10-fold less active as this well-known PDE4 inhibitor rolipram. When lysolipin (**1**) was tested in the same assay, no PDE4 inhibition was detected up to a concentration of 50 μM.

3. Materials and Methods

3.1. Cloning of the Lysolipin Minimal PKS

The genes of the lysolipin minimal PKS II (*llpD*, *llpE*, *llpF*), which are surrounded by the cyclases *llpCI*, *llpCII*, and *llpCIII*, were amplified by PCR using the primers minPKScyc-fw-Hind (aaa gct tga gta gcc aaa cgg gtt c) and minPKScyc-revSs (aag aat tca ata ttg tgc cca cca gta cac) and the template cosmid 4H04 [21] using ProofStart PCR polymerase kit (*Qiagen*). The PCR Program used in an PTC-100 thermocycler (MJ Research, Waltham, MA, USA) was: 95 °C—5 min; 30 cycles with (94 °C—90 s, 62 °C—90 s, 72 °C—4 min); 72 °C—10 min. The PCR product was then cloned into pSETermE*p [24] (Combinature Biopharm AG, Berlin, Germany) via the EcoRI/HindIII restriction sites. The resulting plasmid pCU1 was checked by restriction and DNA sequencing.

The plasmid pCU1 was introduced into *Streptomyces albus* J1074 via a standard intergeneric conjugation protocol as, for example, described in [46].

3.2. Culture Conditions

A pre-culture with medium G20 (600 mL) in six 300 mL Erlenmeyer flasks was inoculated with *S. albus* J1074 and apramycin (50 µg/mL) for 48 h at 28 °C and 180 rpm (B. Braun Certomat HK with shaker B. Braun Certomat U, B. Braun, Melsungen, Germany). The main culture was inoculated with 400 mL of the pre-culture and was grown up in medium M65 (3.6 L) under selection with apramycin (50 µg/mL) in a fermenter (B. Braun Biostat B, B. Braun, Melsungen, Germany) for 96 h at 28 °C and 300 rpm. After 24 h, 15 g/300 mL of sterile XAD-16 was added to the culture. Nutrient solutions: G20 (Glycerol (20 g), malt extract (10 g), yeast extract (4 g) in 1 L of tab water. pH = 7.2). M65 (Malt extract (10 g), yeast extract (4 g), D-glucose (4 g), $CaCO_3$ (2 g) in 1 L of tab water. pH = 7.2).

3.3. Extraction and Isolation

For initial detection, agar plates from *S. albus* incubation were extracted with ethyl acetate, the organic phases evaporated and the extract applied to silica gel TLC analysis (solvent cyclohexane/ethylacetate/methanol 6:8:1, with 1% of trifluoric acetate acid added). For purification, 4 L of culture broth with XAD-16 was filtered over Celite to separate the mycelia from the liquid culture. The filtrate was autoclaved and discarded. The mycelia were extracted two times with acetone/methanol 7:3 and then in acetone/methanol 1:1 in an ultrasonic bath. After filtration, the organic phases were combined, evaporated, water was added, and the pH adjusted to 4–5 with 1 M HCl. Extraction with ethyl acetate and evaporation gave the crude extract. RP silica gel was pretreated with 3–4 column volumes (CV) of pyridine and washed with 3–4 CV of water as a basic activation of the RP phase. After column conditioning with 1–2 CV of the solvent acetone/methanol 1:1 the extract was loaded, and red and violet fractions were selected, accompanied by TLC analysis on silica gel (see above) and LC-ESI-MS analysis (HPLC, Agilent 1100 series. Ion trap, Bruker Daltonic Esquire 3000+, He as reactant gas, with Data Analysis software, Bruker Daltonik, Bremen, Germany). Combined red fractions were dissolved in DMSO and purified with HPLC (Thermo Ultimate 3000 Thermo Scientific, Dreieich, Germany); Column: Dr. Maisch, Ammerbuch-Entringen, Germany, Reprosil 120 C-4, 5 µm, 250 × 20 mm id, pre-colum: Dr. Maisch, standard guard Reprosil 120 C-4, 30 × 20 mm id, flow rate: 13.0 mL/min.; program: 20 min at 45% B, in 5 min to 75% B, 8 min at 75% B, in 2 min to 45% B, 8 min at 45% B; solvent: A = ammonium formate (20 mM) + 0.1% TFA in water; B = acetonitrile). A retention time from 12 to 13 min was observed. After evaporating a Sephadex LH-20 (2 × 2 cm, methanol) and following extraction three times with ethyl acetate and three times with diisopropyl ether was necessary for desalting the sample. This work up procedure gives 3.4 mg lysoquinone-TH1 (**7**) from four liters of culture.

3.4. Feeding Experiment with [1,2-$^{13}C_2$]-Labeled Acetate

For the feeding experiment 2.0 g of the doubly labeled [1,2-$^{13}C_2$] acetate (99% enrichment; Cambridge Isotope Laboratories, Inc., Tewksbury, MA, USA), which corresponds to 5.95 mM end concentration in the fermenter (4 L, B. Braun Biostat B) were added to the culture broth after 32 h of cultivation. The isotope labeled lysoquinone-TH1 (**7**) was purified with same protocol as described above and subjected to NMR-analysis (^{13}C-NMR, ^{1}H-NMR, HMBC, HSQC).

3.5. Biological Activity Assays

Antibacterial assays were carried out with the test strains *Staphylococcus lentus* DSM 6672, *Staphylococcus epidermidis* DSM 20044 and *Propionibacterium acnes* DSM 1897 using a cell viability test based on the reduction of resazurin to resorufin. Details on the cultivation conditions of the strains *S. epidermidis* and *P. acnes*, as well as on the evaluation of cell viability are described by Silber et al. [34]. The experiments with *S. lentus* were performed in the same manner as *S. epidermidis*. The positive control chloramphenicol was applied in a concentration of 10 µM for *S. lentus* and *S. epidermidis* and of 1 µM for *P. acnes*.

The effect of lysoquinone-TH1 (7) on PDE-4B2, a human recombinant cyclic adenosine monophosphate (cAMP) specific phosphodiesterase (BPS Bioscience no. 60042, San Diego, CA, USA) was determined in 96 well plates using the PDELight HTS cAMP Phosphodiesterase Kit (Lonza, LT07-600, Wuppertal, Germany). Lysoquinone-TH1 (7) was diluted in 50 mM Tris-HCl buffer (pH 7.5) containing 8.3 mM $MgCl_2$ and 1.7 mM EGTA. 10 µL of each dilution was transferred to a well. 20 µL PDE-4B2 solution (0.25 U/µL) were added. The reaction was started by adding 10 µL of 12 mM cAMP (Sigma A9501, Taufkirchen, Germany) dissolved in 50 mM Tris-HCl buffer (pH 7.5) containing 8.3 mM $MgCl_2$ and 1.7 mM EGTA to each well of the microtiter plate. PDE-4B2 hydrolysed cAMP to adenosine monophosphate (AMP). After an incubation at 30 °C for 30 min, the reaction was stopped by transferring 30 µL solution containing 10 µL PDELight Stop Solution and 20 µL PDELight AMP detection reagent. The detection reagent converted AMP to ATP and luciferase catalyzed the formation of light from ATP and luciferin. The emitted light is proportional to the level of AMP produced. AMP was quantified after incubation at 30 °C for 10 min by measuring the luminescence using the microtiter plate reader Infinite M200 (Tecan, Crailsheim, Germany) with 0.1 s integration time. The assays were performed in duplicates. Rolipram (4-[3-(cyclopentyloxy)-4-methoxyphenyl]-2-pyrrolidinone) was used as positive control.

4. Conclusions

Lysoquinone-TH1 (7) is a "non-natural natural product", a pentangular aromatic polyketide derived from engineering of the lysolipin biosynthetic pathway. It was produced with *Streptomyces albus* as host expressing the minimal PKS II genes (*llpD-F*) in combination with three cyclases (*llpCI-CIII*) of the lysolipin gene cluster. In a bioactivity profiling study, it was shown that lysoquinone-TH1 (7) only has weak antibacterial activity, but instead is an inhibitor of phosphodiesterase 4 (PDE4) which is a target for treatment of pulmonary diseases. The lysoquinone-TH1 (7) biosynthetic pathway, which was deduced based on NMR data and supported by the new but postulated analogue lysoquinone-TH2 (8) also provides insights on the biosynthesis of lysolipin I (1). Evidence is given for the acetate-derived tridecaketide backbone of 7 in contrast to the dodecaketide malonyl-derived (malonyl- or malonamide CoA) precursor chain of the parent compound lysolipin I (1).

Supplementary Materials: The following are available online at http://www.mdpi.com/2079-6382/7/3/53/s1. Figure S1: Plasmid map of pCU1; Figure S2: HPLC and LC-MS of lysoquinone-TH1 (7) and proposed lysoquinone-TH2 (8); Figure S3: NMR spectra of lysoquinone-TH1 (7); Figure S4: NMR spectra of 13C-enriched lysoquinone-TH1 (7); Figure S5: 2D-NMR data of lysoquinone-TH1 (7); Figure S6: ^{13}C enrichment of 7; Figure S7: PDE-4B2 inhibition assay with lysoquinone-TH1; Table S1: Level of enrichment and specific incorporation of lysoquinone-TH1 (7), resulted from the feeding experiment with doubly labeled [1,2-$^{13}C_2$] acetate.

Author Contributions: T.H. performed strain cultivation and feeding experiments, designed and performed chemical preparative isolation and chemical analyses, wrote the draft manuscript with contributions of all authors. C.E.-M.U. designed and performed cloning of the minimal PKS. J.W. and J.F.I. designed and performed bioactivity studies. W.W., S.G. and T.W. conceived the study, all authors contributed and approved the manuscript.

Funding: This work was supported by the German Ministry of Education and Research [GenBioCom 0315585A] to S.G., T.W. and W.W. T.W. is supported by a grant of the Novo Nordisk Foundation [CFB, grant NNF10CC1016517] and W.W. by a grant from the German Center for Infection Research [DZIF TTU 09.912, FKZ 8020809912].

Acknowledgments: We thank Bruker Daltonics, Bremen, Germany for valuable discussions.

References

1. Hertweck, C. The biosynthetic logic of polyketide diversity. *Angew. Chem. Int. Ed.* **2009**, *48*, 4688–4716. [CrossRef] [PubMed]

2. Kharel, M.K.; Pahari, P.; Shepherd, M.D.; Tibrewal, N.; Nybo, S.E.; Shaaban, K.A.; Rohr, J. Angucyclines: Biosynthesis, mode-of-action, new natural products, and synthesis. *Nat. Prod. Rep.* **2012**, *29*, 264–325. [CrossRef] [PubMed]

3. Zhang, Z.; Pan, H.-X.; Tang, G.-L. New insights into bacterial type II polyketide biosynthesis. *F1000Research* **2017**, *6*, 172. [CrossRef] [PubMed]

4. Tang, Y.; Tsai, S.C.; Khosla, C. Polyketide chain length control by chain length factor. *J. Am. Chem. Soc.* **2003**, *125*, 12708–12709. [CrossRef] [PubMed]

5. Zhou, H.; Li, Y.; Tang, Y. Cyclization of aromatic polyketides from bacteria and fungi. *Nat. Prod. Rep.* **2010**, *27*, 839–868. [CrossRef] [PubMed]

6. Zhang, W.; Watanabe, K.; Wang, C.C.C.; Tang, Y. Investigation of early tailoring reactions in the oxytetracycline biosynthetic pathway. *J. Biol. Chem.* **2007**, *282*, 25717–25725. [CrossRef] [PubMed]

7. Valentic, T.R.; Jackson, D.R.; Brady, S.F.; Tsai, S.C. Comprehensive Analysis of a Novel Ketoreductase for Pentangular Polyphenol Biosynthesis. *ACS Chem. Biol.* **2016**, *11*, 3421–3430. [CrossRef] [PubMed]

8. Kong, L.; Zhang, W.; Chooi, Y.H.; Wang, L.; Cao, B.; Deng, Z.; Chu, Y.; You, D. A Multifunctional monooxygenase XanO4 catalyzes xanthone Formation in xantholipin biosynthesis via a cryptic demethoxylation. *Cell Chem. Biol.* **2016**, *23*, 508–516. [CrossRef] [PubMed]

9. Gullon, S.; Olano, C.; Abdelfattah, M.S.; Brana, A.F.; Rohr, J.; Mendez, C.; Salas, J.A. Isolation, characterization, and heterologous expression of the biosynthesis gene cluster for the antitumor anthracycline steffimycin. *Appl. Environ. Microbiol.* **2006**, *72*, 4172–4183. [CrossRef] [PubMed]

10. Zhang, W.; Ames, B.D.; Tsai, S.C.; Tang, Y. Engineered biosynthesis of a novel amidated polyketide, using the malonamyl-specific initiation module from the oxytetracycline polyketide synthase. *Appl. Environ. Microbiol.* **2006**, *72*, 2573–2580. [CrossRef] [PubMed]

11. Luzhetskyy, A.; Vente, A.; Bechthold, A. Glycosyltransferases involved in the biosynthesis of biologically active natural products that contain oligosaccharides. *Mol. Biosyst.* **2005**, *1*, 117–126. [CrossRef] [PubMed]

12. Drautz, H.; Keller-Schierlein, W.; Zähner, H. Metabolic products of microorganisms, 149. Lysolipin I, a new antibiotic from *Streptomyces violaceoniger* (author's transl). *Arch. Microbiol.* **1975**, *106*, 175–190. [CrossRef] [PubMed]

13. Oki, T.; Konishi, M.; Tomatsu, K.; Tomita, K.; Saitoh, K.; Tsunakawa, M.; Nishio, M.; Miyaki, T.; Kawaguchi, H. Pradimicin, a novel class of potent antifungal antibiotics. *J. Antibiot.* **1988**, *41*, 1701–1704. [CrossRef] [PubMed]

14. Misra, R.; Pandey, R.C.; Silverton, J.V. Fredericamycin A, an Antitumor antibiotic of a novel skeletal type. *J. Am. Chem. Soc.* **1982**, *104*, 4478–4479. [CrossRef]

15. Aoyagi, T.; Aoyama, T.; Kojima, F.; Matsuda, N.; Maruyama, M.; Hamada, M.; Takeuchi, T. Benastatins A and B, new inhibitors of glutathione S-transferase, produced by *Streptomyces* sp. MI384-DF12. I. Taxonomy, production, isolation, physico-chemical properties and biological activities. *J. Antibiot.* **1992**, *45*, 1385–1390. [CrossRef] [PubMed]

16. Yamazaki, T.; Tatee, T.; Aoyama; Kojima, F.; Takeuchi, T.; Aoyagi, T. Bequinostatins C and D, new inhibitors of glutathione S-transferase, produced by *Streptomyces* sp. MI384-DF12. *J. Antibiot.* **1993**, *46*, 1309–1311. [CrossRef] [PubMed]

17. Terui, Y.; Yiwen, C.; Jun-Ying, L.; Ando, T.; Yamamoto, H.; Kawamura, Y.; Tomishima, Y.; Uchida, S.; Okazaki, T.; Munetomo, E.; et al. Xantholipin, a novel inhibitor of HSP47 gene expression produced by *Streptomyces* sp. *Tetrahedron Lett.* **2003**, *44*, 5427–5430. [CrossRef]

18. Chen, Y.; Wendt-Pienkowski, E.; Ju, J.; Lin, S.; Rajski, S.R.; Shen, B. Characterization of FdmV as an amide synthetase for fredericamycin A biosynthesis in *Streptomyces griseus* ATCC 43944. *J. Biol. Chem.* **2010**, *285*, 38853–38860. [CrossRef] [PubMed]

19. Kim, B.C.; Lee, J.M.; Ahn, J.S.; Kim, B.S. Cloning, sequencing, and characterization of the pradimicin biosynthetic gene cluster of *Actinomadura hibisca* P157-2. *J. Microbiol. Biotechnol.* **2007**, *17*, 830–839. [PubMed]

20. Das, A.; Szu, P.-H.; Fitzgerald, J.T.; Khosla, C. Mechanism and engineering of polyketide chain initiation in fredericamycin biosynthesis. *J. Am. Chem. Soc.* **2010**, *132*, 8831–8833. [CrossRef] [PubMed]

21. Lopez, P.; Hornung, A.; Welzel, K.; Unsin, C.; Wohlleben, W.; Weber, T.; Pelzer, S. Isolation of the lysolipin gene cluster of *Streptomyces tendae* Tü 4042. *Gene* **2010**, *461*, 5–14. [CrossRef] [PubMed]

22. Zhang, W.; Wang, L.; Kong, L.; Wang, T.; Chu, Y.; Deng, Z.; You, D. Unveiling the post-PKS redox tailoring steps in biosynthesis of the type II polyketide antitumor antibiotic xantholipin. *Chem. Biol.* **2012**, *19*, 422–432. [CrossRef] [PubMed]

23. Lackner, G.; Schenk, A.; Xu, Z.; Reinhardt, K.; Yunt, Z.S.; Piel, J.; Hertweck, C. Biosynthesis of pentangular polyphenols: Deductions from the benastatin and griseorhodin pathways. *J. Am. Chem. Soc.* **2007**, *129*, 9306–9312. [CrossRef] [PubMed]

24. Menges, R.; Muth, G.; Wohlleben, W.; Stegmann, E. The ABC transporter Tba of *Amycolatopsis balhimycina* is required for efficient export of the glycopeptide antibiotic balhimycin. *Appl. Microbiol. Biotechnol.* **2007**, *77*, 125–134. [CrossRef] [PubMed]

25. Uosaki, Y.; Yasuzawa, T.; Hara, M.; Saitoh, Y.; Sano, H. Sapurimycin, new antitumor antibiotic produced by *Streptomyces*. Structure determination. *J. Antibiot.* **1991**, *44*, 40–44. [CrossRef] [PubMed]

26. Zhang, M.M.; Wong, F.T.; Wang, Y.; Luo, S.; Lim, Y.H.; Heng, E.; Yeo, W.L.; Cobb, R.E.; Enghiad, B.; Ang, E.L.; et al. CRISPR-Cas9 strategy for activation of silent *Streptomyces* biosynthetic gene clusters. *Nat. Chem. Biol.* **2017**, *13*, 607–609. [CrossRef] [PubMed]

27. Zhan, J.; Watanabe, K.; Tang, Y. Synergistic actions of a monooxygenase and cyclases in aromatic polyketide biosynthesis. *Chembiochem* **2008**, *9*, 1710–1715. [CrossRef] [PubMed]

28. Yasuzawa, T.; Yoshida, M.; Shirahata, K.; Sano, H. Structure of a novel Ca^{2+} and calmodulin-dependent cyclic nucleotide phosphodiesterase inhibitor KS-619-1. *J. Antibiot.* **1987**, *40*, 1111–1114. [CrossRef] [PubMed]

29. Ogasawara, Y.; Yackley, B.J.; Greenberg, J.A.; Rogelj, S.; Melançon, C.E. Expanding our understanding of sequence-function relationships of Type II polyketide biosynthetic gene clusters: Bioinformatics-guided identification of frankiamicin a from *Frankia* sp. EAN1pec. *PLoS ONE* **2015**, *10*, 1–25. [CrossRef] [PubMed]

30. Scott, A.I.; Townsend, C.A.; Okada, K.; Kajiwara, M.; Cushley, R.J.; Whitman, P.J. Biosynthesis of corrins. II. Incorporation of 13C-labeled substrate in vitamins B12. *J. Am. Chem. Soc.* **1974**, *96*, 8069–8080. [CrossRef] [PubMed]

31. Bockholt, H.; Udvarnoki, G.; Rohr, J.; Mocek, U.; Beale, J.M.; Floss, H.G. Biosynthetic studies on the xanthone antibiotics lysolipins X and I. *J. Org. Chem.* **1994**, *59*, 2064–2069. [CrossRef]

32. Fu, H.; Ebert-Khosla, S.; Khosla, C.; Hopwood, D.A. Relaxed Specificity of the oxytetracycline polyketide synthase for an acetate primer in the absence of a malonamyl primer. *J. Am. Chem. Soc.* **1994**, *116*, 6443–6444. [CrossRef]

33. Xu, Z.; Schenk, A.; Hertweck, C. Molecular analysis of the benastatin biosynthetic pathway and genetic engineering of altered fatty acid-polyketide hybrids. *J. Am. Chem. Soc.* **2007**, *129*, 6022–6030. [CrossRef] [PubMed]

34. Winter, D.K.; Sloman, D.L.; Porco, J., Jr. A. Polycyclic xanthone natural products: Structure, biological activity and chemical synthesis. *Nat. Prod. Rep.* **2013**, *30*, 382–391. [CrossRef] [PubMed]

35. Silber, J.; Ohlendorf, B.; Labes, A.; Erhard, A.; Imhoff, J.F. Calcarides A–E, antibacterial macrocyclic and linear polyesters from a calcarisporium strain. *Mar. Drugs* **2013**, *11*, 3309–3323. [CrossRef] [PubMed]

36. Matsuda, Y.; Kase, H. KS-619-1, a new inhibitor of Ca^{2+} and calmodulin-dependent cyclic nucleotide phosphodiesterase from *Streptomyces californicus*. *J. Antibiot.* **1987**, *40*, 1104–1110. [CrossRef] [PubMed]

37. Matsuda, Y.; Asano, K.; Kawamoto, I.; Kase, H. K-259-2, a new inhibitor of Ca^{2+} and calmodulin-dependent cyclic nucleotide phosphodiesterase from *Micromonospora olivasterospora*. *J. Antibiot.* **1987**, *40*, 1092–1100. [CrossRef] [PubMed]

38. Yasuzawa, T.; Yoshida, M.; Shirahata, K.; Sano, H. Structure of a novel Ca^{2+} and calmodulin-dependent cyclic nucleotide phosphodiesterase inhibitor K-259-2. *J. Antibiot.* **1987**, *40*, 1101–1103. [CrossRef] [PubMed]

39. Schulz, D.; Beese, P.; Ohlendorf, B.; Erhard, A.; Zinecker, H.; Dorador, C.; Imhoff, J.F. Abenquines A–D: Aminoquinone derivatives produced by *Streptomyces* sp. strain DB634. *J. Antibiot.* **2011**, *64*, 763–768. [CrossRef] [PubMed]

40. Houslay, M.D.; Schafer, P.; Zhang, K.Y.J. Keynote review: Phosphodiesterase-4 as a therapeutic target. *Drug Discov. Today* **2005**, *10*, 1503–1519. [CrossRef]

41. Boswell-Smith, V.; Spina, D.; Page, C.P. Phosphodiesterase inhibitors. *Br. J. Pharmacol.* **2009**, *147*, S252–S257. [CrossRef] [PubMed]

42. Millar, J.K.; Pickard, B.S.; Mackie, S.; James, R.; Christie, S.; Buchanan, S.R.; Malloy, M.P.; Chubb, J.E.; Huston, E.; Baillie, G.S.; et al. DISC1 and PDE4B are interacting genetic factors in schizophrenia that regulate cAMP signaling. *Science* **2005**, *310*, 1187–1191. [CrossRef] [PubMed]

43. Park, S.-J.; Ahmad, F.; Philp, A.; Baar, K.; Williams, T.; Luo, H.; Ke, H.; Rehmann, H.; Taussig, R.; Brown, A.L.; et al. Resveratrol ameliorates aging-related metabolic phenotypes by inhibiting cAMP phosphodiesterases. *Cell* **2012**, *148*, 421–433. [CrossRef] [PubMed]

44. Kanes, S.J.; Tokarczyk, J.; Siegel, S.J.; Bilker, W.; Abel, T.; Kelly, M.P. Rolipram: A specific phosphodiesterase 4 inhibitor with potential antipsychotic activity. *Neuroscience* **2007**, *144*, 239–246. [CrossRef] [PubMed]

45. Houslay, M.D.; Baillie, G.S.; Maurice, D.H. cAMP-Specific phosphodiesterase-4 enzymes in the cardiovascular system: A molecular toolbox for generating compartmentalized cAMP signaling. *Circ. Res.* **2007**, *100*, 950–966. [CrossRef] [PubMed]

46. Musiol, E.M.; Härtner, T.; Kulik, A.; Moldenhauer, J.; Piel, J.; Wohlleben, W.; Weber, T. Supramolecular templating in kirromycin biosynthesis: The acyltransferase KirCII loads ethylmalonyl-CoA extender onto a specific ACP of the trans-AT PKS. *Chem. Biol.* **2011**, *18*, 438–444. [CrossRef] [PubMed]

Permissions

List of Contributors

Sinead Duane, Paula Beatty and Andrew W. Murphy
Discipline of General Practice, School of Medicine, National University of Ireland Galway, Galway, Ireland

Akke Vellinga
Discipline of General Practice, School of Medicine, National University of Ireland Galway, Galway, Ireland
Discipline of Bacteriology, School of Medicine, National University of Ireland Galway, Galway, Ireland

Hani T. Fadel
Dental College and Hospital, Taibah University, Al Madinah Al Munawwarah 42353, Saudi Arabia

Najla Dar-Odeh and Osama A. Abu-Hammad
Dental College and Hospital, Taibah University, Al Madinah Al Munawwarah 42353, Saudi Arabia
Faculty of Dentistry, University of Jordan, Amman 11942, Jordan

Shaden Abu-Hammad
Faculty of Dentistry, University of Jordan, Amman 11942, Jordan

Ruáa Abdeljawad
Department of Pediatrics, Ibn Alhaitham Hospital, Amman 11942, Jordan

Natalia Veneranda Ortiz Zacarías, Jacobus Burggraaf, Jasper Stevens and Ingrid Maria Catharina Kamerling
Centre for Human Drug Research, Leiden, 2333 CL, The Netherlands

Anneke Corinne Dijkmans
Centre for Human Drug Research, Leiden, 2333 CL, The Netherlands
Department of Medical Microbiology, Albert Schweitzer Hospital, Dordrecht, 3318 AT, The Netherlands

Johan Willem Mouton
Department of Medical Microbiology, Radboud University Medical Center, Nijmegen, 6500 HB, The Netherlands
Department of Medical Microbiology and Infectious Diseases, Erasmus Medical Center, Rotterdam, 3015 CN, The Netherlands

Erik Bert Wilms
Hospital Pharmacy, The Hague Hospitals, The Hague, 2545 AB, The Netherlands

Cees van Nieuwkoop
Department of Internal Medicine, Haga Teaching Hospital, The Hague, 2566 MJ, The Netherlands

Daniel Johannes Touw
Groningen Research Institute for Asthma and COPD, Department of Clinical Pharmacy and Pharmacology, University Medical Center Groningen, University of Groningen, Groningen, 9713 GZ, The Netherlands

Sushovan Dam, Jean-Marie Pagès and Muriel Masi
UMR_MD1, Aix-Marseille Univ and Institut de Recherche Biomédicale des Armées, 27 Boulevard Jean Moulin, 13005 Marseille, France

Marta Maciejewska, Delphine Adam, Igor S. Pessi and Sébastien Rigali
InBioS—Centre for Protein Engineering, Institut de Chimie B6a, University of Liège, B-4000 Liège, Belgium

Magdalena Całusińska and Philippe Delfosse
Environmental Research and Innovation Department, Luxembourg Institute of Science and Technology, Belvaux, Luxembourg; Magdalena

Luc Cornet and Denis Baurain
InBioS—PhytoSYSTEMS, Eukaryotic Phylogenomics, University of Liège, B-4000 Liège, Belgium

Sandrine Malchair and Monique Carnol
InBioS—Plant and Microbial Ecology, Botany B22, University of Liège, B-4000 Liège, Belgium

Hazel A. Barton
Department of Biology, University of Akron, Akron, OH 44325, USA

Julia Deibert and Elif Koeksoy
Interfaculty Institute of Microbiology and Infection Medicine Tübingen (IMIT)—Microbial Genetics, University of Tuebingen, Auf der Morgenstelle 28 E, 72076 Tuebingen, Germany

Daniel Kühner and Ute Bertsche
Interfaculty Institute of Microbiology and Infection Medicine Tübingen (IMIT)—Microbial Genetics, University of Tuebingen, Auf der Morgenstelle 28 E, 72076 Tuebingen, Germany
Interfaculty Institute of Microbiology and Infection Medicine Tübingen (IMIT)—Infection Biology, University of Tuebingen, Auf der Morgenstelle 28 E, 72076 Tuebingen, Germany

Mark Stahl
Center for Plant Molecular Biology (ZMBP), University of Tuebingen, Auf der Morgenstelle 32, 72076 Tuebingen, Germany

Nanna Rørbo and Mathias Middelboe
Marine Biological Section, University of Copenhagen, 3000 Helsingør, Denmark

Panos G. Kalatzis
Marine Biological Section, University of Copenhagen, 3000 Helsingør, Denmark
Institute of Marine Biology, Biotechnology and Aquaculture, Hellenic Centre for Marine Research, 71003 Heraklion, Greece

Anita Rønneseth and Heidrun Inger Wergeland
Department of Biology, University of Bergen, 5020 Bergen, Norway

Bastian Barker Rasmussen and Lone Gram
Department of Biotechnology and Biomedicine, Technical University of Denmark, 2800 Kongens Lyngby, Denmark

Kirsten Engell-Sørensen
Fishlab, 8270 Højbjerg, Denmark

Hans Petter Kleppen
ACD Pharmaceuticals AS, 8376 Leknes, Norway

Marte Meyer Walle-Hansen
Bærum Hospital, Vestre Viken Hospital Trust, 3019 Drammen, Norway

Sigurd Høye
Antibiotic Centre for Primary Care, Department of General Practice, Institute of Health and Society, University of Oslo, 0315 Oslo, Norway

Ulugbek A. Abdufattaev
State Institution "Republican Specialized Scientific-Practical Medical Center of Urology", Tashkent 100109, Uzbekistan

Jakhongir F. Alidjanov
State Institution "Republican Specialized Scientific-Practical Medical Center of Urology", Tashkent 100109, Uzbekistan
Clinic of Urology, Pediatric Urology, and Andrology, Justus Liebig University, 35392 Giessen, Germany

Adrian Pilatz and Florian M. Wagenlehner
Clinic of Urology, Pediatric Urology, and Andrology, Justus Liebig University, 35392 Giessen, Germany

Kurt G. Naber
Department of Urology, School of Medicine, Technical University of Munich, 80333 Munich, Germany

Lucía Fernández, Susana Escobedo, Diana Gutiérrez, Silvia Portilla, Beatriz Martínez, Pilar García and Ana Rodríguez
Instituto de Productos Lácteos de Asturias (IPLA-CSIC), Paseo Río Linares s/n, Villaviciosa, 33300 Asturias, Spain

Dubravko Jelić
Fidelta Ltd., Prilaz baruna Filipovi´ca 29, HR-10000 Zagreb, Croatia

Roberto Antolović
Department of Biotechnology, University of Rijeka, Radmile Matej˘ci´c 2, HR-51000 Rijeka, Croatia

Marianna Iorio, Arianna Tocchetti, Giancarlo Del Gatto, and Sonia Ilaria Maffioli
NAICONS Srl, Viale Ortles 22/4, 20139 Milano, Italy

Margherita Sosio and Stefano Donadio
NAICONS Srl, Viale Ortles 22/4, 20139 Milano, Italy
KtedoGen Srl, Viale Ortles 22/4, 20139 Milano, Italy

Joao Carlos Santos Cruz and Cristina Brunati
KtedoGen Srl, Viale Ortles 22/4, 20139 Milano, Italy

Kayla M. Socarras ID, Priyanka A. S. Theophilus, Jason P. Torres, Khusali Gupta and Eva Sapi
Lyme Disease Research Group, Department of Biology and Environmental Science, University of New Haven, West Haven, CT 06519, USA

Jie Feng, Shuo Zhang, Wanliang Shi and Ying Zhang
Department of Molecular Microbiology and Immunology, Bloomberg School of Public Health, Johns Hopkins University, Baltimore, MD 21205, USA

James Gilkerson
Asia-Pacific Centre for Animal Health, Department of Veterinary Biosciences, Faculty of Veterinary and Agricultural Sciences, Melbourne Veterinary School, University of Melbourne, Parkville, VIC 3050, Australia

Laura Hardefeldt, Helen Crabb and Glenn Browning
Asia-Pacific Centre for Animal Health, Department of Veterinary Biosciences, Faculty of Veterinary and Agricultural Sciences, Melbourne Veterinary School, University of Melbourne, Parkville, VIC 3050, Australia
National Centre for Antimicrobial Stewardship, Peter Doherty Institute, Grattan St, Carlton, VIC 3050, Australia

Torben Nielsen
School of Animal and Veterinary Sciences, University of Adelaide, Roseworthy, SA 5371, Australia

Richard Squires
College of Public Health, Medical and Veterinary Sciences, James Cook University, Townsville, QLD 4810, Australia

Jane Heller
School of Animal and Veterinary Sciences, Charles Sturt University, Wagga Wagga, NSW 2650, Australia

Claire Sharp
School of Veterinary and Life Sciences, Murdoch University, Perth, WA 6150, Australia

Rowland Cobbold
School of Veterinary Science, University of Queensland, Gatton, QLD 4343, Australia

Jacqueline Norris
Sydney School of Veterinary Science, University of Sydney, Sydney, NSW 2006, Australia

Sumanth Gandra
Center for Disease Dynamics, Economics and Policy, New Delhi 110020, India

Ramanan Laxminarayan
Center for Disease Dynamics, Economics and Policy, New Delhi 110020, India
Princeton Environmental Institute, Princeton University, Princeton, NJ 08544, USA

Sanjeev K.Singh and Anil Kumar Vasudevan
Department of Infection Control and Microbiology, Amrita Institute of Medical Sciences, Amrita University, Ponekkara, Kochi 682041, India

Dasaratha R. Jinka and Gerardo Alvarez-Uria
Department of Infectious Diseases and Department of Paediatrics, Rural Development Trust Hospital, Bathalapalli 515661, India

Ravishankar Kanithi and Akhila Akula
Department of Paediatrics, Sowmya Children's Hospital, Hyderabad 500038, India

Ashok K. Chikkappa and Onkaraiah Tunga
Department of Paediatrics, Rural Development Trust Hospital, Kalyanadurgam 515761, India

Anita Sharma and Garima Garg
Department of Microbiology and Department of Paediatric Intensive Care Unit, Fortis Hospital, Mohali 160062, India

Dhanya Dharmapalan
Department of Paediatrics, Dr Yewale's Multispeciality Hospital for Children, Navi Mumbai 400703, India

Yingfen Hsia and Mike Sharland
Paediatric Infectious Diseases Research Group, Institute of Infection and Immunity, St. Georges University, London SW17 0RE, UK

Srinivas Murki
Department of Neonatology, Fernandez Hospital, Hyderabad 500029, India

Torben Hofeditz and Stephanie Grond
Institut für Organische Chemie, Eberhard Karls Universität Tübingen, Auf der Morgenstelle 18, 72076 Tübingen, Germany

Claudia Eva-Maria Unsin
Interfakultäres Institut für Mikrobiologie und Infektionsmedizin, Eberhard Karls Universität Tübingen, Auf der Morgenstelle 28, 72076 Tübingen, Germany

Wolfgang Wohlleben
Interfakultäres Institut für Mikrobiologie und Infektionsmedizin, Eberhard Karls Universität Tübingen, Auf der Morgenstelle 28, 72076 Tübingen, Germany
German Center for Infection Research (DZIF), partner site Tübingen, Auf der Morgenstelle 28, 72076 Tübingen, Germany

Tilmann Weber
Interfakultäres Institut für Mikrobiologie und Infektionsmedizin, Eberhard Karls Universität Tübingen, Auf der Morgenstelle 28, 72076 Tübingen, Germany
The Novo Nordisk Foundation Center for Biosustainability, Technical University of Denmark, Kemitorvet bygning 220, 2800 Kongens Lyngby, Denmark

Jutta Wiese and Johannes F. Imhoff
GEOMAR, Helmholtz-Zentrum für Ozeanforschung Kiel, Düsternbrooker Weg 20, 24105 Kiel, Germany

Index